Urban Sanitation

Urban Sanitation
A Guide to Strategic Planning

Kevin Tayler, Jonathan Parkinson
and Jeremy Colin

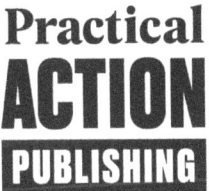

Practical Action Publishing Ltd
25 Albert Street, Rugby, CV21 2SD, Warwickshire, UK
www.practicalactionpublishing.com

Published by ITDG Publishing

© GHK International Ltd 2003

First published in 2003

ISBN 1 85339 558 7
ISBN 13   9781853395581
ISBN Library Ebook. 9781780441436
Book DOI: http://dx.doi.org/10.3362/9781780441436

All rights reserved. No part of this publication may be reprinted or reproduced or utilized in any form or by any electronic, mechanical, or other means, now known or hereafter invented, including photocopying and recording, or in any information storage or retrieval system, without the written permission of the publishers.

A catalogue record for this book is available from the British Library.

The authors, contributors and/or editors have asserted their rights under the Copyright Designs and Patents Act 1988 to be identified as authors of their respective contributions. Since 1974, Practical Action Publishing has published and disseminated books and information in support of international development work throughout the world. Practical Action Publishing is a trading name of Practical Action Publishing Ltd (Company Reg. No. 1159018), the wholly owned publishing company of Practical Action. Practical Action Publishing trades only in support of its parent charity objectives and any profits are covenanted back to Practical Action (Charity Reg. No. 247257, Group VAT Registration No. 880 9924 76).

Typeset by Dorwyn Ltd, Rowlands Castle, Hants

Contents

List of figures	viii
List of tables	x
List of boxes	xi
Preface	xiii
Acknowledgements	xv
Introduction	xvii

1 Urban sanitation – problems and responses — 1
- Rapid urbanization, poor sanitation and their consequences — 1
- Why improve sanitation? — 3
- Current responses to sanitation problems — 5
- Three models of sanitation improvement — 7
- Moving beyond narrowly defined models — 9

2 A strategic framework for urban sanitation planning — 12
- What we mean by the terms 'strategic' and 'strategic planning' — 12
- Three key questions that help to define a strategic process — 13
- Principles for effective strategic planning — 16

3 Strategic sanitation planning in towns and cities — 25
- The development of a strategic model – the Bharatpur pilot process — 25
- Stages in the development of a strategic plan — 31
- Preparing to plan — 32
- Understanding current problems — 33
- Developing solutions — 35
- Developing the city-wide plan — 42
- Next steps — 46

4 Developing a supportive context — 48
- Municipal planning in context — 48
- Four barriers to improved sanitation — 49
- Raising the profile of sanitation — 50
- Developing a commitment to strategic planning — 51
- Developing a supportive policy context — 52
- Increasing capacity to produce and implement strategic plans — 61

5 Developing a strategic process from the local level — 67
Three approaches to planning at the local level — 67
Community initiated sanitation – the case of Pakistan — 68
A process for planning at the local level — 73
Preparation stage — 74
The planning workshop — 77
Developing solutions — 80
The sanitation plan — 83
Moving beyond the local level — 84

6 The role of sanitation and hygiene promotion in developing and informing demand — 88
Sanitation and hygiene promotion and the links between them — 88
Where are we now? Assessing current sanitation and hygiene practice — 89
Planning a promotion campaign — 94
Deciding on appropriate media for promotion — 97
Some points on promotion materials — 97
Implementing the programme — 98
Creating an enabling environment — 99
Funding options for sanitation and hygiene promotion — 100

7 Gathering and using information for strategic planning — 102
Information and planning processes — 102
Types of information — 103
Information requirements — 103
The importance of triangulation — 106
Sources of information — 106
Recording, analysing and presenting information — 107
Information for local and municipal plans — 108
Developing an integrated information base — 118
Information for policy makers and programme planners — 120

8 Choosing an appropriate sanitation technology — 125
Approaches to sanitation selection — 125
Categories of sanitation technology — 126
A step-wise procedure for sanitation choice — 126
Costing viable sanitation options — 132
Estimating the cost of a networked system — 134
Recurrent costs — 135
Willingness to pay for improved sanitation services — 136
Approaches to estimating willingness to pay — 137
Options for reducing costs — 139

9	**Guidelines for holding a participatory workshop**	**144**
	How and when can workshops be used?	144
	Preparing for the workshop	144
	Preparing information to present to the workshop	147
	Workshop logistics	148
	The workshop itself	153
	Recording the outputs of the workshop	156
10	**Implementing the plan**	**158**
	First steps	158
	Developing detailed proposals	159
	Options for supervision and implementation	161
	The need for formal agreements	168
	Monitoring the progress of the plan	169
	Assessment	171
	Sharing experience	172

Appendices
   1 Links between sanitation and health   177
   2 Summary information on sanitation technologies   183
   3 Participatory methods for assessing sanitation conditions   196
   4 Sources of further information   203

Glossary   **213**
References   **215**
Index   **219**

Figures

Figure 1.1	Absolute lack of facilities	2
Figure 1.2	Facilities provided but in poor condition	3
Figure 1.3	Problems caused by poor operation and maintenance	3
Figure 1.4	Problems with formal schemes	6
Figure 2.1	Grounding action in the existing situation	14
Figure 2.2	Information flows required to respond to informed demand	17
Figure 2.3	The role of champions in promoting recognition of local initiatives	21
Figure 3.1	Small-steps approach towards achieving the desired situation	27
Figure 3.2	The strategic process at the municipal level	31
Figure 3.3	Steps in developing solutions	35
Figure 3.4	Problems caused by household level action	38
Figure 3.5	Problems caused by neighbourhood level improvements	38
Figure 3.6	Problems with impacts at the municipal level	39
Figure 3.7	Considering resource requirements	41
Figure 3.8	The typical structure of a municipal sanitation plan	42
Figure 4.1	Municipal planning in context	49
Figure 4.2	Requirements for widespread adoption of strategic planning	50
Figure 4.3	Stages in developing and implementing policy	53
Figure 4.4	The place of testing in developing appropriate standards	59
Figure 5.1	Orangi Pilot Project (RTI) access chamber under construction	72
Figure 5.2	The planning process at local level	74
Figure 5.3	Procedure for assessing appropriate responses to local sanitation problems	79
Figure 6.1	An integrated approach to sanitation and hygiene promotion	89
Figure 6.2	Evidence from transect walks	90
Figure 7.1	Example of problem tree analysis	112
Figure 8.1	Key questions to inform sanitation choice	127
Figure 8.2	On-plot provision does not need much space	128
Figure 8.3	Shared toilets may be appropriate	129
Figure 8.4	Communal facilities in public places	129
Figure 8.5	Algorithm for wastewater disposal from 'wet' sanitation systems	132
Figure 9.1	Participatory planning using plans and scale models	153
Figure 10.1	Poor design and construction inhibits good operation and maintenance	161
Figure 10.2	The need for improved practices	163
Figure 10.3	Links between activities, outputs, purpose and goal	170

Figure A1.1 Faecal–oral disease transmission routes and the role of improved sanitation and hygiene in breaking them   178
Figure A2.1 Simple pit latrine   184
Figure A2.2 Ventilated improved pit (VIP) latrine   185
Figure A2.3 Twin-pit VIP latrine   186
Figure A2.4 'Dry box' latrine   188
Figure A2.5 Single leach pit latrine   189
Figure A2.6 Double-pit or twin leach pit latrine   190
Figure A2.7 Septic tank discharging to a soakaway or drainfield   192
Figure A2.8 Sewered interceptor tank system   194

Tables

Table 6.1	Participatory investigations used in the APUSP	92
Table 7.1	Framework for identification of existing tasks and responsibilities	113
Table 7.2	Bharatpur resource analysis	114
Table 8.1	Categorization of sanitation technologies	127
Table 8.2	Operation and maintenance costs for different technologies	136
Table 9.1	Advantages and disadvantages of the various presentation options	150
Table 10.1	Options for supervising and implementing new works and operation and maintenance tasks	166

Boxes

Box 1.1	Differing objectives – the case of Bharatpur, India	5
Box 2.1	Unbundling technologies – the case of Maseru, Lesotho	18
Box 2.2	Bharatpur – an incremental approach to demand and incentives	23
Box 3.1	Tasks identified during the Bharatpur workshop	30
Box 3.2	Key points stressed during the Bharatpur workshop	37
Box 3.3	Overall framework of the strategic plan	44
Box 3.4	The solid waste management component of the municipal plan	45
Box 4.1	The influence of limited resource availability on operational systems	54
Box 4.2	Principles for the development of appropriate standards and specifications	58
Box 4.3	Provision of materials as an incentive for investing in sanitation	60
Box 4.4	WASPOLA – a project approach to policy development	62
Box 5.1	Saifabad 2, Faisalabad – an area-based scheme	69
Box 5.2	The CKAIP in Hyderabad and the consequences of failing to take a wide view	71
Box 5.3	Sukkur, Pakistan – an example of failure to deal with operating costs	73
Box 5.4	Problem analysis in the Sri Lankan micro-planning process	78
Box 5.5	Points to bear in mind when conducting follow-up negotiations	82
Box 5.6	The Lodhran Project – adapting a local model to the municipal level	86
Box 6.1	Developing solutions on the basis of pooled knowledge	93
Box 6.2	School health clubs in Zimbabwe	95
Box 6.3	Exchange visits in Ouagadougou, Burkina Faso	98
Box 7.1	The value of field observation – an example from India	105
Box 7.2	Field investigations in Quthbullapur, Andhra Pradesh	110
Box 7.3	Investigating local solid waste collection services – Faisalabad, Pakistan	117
Box 7.4	Social and technical mapping – the approach proposed in Bharatpur	119
Box 7.5	Example of pro-forma for neighbourhood profile	121
Box 8.1	Standard bill of quantities type schedule for a VIP latrine	134
Box 8.2	Implicit and explicit subsidies – examples from sewerage schemes in Pakistan	138
Box 8.3	Triangulating the results of 'rule of thumb' and revealed preference methods	140
Box 8.4	Contingent valuation and solid waste disposal in Chennai, India	141
Box 9.1	Options for presenting the results of previous investigations	149
Box 9.2	Sticky cloths – how to prepare and use them	152
Box 10.1	Training for managers and residents in Yoff, Senegal	165

Box 10.2	Community toilets in Pune	167
Box 10.3	Possible contractual arrangements for community-managed schemes	167
Box 10.4	Service provision by local entrepreneurs – a case from South Africa	168
Box 10.5	'Face-to-face' community exchanges	174
Box 10.6	Water and Environmental Sanitation Network (WESNET), Pakistan	175
Box A3.1	Examples of what you might observe in the course of a transect walk	197
Box A3.2	Assessing differences through conventional surveys	201

Preface

This book grew out of research into the practical application of the Water and Sanitation Program's (WSP) Strategic Sanitation Approach (Wright 1997). The UK government's Department for International Development (DFID) funded the research under its Engineering Knowledge and Research programme.

The WSP had already piloted the Strategic Sanitation Approach (SSA) in West Africa and the DFID-funded research was intended to build on this early work. The research explored the practical relevance of the SSA's concepts and principles through short studies of projects and programmes that incorporated some of the SSA principles, detailed investigations of subjects with relevance to aspects of the SSA and a pilot strategic sanitation planning exercise in the Indian town of Bharatpur, in Rajasthan. While this research confirmed the validity of many of the SSA's principles and assumptions, the book is not about the SSA as such, but rather about the importance of tackling sanitation problems and needs in a strategic way.

The research was led by GHK Research and Training, part of the GHK Group, and also involved inputs from the Water, Engineering and Development Centre (WEDC) at Loughborough University, also in the UK, and the Water and Sanitation Program's Regional Office in South Asia (WSP–SA). All three authors were involved in the research, Kevin Tayler as team leader, Jonathan Parkinson as a researcher and Jeremy Colin as the facilitator of the planning process in Bharatpur.

A first draft of a strategic sanitation planning guide was developed and circulated in 2000. The present book has been developed from that first draft following the considerable feedback received from researchers and practitioners.

Acknowledgements

Thanks are due to the UK government's Department for International Development (DFID), which provided funding for the research that led to the book and has also contributed funds for the production of the book itself. Our thanks also go to the Water and Sanitation Program – South Asia (WSP-SA), and in particular to Barbara Evans, Clarissa Brocklehurst and Fiona Fanthome, who provided support and guidance throughout the pilot project in Rajasthan. Special mention should be made of the role played by Dr Godhara and Mr Chaturvedi from Bharatpur Municipal Council and thanks are also due to colleagues from the Asian Centre for Organization, Research and Development (ACORD) and Lupin for their close collaboration and cooperation with the research team.

The authors are also grateful to Dr Andrew Cotton and Dr Darren Saywell from the Water, Engineering and Development Centre (WEDC) who were involved in the early stages of the research study and provided comments on the first draft of the guide.

Albert Wright (previously with the Water and Sanitation Program) played an important part in developing the Strategic Sanitation Approach (SSA), which provided the starting point for our research and provided the conceptual framework for the development of the approach towards strategic planning described in the book. Dr Robert Boydell (former manager of WSP-SA) offered invaluable support to the research team in the early stages of the research process.

In Pakistan, thanks for information, ideas and assistance are due to Sadia Fazli, Akhbar Zaidi and Arif Hasan in Karachi and Mr Ahmed Nazir Wattoo of the NGO Anjuman Samaji Behbood (ASB), Shahid Mahmood of the NGO Community Action Programme (CAP) and the Faisalabad Area Upgrading Project team in Faisalabad. Fayyaz Baqir provided information on the Lodhran project.

Further feedback on strategic processes at the municipal level was obtained from workshops in India and Bangladesh. Thanks for organizing these workshops are due to Mr Satyanarayana, Municipal Commissioner Quthbullapur, Andhra Pradesh, Mr Jayanta Chakrobarty, in Kolkata and Han Heijnen and his team in Dhaka.

Ben Fawcett, Gift Manase and Martin Mulenga at Southampton University provided comments and information on initiatives in Southern Africa. Information on the Yoff project in Senegal was provided by Claudia Bockman Weisburd.

The views expressed are the author's own and do not necessarily represent those of any of the individuals and organizations mentioned above. Useful comments on drafts of the book were made by Tom Carter, Jeremy Ockleford, Bob Reed and Magdalena Banasiak.

The diagrams used to illustrate sanitation technologies in Appendix 2 were produced by Rod Shaw at WEDC.

Introduction

Subject and scope

This book is a guide to strategic options for improving sanitation conditions in the rapidly growing towns and cities of the 'South'. It uses the term sanitation in its widest sense to cover excreta disposal, sullage and stormwater drainage, solid waste management and hygiene, and stresses the need to go beyond a concern with the provision of facilities to consider the services that people receive. The term 'strategic' can have different meanings for different people and will be explored further in the first two chapters. However, two key points deserve mention at this point. First, that the ultimate aim of strategic interventions must be to lead to changes at the level of a city as a whole rather than to create isolated pockets of good practice and, second, that a strategy must concern itself with the way in which a desired outcome is to be achieved as much as with the outcome itself.

Target audience and purpose

The book should be of interest to decision makers and their advisers, working at the international, national, state/provincial and municipal levels, some of whom will be concerned with sanitation alone while, for others, sanitation will be one concern among many. It has two aims. First, it aims to convince readers of the benefits of adopting a strategic approach to sanitation planning, which takes account of both constraints and available resources and recognizes the importance of relevant information to decision making. Second, it aims to provide readers with practical guidance on how they might start to think and act more strategically in whatever situation they find themselves.

Structure of the book

The book is divided into ten chapters and these in turn fall naturally into four groups.

Chapters 1 and 2 set the scene for the rest of the book. Chapter 1 provides a brief overview of urban sanitation problems and possible responses to those problems. Chapter 2 builds on this initial analysis by defining what we mean by 'strategic' and 'planning' and using these definitions as the basis for developing a strategic framework for urban sanitation planning.

Chapters 3–5 are concerned with planning processes and the systems that support them. Chapter 3 deals with the strategic planning process at the municipal level. Chapter 4 deals with the options for developing a supportive context for strategic planning, recognizing that this context must be developed by higher levels of government. Chapter 5 considers the options for acting strategically at the local level when there is little or no commitment to strategic planning at either the national or the municipal level. Readers may suggest that it would be more logical to put the development of a more supportive context first, and in a purely rational world this would indeed be the correct approach. However, the world is not entirely logical and we have found that there is seldom a single 'correct' place from which to start to think and act more strategically. The policies and programmes that emanate from the 'centre' certainly have a profound effect on what is possible at the municipal and local levels. However, it is equally important to recognize that policies and programmes are most likely to be effective if they are firmly based on the practical lessons learnt in the field. Bearing these points in mind, we have structured the chapter along roughly the same lines as those taken by the research, starting at the municipal level and then moving on to consider implications for policy and for local action.

Chapters 6–9 provide additional guidance on issues and subjects that are likely to be key to the strategic planning process. The aim is that readers will find practical guidance within them, supplementing the more process-orientated information provided in Chapters 3–5. Chapter 6 explores the role of sanitation and hygiene promotion in developing and informing the demand that is necessary for any successful attempt to provide improved sanitation. Chapter 7 is concerned with the very important subject of information for strategic planning. The focus is on what level of information collection and analysis is appropriate at each stage of the planning process. Chapter 8 deals with the various aspects of choosing an appropriate sanitation technology, bearing in mind the need for that technology to be suited to local conditions, acceptable to local people and affordable. The processes described in Chapters 3–5 rely on workshops to bring stakeholders together to exchange views and information and to make key decisions. In view of the vital role that these workshops play in the planning process, Chapter 9 provides guidance on preparing for and holding a participatory planning workshop.

The only good plan is a plan that is implemented, but few plans are implemented in full and many are stillborn. Chapter 10 responds to this unfortunate state of affairs by providing guidance on implementing the plan, placing special stress on the vital first steps after the plan has been agreed and accepted by the various stakeholders.

CHAPTER 1
Urban sanitation – problems and responses

THIS CHAPTER BEGINS with a brief review of the impact of rapid urbanization in the developing world on access to sanitation, going on to show that sanitation problems are not only about an absolute lack of services. Reasons for improving sanitation facilities are explored, as are the views of different stakeholders. Current responses to sanitation deficiencies are then considered and their strengths and weaknesses are briefly explored.

Three commonly accepted models for sanitation improvement are introduced and briefly assessed. The scope for developing a hybrid approach to sanitation provision, building on the best features of each of the three models, is considered, with special reference to the Water and Sanitation Program's Strategic Sanitation Approach, which provides the starting point for the approach to urban sanitation developed in the book.

Rapid urbanization, poor sanitation and their consequences

Rapid urbanization is occurring throughout the developing world, creating a demand for housing, infrastructure and services, including excreta disposal, sullage and surface water drainage and solid waste management. The World Bank estimates that almost 26% of the world's urban population, over 400 million people, lack access to the simplest latrines (World Bank 2000, p.140), while drainage and solid waste collection are either absent or inadequate in many low-income settlements.[1]

Sanitation is often at its worst in the informal areas – the areas built outside formal rules and regulations in which most poor people live. In many countries, the informal sector is now the main provider of urban housing, but informal developers seldom provide their schemes with anything more than the most basic services and subsequent sanitation provision often lags behind that of electricity and water supply.

Poor sanitation has serious consequences for health (WHO/UNICEF 2000). It has been estimated that 2.2 million people, mostly children under the age of five, die each year from diarrhoeal diseases, which are associated with polluted drinking water, poor sanitation and poor domestic hygiene (Murray and Lopez 1996). The same source suggests that intestinal worms, which can be controlled by the introduction of improved sanitation, infect about 10% of the population of the developing world. Worldwide, around 200 million people are infected with schistosomiasis and 20 million of these suffer severe consequences (Esrey et al. 1991). Further information on the links between sanitation and health is given in Appendix 1.

Sanitation deficiencies can take a number of forms as listed and briefly discussed below.

1. There may be an absolute lack of sanitation facilities. This situation is commonly but not exclusively found in rapidly growing 'informal' settlements on the urban fringe. It may also be found where

2 URBAN SANITATION

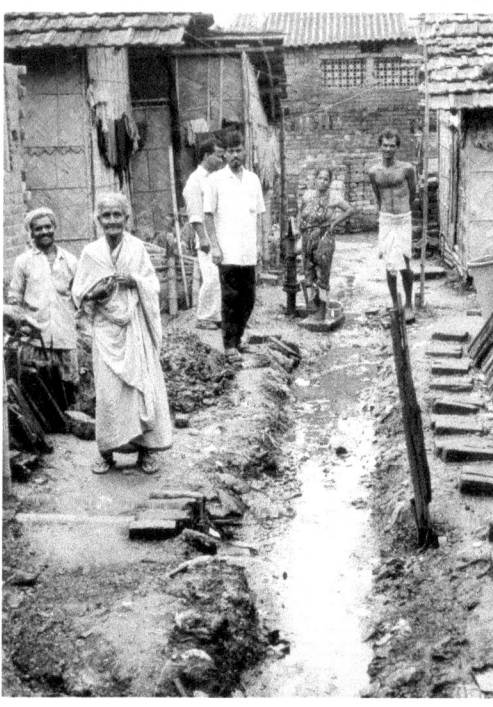

Figure 1.1 Absolute lack of facilities
In this 'refugee settlement' in Kolkata, India, people do not have legal tenure and are therefore denied access to basic sanitation and drainage improvements. The first priority in such situations must be to formalize the community's tenure in some way.

people have no legal right to occupy the land on which they live (see Figure 1.1). Examples of such people include pavement dwellers and squatters on land alongside railways and canals. In fringe areas, an absolute lack of facilities is likely to be replaced in time by one of the following situations.

2. Sanitation facilities are provided, but in poor condition so that they are inconvenient, unpleasant and/or unhygienic (see Figure 1.2). Examples include over-used and poorly maintained communal latrines and bucket latrine systems. In some cases, such facilities continue to be used by people even though their use has been officially discontinued.

3. Some people have limited access to existing sanitation facilities. A person's access to a facility or service may be influenced by his or her status and what he or she can pay. The fact that a sanitation facility exists does not mean that everyone will be allowed to use it. 'Slum' landlords may reserve the best facilities for their own use, leaving large numbers of tenants to share the remaining facilities.

4. Sanitation facilities have been provided but suffer from poor operation and maintenance, which shortens their useful life, and at worst, results in complete system failure. Communal sanitation facilities can be particularly vulnerable to poor operation and maintenance. As shown in Figure 1.3, poor solid waste management is a particular problem which affects wastewater drainage systems.

5. Solutions to local problems result in environmental problems elsewhere. Sewerage, solid waste collection and drainage schemes remove wastes from the areas that they serve but do not remove the wastes from the environment. The result is pollution of the

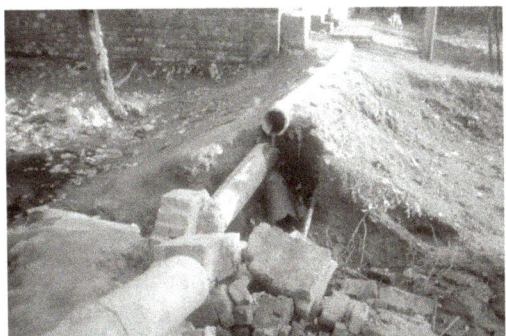

Figure 1.2 Facilities provided but in poor condition
This community-built sewer in Lahore, Pakistan has failed because of poor design and lack of maintenance.

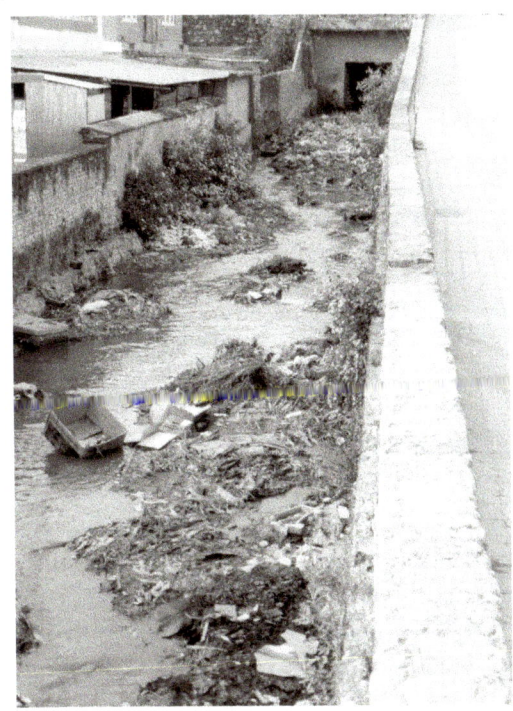

Figure 1.3 Problems caused by poor operation and maintenance
This drain in Kathmandu, Nepal, is becoming blocked by uncollected solid waste. Poor solid waste management can lead to flooding by faecally polluted water during the rainy season.

natural aquatic environment (rivers, lakes, groundwater, and marine waters). Householders living in areas with poor sanitation and drainage tend to focus on their own local environment and are understandably less concerned about the needs of the wider environment.

Why improve sanitation?

Sanitation is just one of the issues that vie for the attention of politicians and other decision makers. Why should it be given priority and why is urban sanitation particularly important? Several answers to these questions are listed below.

○ Health. Good sanitation is a prerequisite for healthy cities, protecting people from a range of excreta-related diseases. These are likely to be chronic in some areas and have the potential to reach epidemic proportions in the absence of adequate household waste disposal arrangements. The health risks of poor sanitation are likely to be higher in densely populated low-income urban areas, where it is not uncommon for one child in five to die before the age of five.

○ Convenience and privacy. Sanitation facilities in or close to the house provide greater privacy and increased convenience for users. Women in particular are likely to value the opportunity of being able to defecate and urinate in privacy and comfort at a place in or close to their homes at any time of the day.

○ The environment. When untreated wastes are discharged to the environment, they can cause damage which, once started, is difficult and expensive to correct. This is a particular problem in the large and rapidly growing cities of the South. So, failure to develop sanitary solutions to waste disposal problems can result in massive environmental problems, which will be difficult to deal with in the future.

- Livelihoods. Healthy people are stronger and less likely to be absent from work because of sickness. They therefore benefit from increased earning power and reduced expenditure on health care. So, through their health impacts, sanitation improvements can have a positive impact upon livelihoods, particularly on those of the poor.

- The economy. The positive impacts of improved sanitation on individual livelihoods and the environment are likely to feed through to the wider economy so that improved sanitation has potential benefits for the economy as a whole.

- Social capital. Failure to provide sanitary conditions in low-income areas contributes to inequality, which in turn can undermine social capital – the relationships of trust and confidence that exist within society. Without it, a society is likely to be weak and unstable, with limited capacity to respond effectively to adverse conditions.

- Equity. An unequal society is also an unjust society, particularly when the inequality relates to basic human needs such as that for clean and healthy living conditions.

Different groups are likely to have different reasons for wanting better sanitation.

While householders are likely to have some understanding of the health risks of poor sanitation, their main concern will often be with convenience and improvements in their immediate environment.

Health professionals will naturally emphasize health benefits and, in particular, the role of sanitation in preventing people from coming into contact with potentially harmful pathogens (disease-causing microorganisms).

Engineers tend to be more concerned with the wider environmental aspects of wastewater disposal, particularly biological and chemical degradation of surface water and groundwater. This is partly because engineering education draws on experience in western industrialized countries, where the main task over the last 100 years has been to deal with the legacy created by the provision of household sanitation and sewers without adequate provision for wastewater disposal.

Politicians and local councillors are usually aware of the above, and some may have a vision of a more equitable society. Most will recognize that improvements in infrastructure and services in their constituencies can increase the number of people who vote for them.

Economists argue that improvements in health, the environment and convenience are only steps towards improving the economy as a whole.

Social development specialists are likely to be concerned with livelihoods, social capital and equity.

Box 1.1 provides an example from Bharatpur, in Rajasthan, India, of what some of these different perspectives can mean in practice.

The various viewpoints can be brought together to suggest two overarching reasons to improve sanitation – to ensure that:

- people lead healthy and productive lives
- the natural environment is protected.

Achievement of these objectives helps to create the economic and social capital required for a well ordered society.

The relative importance given to the two overarching objectives will be influenced by the local situation and by the concerns of the different stakeholders. In particular, some stakeholders will focus mainly on the needs of people while others will wish to protect the wider environment.

Box 1.1 Differing objectives – the case of Bharatpur, India

Bharatpur is a small town in Rajasthan, India. In 1997, it was selected as the location for the development of a pilot strategic sanitation planning process. Early in the process, it became clear that different stakeholders had different objectives.

Representatives of the Water and Sanitation Program – South Asia (WSP-SA), an international organization with links to the World Bank and UNDP, were concerned that services were heavily subsidized and looked for ways of ensuring that sanitation users would pay at least something towards the cost of sanitation services.

The main concern of municipal officials was with the pollution of the Sujan Ganga, the moat that encircles the historic fort at the centre of the town. This was originally fed by clean water from outside the town but over the years has become grossly polluted, serving now as a receptacle for most of the liquid wastes generated in the central part of the town. Officials saw the pollution of the moat as a deterrent to tourism and hence a negative influence on the economic development of the town.

Residents of low-income areas and representatives of the non-governmental organizations working with them were, not surprisingly, more concerned with improvements to their own sanitation facilities and the effect that these might have in affording them greater convenience and improving the local environment.

Where resources are scarce, it will be difficult to achieve everyone's objectives at the same time. This suggests that planning processes must be able to mediate between different objectives in order to identify agreed goals that are acceptable to everyone. This will often require negotiation, which will only be possible if:

o all stakeholders are involved, or at least represented, in the process from the start

o the processes by which decisions are made are as transparent as possible.

The difficulty is to ensure that these requirements are applied in practice and this is one of the key issues addressed later in this book.

Current responses to sanitation problems

Acceptance that good sanitation is important does not necessarily lead to effective provision. Indeed, the information given at the start of this chapter suggests that the number of urban dwellers without adequate sanitation is actually increasing as efforts to provide sanitation services fail to keep pace with the remorseless growth in urban populations throughout the developing world. In exploring the reasons for this failure, it is important to be aware of the strengths and weaknesses of current responses, both formal and informal, to sanitation problems.

Formal responses

Formal government-led or sanctioned attempts to deal with sanitation deficiencies at the city level tend to take a centralized approach, focusing first on the production of overall 'master plans' and then on the provision of trunk sewers, main drains and city-wide solid waste collection services (see Figure 1.4). Most of these schemes have failed to meet their objectives with the result that formally provided services are limited in extent, serving only higher income areas that are relatively close to city centres (Swyngedouw 1995).

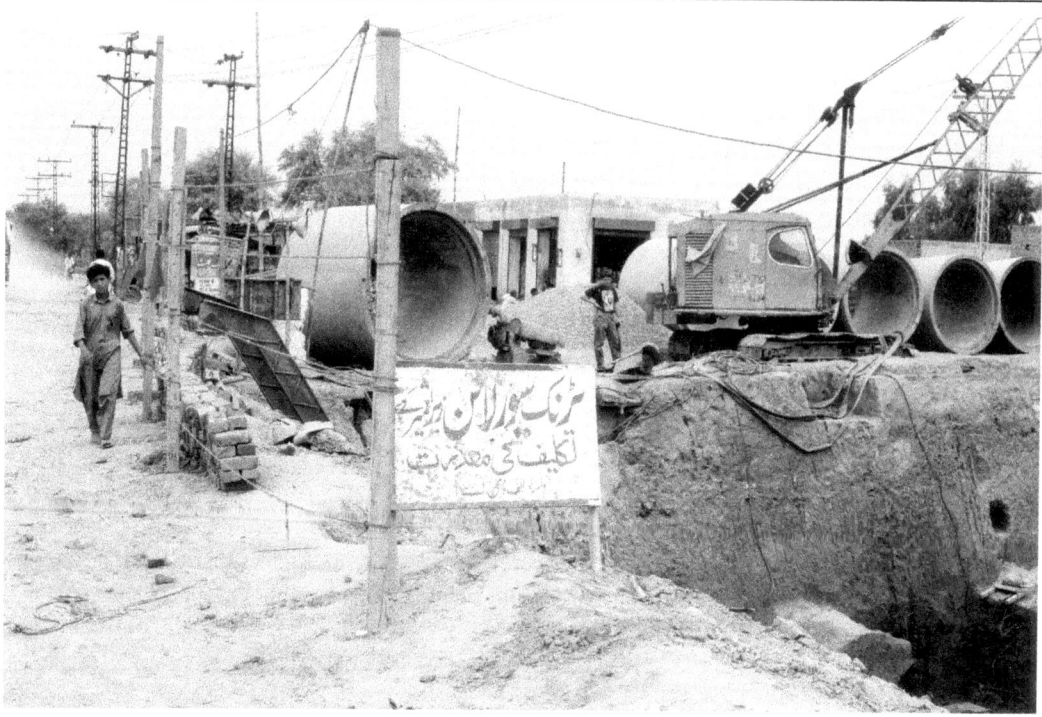

Figure 1.4 Problems with formal schemes
Large-scale sewerage schemes require large investments and are often delayed by financial and technical constraints. These sewer pipes in Faisalabad, Pakistan, have waited for over 10 years to be laid in the ground. The overall sewerage plan is now many years behind schedule.

In some countries, programme approaches, involving the provision of a large number of small-scale facilities to individual communities and/or householders, have also been tried. Examples include the Indian government's Integrated Low Cost Sanitation scheme and efforts to promote the use of pit latrines in Africa. Programme approaches tend to be more directly poverty-focused than 'master plans'.

Formal efforts to improve infrastructure services in low-income areas have often taken the form of projects, many of which have been externally funded and most of which have remained as one-off initiatives. These have invariably focused upon the construction of new facilities. Many of these initiatives have taken little account of the need to integrate services in low-income areas with city-wide services. At worst, the organizations responsible for operating and maintaining sewerage, drainage and water supply facilities have never formally adopted the facilities provided. Another problem is the failure of externally funded projects to have any significant impact upon the ways in which government departments and other local stakeholders seek to provide services.

Few of these projects and programmes have made a significant impact upon the sanitation needs of cities as a whole. The reasons for this include the following.

○ Sanitation often has a low profile – too few senior officials and politicians see sanitation as important in relation to other economic concerns and political pressures.

○ Projects and programmes tend to be supply driven – they provide what professionals think is needed while ignoring the concerns of users, with the result that facilities are not always used as intended or are not used at all.

○ The focus on capital investment is seldom matched by a practical concern for better operation and maintenance. Sanitation planners often talk about the need for better operation and maintenance but words are rarely matched with actions.

○ There are few incentives to 'institutionalize' initiatives so that the approach that they embody becomes the norm rather than being confined to isolated, often externally financed, projects and programmes.

A particular problem with programme schemes is the difficulty of managing the provision of a large number of small-scale facilities. Faced with the need to meet ambitious targets, executing agencies may feel pressured to decide where and when facilities will be provided rather than responding to user demand. Household members may then misuse facilities or even fail to use them at all. This is a particular example of a more general problem; the tendency for actual systems and procedures to be different from those enshrined in codes and instruction manuals.

Informal responses

Local stakeholders, including local government, community groups and individual households, often respond to the absence or failure of planned schemes by providing their own local facilities. While these small-scale schemes may be responsive to the immediate needs of users, many suffer from:

○ a tendency to shift problems from the local level to the wider environment rather than solving them completely

○ poor technical standards, specifications and construction details, which reduce performance and can often lead to premature failure of facilities

○ lack of coordination, both horizontally, between different local initiatives, and vertically, between local schemes and the higher-order facilities provided by central providers.

National planners and international agencies tend to dismiss this form of activity because of its limitations. However, the overall scale and impact of small-scale activity can be significant and for this reason it cannot be ignored in any strategic approach to sanitation provision.

Three models of sanitation improvement

It is possible to identify three idealized models for local environmental improvement, each of which provides a possible response to the problem of inadequate environmental services, including sanitation (McGranahan et al. 2001, Chapter 5).

○ The planning model, built around bureaucratic mechanisms and implemented by administrators, engineers and public officials. This is target orientated, guided by regulations and technical standards and sanctioned by state authority, backed up where necessary by coercion. City-wide masterplans and 'officially' sponsored projects to upgrade low-income areas both follow this model.

○ The market model, which views people as consumers of services. Each household is assumed to be in the best position to make informed choices about the level and type of service that best suits it. It makes decisions on the basis of its own perceived interests, bearing in mind price signals and the need to make the most efficient use of household resources to maximize personal utility. In recent years, the market model has been strongly promoted by some international agencies.

o The local collective action model, implemented through voluntary associations and seeking to further the interests of their members and the visions of their leaders. Advocates of the model suggest that self-managed services can often be significantly cheaper than those provided by government departments.² The fact that low-income areas are often 'invisible' to the rest of the city, including the government officials who are responsible for providing services, can be an added argument for advocating local collective action. The local responses to the failure of 'official' plans, projects and programmes introduced in the previous subsection clearly follow this model.

These are idealized models and the real world is invariably rather more complex than can be represented by a simple model. Nevertheless, they provide a useful starting point for analysis.

Each of the models has both strengths and weaknesses.³ The planning model, at least in theory, makes use of specialist knowledge to provide a logical approach to sanitation problems. This is a strength that has perhaps been downplayed in recent years. This book starts from the assumption that planning has an important place in sanitation provision. However, the planning model is essentially top down and pays little attention to the opinions and needs of the intended users of sanitation services. Where resources are scarce, the immediate pressure to provide improved services in higher-income areas and/or in areas inhabited by groups with political 'clout' invariably over-rides long term planning objectives, with the result that plans are at worst ignored and at best only partially implemented. Invariably, the rich and well connected benefit, while the poor are left out. Interventions in low-income areas are hampered by a lack of local knowledge and often take little account of local conditions, producing schemes that perform badly and, at worst, are not used at all.

Proponents of a pure version of the market model argue that market forces are more likely than central planning to provide the services that people need. At worst, this can be a rather ideological viewpoint, which pays little attention to what actually happens in the real world. Less ideological advocates of the model suggest that it ensures that prices for services are realistic, thus doing away with the need for unaffordable and unsustainable subsidies. They argue for an increased role for the private sector, which in the right circumstances and at the right scale can deliver services more effectively than an inefficient public sector. On the other hand, the market model's focus on individual choice ignores the fact that waste disposal choices made by individual households may affect the health of their neighbours and that of the community at large. The model also pays insufficient attention to the fact that choices are not made in a vacuum but are influenced by the facilities that already exist and by the knowledge of potential service users. For example, a household's strategy for dealing with liquid or solid waste will be influenced by the availability or otherwise of a sewer and/or a solid waste collection service in the vicinity and by what it knows about the available options.

Perhaps the most telling criticism of the market model is its historical failure to provide adequate sanitation services in rapidly growing 'western' cities. In the late nineteenth-century, these cities faced similar situations to those now faced by cities in the 'South' but generally on a smaller scale and with greater access to financial resources. The western experience was that market forces on their own were insufficient to either guarantee improved sanitation facilities in low-income areas or to protect the environment. Improvements in sanitation facilities required the introduction and enforcement of public health legislation, backed up by considerable public expenditure. Environmental improvements often had to wait until late in the twentieth century and were also heavily dependent on legislation and public expenditure. Given this failure of market forces to deliver improved sanitation and environmental conditions in western cities, there must be considerable doubt about their ability to do better in 'southern' cities faced with unprecedented rates of growth and high levels of poverty.

Like the market model, the local collective action model starts with the concerns of residents rather than the opinions and assumptions of 'experts'. The action that flows from it is likely to reflect a common agenda rather than the concerns of individuals, thus overcoming one of the basic problems with the market model. As already indicated, it has been effective in achieving local improvements, particularly in informal areas where other approaches have failed to deliver services.

Unfortunately, the model also has weaknesses. It relies heavily on local knowledge and this, no less than that of external professionals, can be partial and misdirected. The model also suffers from two types of boundary problem. First, there may be difficulties in deciding where one collective initiative should finish and its neighbour should begin. Second, one area's solution to its wastewater disposal problem may well become another area's problem. Another major limitation of local collective action lies in its unreliability – both in the sense that it may take root in one place but not in another and that there is no guarantee that initiatives will endure over time. One of the biggest problems faced by community groups and NGOs working at the local level has been that of linking local facilities provided through local collective action with the higher-level facilities provided by 'official' service providers. For instance, it is quite rare for sewerage authorities in India and Pakistan to formally accept connections from sewers built through local collective action. These limitations mean that it is difficult to see how local initiatives on their own can provide a comprehensive response to sanitation problems.

Moving beyond narrowly defined models

This brief review of existing models and approaches suggests that no single model of sanitation improvement, whether it is based on planning, the market or local collective action, can tackle all aspects of sanitation problems. On the other hand, an approach that does not include elements of all three is unlikely to be successful. Many human activities involve planning, which, at its most basic, is nothing more than thinking in advance about how to solve a problem or achieve an objective. Indeed, planning is essential in any situation that requires making the best use of limited resources – in other words in almost every situation faced by those responsible for the management of rapidly growing cities. The issue is not whether to plan but rather how and over what period to plan. Similarly, while a focus on either markets or local collective action will not in itself solve sanitation problems, each has a place in an overall sanitation improvement strategy.

If this is accepted, the question then becomes how to combine elements of the three models outlined above in ways that provide the best prospects for improved sanitation provision. Various attempts have been made to answer this question, one of which is the Strategic Sanitation Approach (SSA). This was developed by the then UNDP – World Bank Water and Sanitation Program, now simply the Water and Sanitation Program (WSP). It was developed in the mid-1990s and was initially piloted in Ouagadougou and Kumasi in West Africa (Wright 1997; Whittington et al. 1992; Saidi-Sharouze 1994). The principles of the SSA are elaborated and discussed in detail by Saywell and Cotton (1998). This book grew out of research into the practical application of the SSA.

The SSA combines a commitment to planning with guiding principles that are normally associated with market-based approaches to sanitation provision. Some of these guiding principles are also compatible with an increased role for local collective action. The two fundamental principles relate to the need for:

o a demand orientation, which focuses on the services that people want and for which they are willing to pay

o appropriate incentives, designed to ensure that providers and users act in ways that bring about improvements in sanitation services.

In support of these key principles, the SSA also stresses the need for:

o sound finances, which it links to the need for a demand responsive approach and the importance of appropriate financial incentives

o a concern with cities as a whole rather than discreet projects

o a wide view of sanitation, encompassing human waste disposal, sullage disposal, stormwater drainage and solid waste management

o horizontal unbundling of technologies – the use of different sanitation options in different areas within a city

o unbundling of responsibilities – in essence the division and devolution of responsibilities so that one organization does not take responsibility for all aspects of sanitation provision

o the use of a small steps approach, which focuses on the process of sanitation provision rather than a limited number of large projects.

The research upon which this book is based concluded that, while many of the principles that underpin the SSA are sound, the SSA itself has practical limitations. There are two reasons for this. First, it focuses mainly on action at the municipal level, paying little attention to the need to develop and sustain the political and administrative systems that are required to support strategic planning. Second, its strong focus on principles, applied rather rigidly, makes it very far removed from the actual situations found in most towns and cities. For instance, its approach to demand relies heavily on contingent valuation studies, which are neither appropriate nor useful in every situation. This focus on externally determined, rigorously applied principles means that the SSA does not always relate closely to the needs and aspirations of local institutional stakeholders. It says 'this is where you should be' but provides little guidance on how to get there. Wright (1997) suggests that the SSA is only possible if adaptable and flexible institutional systems already exist, but the reality is that this condition is not met in many towns, cities and countries.

What then is the way forward? In Chapter 2, we develop an overall framework for answering this question. We do not claim that this will provide a single all-encompassing model. Rather, it provides the ground rules upon which context-specific responses to sanitation problems can be developed. Subsequent chapters provide guidance on how this framework might be applied in practice.

Key points in this chapter

1. Rapid urbanization is creating an increasing need for improved sanitation services, particularly those to serve the urban poor.

2. Sanitation services can be deficient in a number of ways. The problem is not just one of an absolute lack of facilities.

3. Different people may have different reasons for wanting to improve sanitation. It is important to be aware of these reasons and reach consensus on objectives when developing a sanitation programme. Where resources are scarce, it may be necessary to negotiate in order to agree on ways in which the objectives of different stakeholders can be reconciled.

4. Until now, efforts to provide improved sanitation services have proved to be inadequate, whether made 'officially' by government or 'unofficially' by local stakeholders.

5. It is possible to identify three broad models for sanitation improvement, based on central planning, the market and local collective action respectively. These are idealized models with weaknesses as well as strengths, and none is likely, in itself, to provide a comprehensive response to the urgent need for improved urban sanitation provision.

6. The way forward must be to combine elements of these three models in ways that are appropriate to local situations. The challenge is to develop guidelines for the ways in which this can be achieved in practice for any given situation.

Chapter 1 endnotes

1 The health implications of poor housing and living conditions in urban areas of the Third World are described in detail by Cairncross et al. (1990). Black (1994) describes the scale of the problem in relation to the problems associated with a lack of sanitation.
2 For instance, the Orangi Pilot Project in Pakistan suggests that the cost of community-managed local sewers in Karachi is approximately one quarter of the cost of sewers provided by government agencies.
3 Our brief summary of the strengths and weaknesses of the various approaches draws on the points made by McGranahan et al. (2001), who explore the issues in some detail.

CHAPTER 2
A strategic framework for urban sanitation planning

THIS CHAPTER PROVIDES the framework for the material contained in later chapters in the book. It establishes the meaning of the terms 'strategic' and 'strategic planning', stressing the fact that strategies need to be flexible if they are to respond to changes in conditions and the increased availability of information. They must be grounded in the existing situation and concerned not only with overall objectives but also with the ways in which those objectives might be achieved.

Six key principles, which will help to ensure that any strategy will stay on course, are introduced and examined later in the chapter. They should be interpreted in the light of the local situation rather than applied rigidly. The importance of some or all of them may not be generally recognized at the start of the planning process. Where this is the case, an early planning objective should be to achieve increased awareness of their relevance.

What we mean by the terms 'strategic' and 'strategic planning'

We must first define what we mean by the terms 'strategic', 'plan' and 'strategic plan'. At the most basic level, a *strategy* may be defined as *a way of tackling a problem or working towards an objective* (Kneeland 1999). In theory, the term is equally relevant to a 'high level' task such as tackling the sanitation needs of a whole city, and a relatively 'low level' task such as planning for improved sanitation and drainage in a particular neighbourhood. In practice, it is usually reserved for efforts to achieve higher level goals. For instance, the Food and Agriculture Organization (FAO) has defined strategy as 'a *set of chosen short-, medium- and long-term actions to support the achievement of development goals and implement water-related policies*' (FAO 1995).

In essence, to plan is to think ahead about a problem and the way in which it is to be tackled. People normally think of planning as a formal activity, involving written documents, and this is the way in which we will use it. However, readers should be aware that many types of human activity involve planning, much of it informal and held in people's heads rather than written down.

Taking this definition of planning together with the FAO definition of a strategy, we can say that a strategic plan should be a written document that defines overall goals and also identifies a series of actions that might be taken to achieve these goals.

Unfortunately, this description says little about the ways in which goals and the actions designed to lead to them are decided. If the goals and actions are set out at beginning of the planning process and followed rigidly, the strategy begins to look suspiciously like an old-fashioned master plan. This 'blueprint' approach to planning can work well when there is good initial information on physical circumstances and the views and responses of the various people who will be involved in or affected by the plan. However, these conditions will rarely apply in the complex situations found in rapidly growing cities. In such circumstances, there is a need for a flexible approach, which allows plans to be adapted to suit changing circumstances and the availability of new and improved information. Rondinelli (1993)[1] suggests that strategic planning in such circumstances should *'start with what is known and attempt to broaden the base of knowledge and to formulate alternative interventions that will set other changes in motion'*. He contrasts this approach with attempts to bring about sweeping and comprehensive reforms, the effectiveness of which cannot be predicted.

This 'adaptive' approach to strategic planning underlies the thinking set out in this book. Acceptance of it leads to recognition that longer-term actions and programmes will usually have to be modified in the light of the experience gained from their shorter-term counterparts.

Acceptance of the approach also has implications for thinking on where strategic processes can start and who should be responsible for them. In contrast to 'blueprint' plans, which are invariably prepared by professionals on behalf of government, adaptive planning processes should seek to build on experience from a variety of sources. While senior government decision makers are likely to be involved in developing strategic plans, strategies for municipal sanitation provision can and do emerge from the activities and ideas of non-government stakeholders acting more locally. We will consider this point in more detail in Chapter 5.

Bearing in mind these general points, we now explore the strategic process in more detail.

Three key questions that help to define a strategic process

Any strategic programme or initiative must concern itself with three basic questions.

○ What is the current situation or where are we now?

○ What are the objectives of the planning process or where do we want to go?

○ What options exist for moving from the first to the second or how do we get from here to there?

Each of these is now explored in more detail.

Where are we now? Grounding plans in the current situation

To be grounded in the existing situation, a sanitation plan or programme must:

○ take account of what already exists, recognizing that existing facilities, including those provided by individual householders, community groups and the private sector, represent a considerable investment (see Figure 2.1)

○ respond to actual problems and deficiencies, recognizing that sanitation problems are as likely to stem from management deficiencies, inadequate operation and maintenance and poor coordination between stakeholders as from an absolute lack of facilities.

Unless plans are grounded in this way they risk finding solutions to problems that do not exist while failing to address real problems and needs.

At a deeper level, plans that do not take account of the ways in which people think are unlikely to be implemented as intended. There are two aspects to this.

○ Sanitation strategies must take account of the attitudes, assumptions and behaviour of the people that they target. The most theoretically sound sanitation technology will provide no benefits if it is not used as intended, or worse not used at all. This

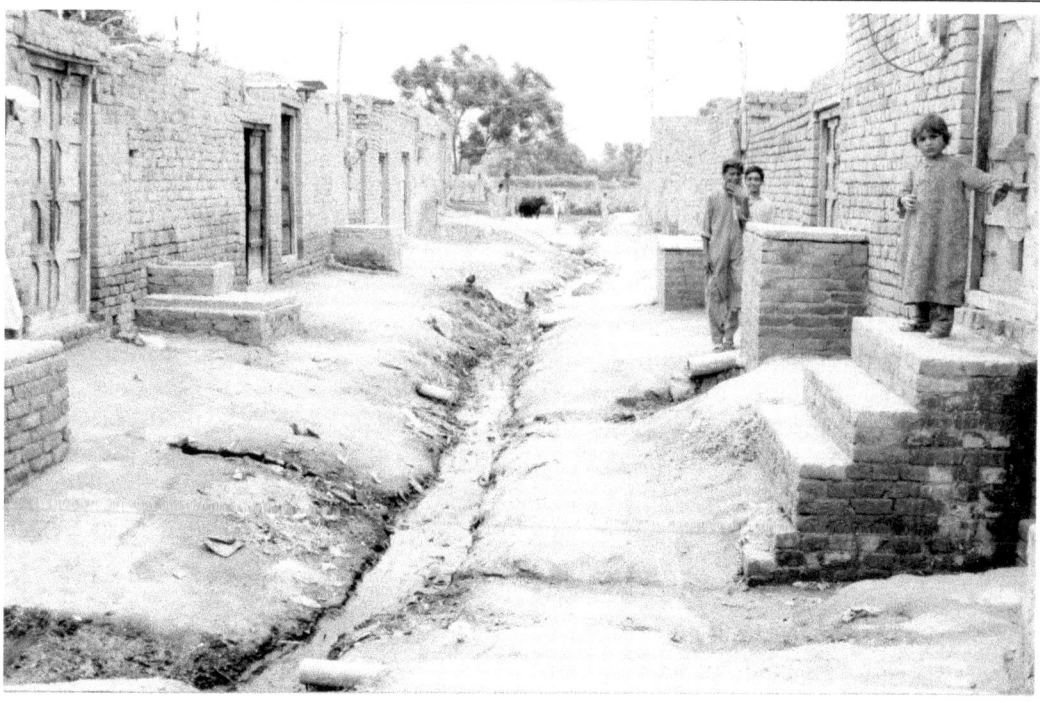

Figure 2.1 Grounding action in the existing situation
Do not assume that there are no existing sanitation facilities. The brick septic tanks located along the sides of the street show that householders have already invested in sanitation facilities. These tanks could be linked to a small-bore sewer.

suggests that efforts to install latrines, provide drainage and introduce improved solid waste management services must be accompanied by efforts to educate users and improve personal and collective hygiene.

o Sanitation strategies must consider the way in which institutions operate and the assumptions that underlie existing practices. We normally think of institutions in terms of their structures and systems but their performance is also strongly influenced by the way in which the people within them routinely think. For instance, many people in government institutions think only in terms of official provision, ignoring the contribution to sanitation services made by 'informal' providers. We will see in Chapter 3 that strategies to improve sanitation will often need to involve efforts to foster new ways of thinking and acting within the organizations that provide sanitation services.

Grounding plans in the existing situation requires attention to the context within which initiatives at the municipal and local levels take place. This may have implications for where a strategic process should start and who should start it. As we will see in more detail in Chapter 5, it is possible for non-government stakeholders to develop more or less strategic sanitation initiatives in specific areas and in doing so to influence the attitudes and assumptions of government. Where there is little initial official interest in strategic planning, this may the only way in which a strategic process can be started.

Where do we want to go? The objectives of the planning process

This question can be answered at several levels, depending on just how objectives are defined.

At the most basic level, it is useful to develop a shared vision of the future sanitation situation in a town or city as a whole. The vision should be:

o *equitable* in that it is concerned with the needs of all, including the urban poor – a concern with equity will normally require that the strategy pays particular attention to the areas in which low-income people live

o *environmentally acceptable* in that solutions to local problems do not cause deterioration of the wider environment or use resources that cannot be replaced[2]

o *sustainable* in that it continues to address needs over time – this means that its focus should be on services, covering not just the provision of facilities, but also their subsequent operation and maintenance.

While a vision provides guidance on the general direction to be taken, it does not define specific objectives and indeed may say little about the forms that those objectives might take. These more concrete objectives of the strategy, which may be described as its goals, may be difficult to define at the beginning of the planning process, particularly when information is limited. This is not necessarily a problem, provided that the strategy has an explicit commitment to define them over time.

There are likely to be situations in which resource limitations mean that achieving change at the level of the city as a whole appears to be an almost unattainable dream. Alternatively, it may be that an individual or group has a strategic vision but no remit to work beyond a particular area. In such circumstances, immediate objectives may have to be defined in relation to a more limited area. Where this is the case, it will be important to consider the ways in which the approach adopted can later be scaled up to cover other similar areas. Without this 'city-wide' perspective, it will be all too easy to accept non-replicable features in the solutions adopted, not least high levels of subsidy. Where such features are accepted, improved services are likely to be confined to limited areas so that they have no impact on the vast majority of the population.

How do we get from here to there? Deciding on the action to be taken

We have already noted that in an uncertain world, strategic plans need to be flexible and adaptable, with later interventions influenced by the outcomes of earlier activities. This suggests the need for a stepwise approach to setting, refining and working towards objectives. Early activities provide opportunities to gain an improved understanding of problems and possibilities, allowing intermediate objectives to be defined and/or refined. As the process develops, the overall vision can be developed into a more concrete set of goals. Even after the individual components of the strategic plan have been decided, there will be a need to review longer term actions and objectives in the light of the experience gained as the plan unfolds.

The problem with the approach is that it will sometimes be difficult to determine whether a particular action will take us where we want to go. There is a real danger that the approach will have no clear focus and deteriorate into a series of isolated initiatives, which lead nowhere in particular. The principles that are introduced and discussed in the remainder of this chapter help to avoid this danger by providing a framework for assessing whether or not efforts to improve sanitation services are moving in the right direction.

Principles for effective strategic planning

We have identified six principles for effective strategic planning. These are broadly based on those identified in the original Strategic Sanitation Approach (SSA), as described by Wright (1997), but have been modified as necessary to take account of important issues that emerged in the course of research into its implementation in practice.

Principle 1 Respond to informed demand

Until fairly recently, efforts to improve service provision focused on *supply,* i.e. what the organization responsible for provision could deliver. Purely supply-driven approaches are based on the knowledge and assumptions of outsiders and pay little attention to what users want and their willingness to pay for services. Their failure to take account of the local situation and people's needs can lead to premature failure of services. At worst, they can deliver facilities and services that are not used because they are not what people want.

In response to these deficiencies, the current 'received wisdom' emphasizes the need to respond to *demand* so as to provide the services that people want and for which they are willing to pay. While clearly an improvement on the old supply-driven approach, a purely demand-responsive approach to planning presents the following problems.

○ It is based solely on what the intended service users know, thus limiting the scope for the introduction of new ideas and hence for change and innovation.

○ In implicitly accepting that people's main concerns are likely to relate to their immediate surroundings, it tends to favour local improvements at the expense of the wider environment.

○ In equating demand with willingness to pay, it may downplay the fact that the main problem may be either the unwillingness of service providers to charge users for the full cost of the services or the inability of poor people to pay the full cost of the services on offer.

○ It pays insufficient attention to the capacity of service deliverers to respond to demand. Where this capacity is limited, there is a real danger that demand for a service will be increased without any realistic prospect that service providers can respond to that demand.

These points suggest that, rather than a pure demand- or supply-based approach, the need is for a process that first *establishes* demand, then *informs* it and finally *responds* to the informed demand in an effective way.

The point about informing demand is particularly important. We will see in Chapter 8 that the choice of sanitation technology should be guided by objective assessment of local conditions. Those who guide this process of choice, whether they are professionals or local activists, can help to ensure that demand is informed.

This does not mean that the flow of information should all be in one direction. Figure 2.2 illustrates the point that, to be informed, sanitation choices must also take account of the knowledge and views of the intended users of sanitation facilities. Like all diagrams, this is a simplification of reality and planners should be aware that technical information does not rest solely with official providers. For instance, in Pakistan, NGOs and CBOs, rather than government authorities, are the main promoters of sewerage to serve informal areas.

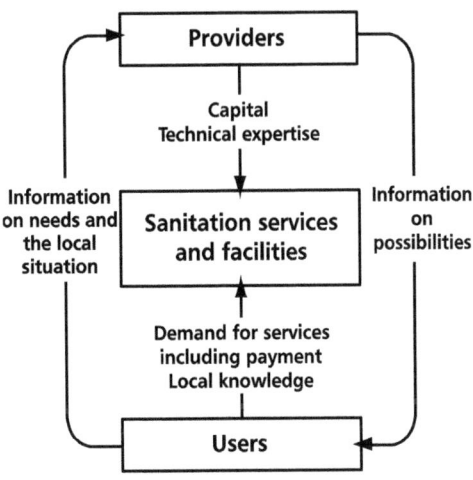

Figure 2.2 Information flows required to respond to informed demand

studies may provide useful information on the demand for services, they are unlikely to yield results that are commensurate with the effort required to conduct them unless there is a basic acceptance of the need to charge for services. Further information on methods of assessing willingness to pay and their potential uses is given in Chapter 8.

Where does willingness to pay fit into this scenario? Economists often start from the assumption that there can be no demand for a service unless users are willing to pay for it. This assumption is reasonable in an ideal world in which everyone pays the full cost of the services that they receive. However, there is evidence from many countries that governments rarely recover the full cost of the services that they provide selectively to higher-income groups. Where this is the case, insistence on recovering the full cost of services from poor people is inequitable and probably unrealistic. Where the rich receive subsidies it is arguable that poor people can quite legitimately demand services even when they are unwilling to pay the full cost of those services. The key issue here is whether the charges collected from users are sufficient to cover the ongoing operation and maintenance of services and hence ensure their sustainability over time. We will return to this point shortly.

This brief discussion of the issues surrounding demand and willingness to pay suggests that, while willingness to pay

Principle 2 Focus on sound finances

Expansion of sanitation systems will not be possible unless an institution or group of individuals, preferably the intended users, is willing to pay for the new facilities required. Even when facilities have been provided, they will fail sooner or later unless funds are available to cover their ongoing operation and maintenance. So, it will be impossible to first provide and then sustain services to cities as a whole without ensuring that the finances of sanitation service providers are sound.

Progress towards achieving sound finances can be made by increasing the amount that sanitation users pay for services, always assuming that these increases are related to the quality of service provided.[3] However, this is only one side of the equation. It is equally important to consider the ways in which the cost of sanitation services can be reduced. Options in this respect include the following.

o Choose an affordable technology, as in many situations, on-site or local sanitation facilities will be a lot cheaper to build and operate than centralized sewerage. When considering the affordability of a technology, do not consider only its capital cost but also the amount that will be required to operate and maintain it over time.

o Select an appropriate level of service, for instance designing drainage systems to deal with the rainfall that occurs on average once every six months (in technical terms a six month return period storm) rather than that which occurs on average once in every 10 years. While the latter may be the ideal, in that it reduces the frequency and intensity of flooding, the former may be all that can be afforded in the short term.

o Use appropriate technical standards, taking account of the local situation and the function that the facility is intended to perform. The standards that are appropriate for low-income areas may be very different from generally accepted norms, which are often based, with little amendment, on those used in western industrialized countries. For example, shallow sewers with inspection chambers rather than manholes may be appropriate under pavements and in narrow lanes that do not carry heavy traffic. A note of caution is needed here. There is no point in reducing standards in order to reduce capital costs if the result is a greatly increased need for maintenance, significantly shortened facility life or both.

o Improve management efficiency, perhaps by encouraging the involvement of private sector and/or civil society organizations in aspects of sanitation provision, thus reducing costs and helping to make services more affordable. Involvement of civil society organizations and local entrepreneurs is likely to be particularly appropriate for local services, and we will return to this issue when we consider the options for devolving responsibility for such services.

These objectives are not mutually exclusive and there will normally be a need for integrated action involving more than one of them. In particular, increased tariffs will tend to exclude the poorest and there will often be a need to explore ways in which they can be provided with an adequate but sustainable service. One option in this respect will be to consider the use of different technologies in different areas. For instance, on-site excreta disposal may be the best option in relatively low-density low-income areas on the urban periphery, even when sewers are provided in the town or city centre. This is what the SSA describes as unbundling of sanitation technologies (see Box 2.1)

Principle 3 Develop incentives for good practice

Incentives encourage individuals and organizations to act in certain ways and in doing so help to provide the context within which efforts to improve sanitation services take place. They can apply both to individual san-

---

Box 2.1 Unbundling technologies – the case of Maseru, Lesotho

Maseru, the capital of Lesotho in Southern Africa, has a population of just over 200 000. It is a low-density city that has spread far beyond the limits of the original colonial town. The central business district and adjacent areas are sewered and the sewers discharge to a waste stabilization pond treatment system. While this system functions effectively, the cost of extending it to the whole of the sprawling city would be enormous and clearly unaffordable to the mainly low-income people who live in outlying areas. Because of the lack of house water connections and low density, sewerage would be technically inappropriate for these areas in any case. In fact, most people in these outlying areas have solved their own excreta disposal needs by building pit latrines, most of which serve individual households although 'row tenements' – groups of single-room dwellings built for rent – are served by shared facilities. In Maseru, unbundling has happened in practice, with or without formal plans.

itation users and to the organizations that provide sanitation services. Incentives for service providers and their employees to improve their performance have a particularly important role in providing the context for strategic planning. They can take the form of:

o *rewards for good performance* – for instance, increased funding for municipalities that succeed in implementing effective sanitation programmes

o *sanctions against harmful actions and/or failure to act* – for instance, a ban, supported by fines, on the use of untreated sewage to irrigate crops.

Incentives will only be effective if there are clear rules for implementing them and referees to see that the rules are enforced. Referees, in the form of regulatory bodies, will be particularly important when the private sector is given a large role in sanitation provision. At the local level, informed and organized users may be the best guarantors of effective services.

It is often assumed that incentives should be applied at the city level by the municipal authorities and other local stakeholders. However, incentive structures are often decided at the 'centre' by higher levels of government, while local governments tend to follow the rules and regulations handed down to them from above. In most countries, this situation is unlikely to change greatly in the near future, despite the widespread talk of decentralization. The clear implication is that efforts to introduce incentives for the adoption of strategic planning approaches will often have to be made by higher levels of government. In particular, strategic planning is unlikely to be widely practised unless government rules and procedures require it. We will return to this issue in Chapter 4.

Principle 4 Involve stakeholders in appropriate ways

Stakeholders are people, groups and organizations with an interest in some particular subject, in this case sanitation. They include the following:

o Primary stakeholders – individuals, groups and institutions that the planned activity is likely to affect, either positively or negatively. In addition to individuals and households, they include the community groups and community-based organizations (CBOs) that represent them. Primary stakeholders are not just passive receivers of services. Individual households will usually be involved in some way in providing their own facilities while CBOs may be involved in lobbying for improved services and initiating and managing small- to medium-sized sanitation improvement initiatives.

o Secondary stakeholders – all others who are involved in aspects of sanitation provision. These include the government and international organizations that develop and/or advise on sanitation policies and provide finance for sanitation programmes, service delivery organizations in the public, private and civil society sectors and organizations that act as intermediaries between service providers and service users.

Stakeholders may be involved in planning for improved sanitation provision and later in managing aspects of sanitation provision, operation and maintenance.

The key to successful stakeholder involvement in planning lies in ensuring that the various stakeholders are involved in ways that are appropriate to their interests, capabilities and responsibilities. For example, members of a particular community are more likely to be interested in discussing options for solid waste collection services to serve their area than they are in the location of the municipal landfill (unless of course the latter is close to where they live).

The key to realistic assessment of the possible roles for different stakeholders in provision, operation and maintenance lies in recognition of the possibility of 'unbundling' of responsibilities. All this means is that it is possible for responsibilities for sanitation provision to be divided and devolved, with different groups taking responsibility for services in different areas (horizontal unbundling) and/or at different levels in the service hierarchy (vertical unbundling). In most situations, there will already be some division of responsibilities, with various individuals and groups taking responsibility for aspects of sanitation provision, albeit in some cases informally. The challenge for planners will often be to integrate this more or less informal, local activity into the mainstream. This will require:

○ recognition of the validity of stakeholder efforts

○ agreement on roles and responsibilities

○ provision for improved coordination between different stakeholders.

Each of these important requirements is now explored.

Recognising the validity of stakeholder efforts

The main problem here is that many of the activities undertaken by individuals and groups to improve sanitation conditions are informal in the sense that they take place outside official rules and procedures. Almost by definition, these efforts go unrecognized by government and yet they represent a valuable resource. Demonstration projects can be used to show the viability of community-led initiatives. However, government officials may not be prepared to recognize the findings of such projects.

Champions of local stakeholder involvement can help to overcome these problems, particularly if they have at least one foot in the government camp so that they act as a bridge between the government and informal stakeholders. Figure 2.3 shows one initiative that benefited from, and indeed was initiated by, a local champion.

Agreement on roles and responsibilities

The starting point for agreement on roles and responsibilities is recognition that sanitation services are often provided through more or less hierarchical systems, the components of which are linked so that performance at one level of the system depends on the adequacy or otherwise of the services provided at other levels. This point is clearly illustrated by sewerage, which normally includes the following:

○ household facilities (WCs, washing facilities, etc.) connected to

○ tertiary or street sewers, which in turn connect to

○ secondary or collector sewers, serving local neighbourhoods and larger districts. Unless systems are decentralized with local treatment facilities, these in turn must connect to

○ primary facilities, trunk sewers and sewage treatment facilities.

While the hierarchy may not be so obvious for other services, it is usually there. For instance, on-site sanitation may appear to involve only on-site facilities but there will usually be a need for 'higher level' pit emptying and sludge disposal services. Once this hierarchy is recognized, it is possible to match roles and responsibilities to the interests and abilities of the various stakeholder

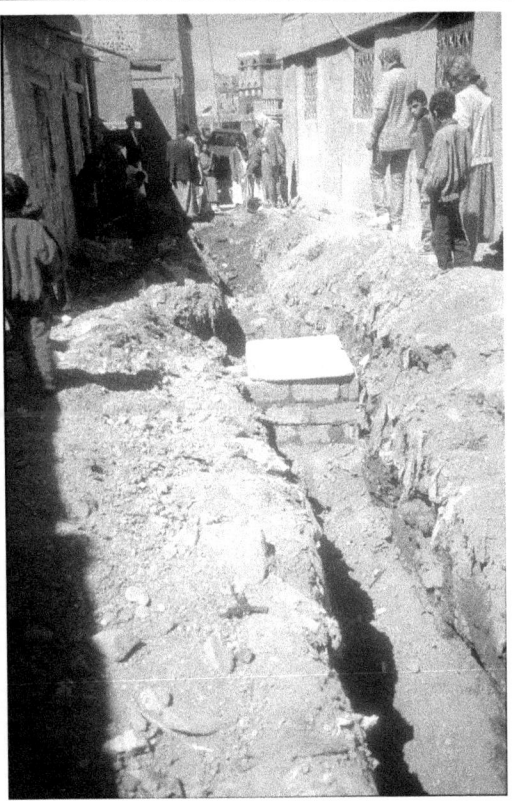

Figure 2.3 The role of champions in promoting recognition of local initiatives

This sewer under construction in Noqom, on the outskirts of Sana'a, Yemen, is part of an initiative started by a local member of parliament and funded by local people. The overall design was carried out by the National Water and Sanitation Agency (NWASA), for whom the member of parliament had previously worked. Later extensions have been funded through the World Bank-supported Public Works Program, suggesting that the approach has, at least in part, been 'institutionalized'.

groups and organizations, using the following broad guidelines.

○ Households should normally be responsible for managing facilities within their plot boundaries (as is normally the case already).

○ Community organizations, ward councillors, local NGOs, local entrepreneurs and local branches of municipal government and/or specialist service providers may be involved in the management of relatively simple local systems. Their direct interest in the functioning of these services means that they may carry out management tasks more effectively than would a remote government department.

○ Larger, more formally structured organizations will be required to manage higher-order services. Most will be government organizations, although recent years have seen increased interest in the involvement of the private sector in the management of municipal services.

In Chapter 5, we record how one organization, the Karachi based Orangi Pilot Project (OPP) has developed an approach to the assignment of roles and responsibilities that is in close agreement with these general principles.

Coordinating stakeholder efforts

The downside of unbundling is that it often leads to fragmented responsibilities and thus creates an increased need for effective coordination between different organizations. Indeed, lack of coordination between the various individuals, groups and organizations with an involvement in sanitation provision is often one of the biggest obstacles to the introduction of improved services. In many situations, the priority will be to improve coordination between the various stakeholders rather than to encourage further unbundling of responsibilities. The practical ways in which this might be achieved will be considered further in later chapters.

Principle 5 Take a wide view of sanitation

Sanitation strategies should look beyond local solutions to narrowly defined problems to recognize the importance of hygiene and the links between different sanitation services. Excreta disposal, solid waste management and drainage are interrelated and the impact of improvements in one may be reduced if they are carried out in isolation from improvements in the others. For instance, plans to replace existing drains with sewers must make allowance for the dual role of existing drains as carriers of both foul and storm water. Uncollected solid waste tends to find its way to drains and sewers, greatly increasing maintenance requirements. Some excreta disposal methods (for instance, pit latrines) may require separate provision for sullage disposal.

There is a second aspect to taking a wide view of sanitation. This concerns the need to go beyond local solutions to local problems to consider the wider environmental impacts of proposed initiatives. We have already noted that, while local initiatives can have a significant impact upon health and environmental conditions in low-income communities, they can create problems for the wider environment. For instance, while sewerage will improve conditions in the areas that it serves, the sewage that it carries may pollute the surface water bodies to which it is discharged, resulting in fish kills that may affect the livelihoods of fishermen. Health impacts, in particular the transmission of intestinal nematodes such as roundworm (*ascaris*) and hookworm may be a concern where wastewater is used for irrigation.[4]

One response to this need to consider the wider implications of sanitation initiatives is to seek to retain excreta on or near the plot, allowing it to decompose naturally in a pit or tank and thus reducing the danger of surface water pollution. There is also much to be said for considering the options for keeping 'black' and 'grey' water separate so as to reduce the volume of high strength waste to be treated. Chapter 8 and Appendix 2 provide further information on sanitation options and the factors that affect sanitation choice.

Principle 6 Take manageable steps towards securable intermediate objectives

This last principle is closely linked with the adaptive approach to the development and implementation of strategies introduced earlier in this chapter. It is based on recognition of the fact that it will often be possible to convert large and complex problems into smaller disaggregated ones that can be dealt with incrementally through what the SSA referred to as a 'small steps' approach (see Chapter 3).

In order to achieve a sustainable objective and hence bring about lasting benefits, each step must be large enough to overcome the fundamental problem that it sets out to solve. So, for instance, the provision of local solid waste collection services may not work if simultaneous provision is not made for the secondary collection services to which they will connect. For this reason, we prefer to use the term 'manageable steps' because not all the steps can or should be small. The challenge for planners is therefore to identify manageable steps towards achievable objectives that:

- are consistent with the need to move towards overall goals
- once achieved, can be sustained so that they result in lasting benefits
- are framed in the light of existing systems and resources (where we are now)
- help to change systems and develop resources in a way that enables more ambitious follow-on steps to be taken in the future.

There will always be some tensions between the need to achieve sustainable benefits and that to move in manageable steps. Resolving these tensions is perhaps the most difficult and yet most important task required of strategic planners.

One option for responding to these tensions is to first examine the extent to which problems can be solved locally, only going on to consider the wider context when initial analysis shows that local action alone cannot address a particular problem. This is the basic philosophy underlying what has come to be known as the household-centred approach.

It may be that key stakeholders do not recognize the need to follow one or more of the other strategic principles. For instance, sanitation services are often heavily subsidized. In such circumstances, the concept of demand, in the sense of establishing willingness to pay something approaching the full cost of services, may mean little to the various stakeholders. Where this is the case, it may be necessary to look at options for moving in manageable steps towards full acceptance of the principle. In the case of demand, the first step might be to persuade sanitation providers that the poor do pay for services. This might be followed by attempts to obtain full cost recovery on operation and maintenance costs and finally to attempts to recover something close to the full cost of providing and maintaining services. Box 2.2 provides an example of how this approach was applied in Bharatpur.

Key points in this chapter

1. The ultimate aim of sanitation strategies should be to provide effective sanitation services to towns and cities as a whole. In the short term, there may be a need to focus on more local action, but this should have the potential to be scaled up to a city-wide scale.

2. In the interests of equity, special attention should be given to the sanitation needs of low-income areas.

Box 2.2 Bharatpur – an incremental approach to demand and incentives

The fieldwork in Bharatpur revealed very little commitment to a demand-based approach. Municipal officials felt strongly that services for the poor should be either free or heavily subsidized. In theory, households were required to provide a small contribution to the cost of latrines provided under the Indian government's Integrated Low Cost Sanitation (ILCS) programme. In practice, this contribution was not collected, partly because the state government made no attempt to recover costs from municipalities so that the latter had no incentive to recover them from households. In the light of this situation, the WSP team that supported the process focused on incremental improvements, advocating the introduction of hygiene promotion to increase demand for sanitation and encouraging the state government to start to collect the municipal contribution to the ILCS scheme.

3. Plans should focus on providing sustainable services rather than facilities alone, paying particular attention to operation and maintenance.

4. Plans should be grounded in the existing situation and respond to actual rather than assumed problems and deficiencies. In particular, they should address any problems with the management of existing facilities.

5. Sanitation strategies should be flexible, allowing for later activities to be amended in the light of feedback from earlier activities.

6. Sanitation providers should recognize the need to first inform and then respond to user demand.

7. Action must be matched to available resources and so plans need to consider the financial implications of sanitation choices and pay attention to the need for sound finances.

8. Incentives help to provide the context within which sanitation initiatives take place and so can have an important impact on the success of sanitation plans. They will normally have to be created by higher levels of government.

9. It is neither necessary nor desirable for one organization to be responsible for all aspects of sanitation provision. Some division and devolution of responsibilities will often be appropriate. Conversely, there will be situations in which the priority is improved coordination between the various stakeholders.

10. Different sanitation technologies may be required in different locations in the same town or city.

11. Sanitation strategies should take account of the links between different services, the impact of local action on the wider environment and the dependence of local services on higher-order facilities.

12. A sanitation strategy is more likely to be achievable and adaptable to circumstances if it focuses on identifying intermediate objectives and taking manageable steps towards those objectives.

Chapter 2 endnotes

1 Rondinelli's argument draws on the earlier work of Lindblom (1965).
2 There may sometimes have to be short-term trade-offs between solutions to people's pressing needs and a concern with the environment as a whole, but sanitation planners should be aware of those trade-offs and look for solutions to problems that minimize adverse environmental impacts.
3 In some cases, existing tariffs for sewerage and drainage are so low that tariff increases must be the first step. However, even in such cases, long-term plans must take account of the link between providing an adequate quality of service and maintaining tariffs at satisfactory levels.
4 Blumenthal et al. (2000), Edwards (1992), Shuval et al. (1986) and Strauss and Blumenthal (1990) provide detailed documentation of the health implications of reuse of excreta and wastewater for irrigation and aquaculture and the strategies for mitigation of the health risks.

CHAPTER 3
Strategic sanitation planning in towns and cities

IN THIS CHAPTER, we are concerned with how a strategic approach to planning can be translated into action at the municipal level. Sanitation problems vary from place to place and so the intention is not to provide a blueprint for dealing with every type of problem in every type of situation. Rather, we suggest a step-wise approach to analysing and solving problems.

The first part of this chapter describes the pilot planning process carried out in the town of Bharatpur in the Indian state of Rajasthan. Following this, a conceptual approach to planning at the municipal level, based on the Bharatpur experience, is introduced and explored.

The development of a strategic model – the Bharatpur pilot process

The background

Bharatpur is a town with a population of about 200 000, located some 150 km south of Delhi. It is a fairly typical medium-sized Indian town. There is no sewerage and most households discharge wastewater to open drains via septic tanks. The town centres on a large fort, which is surrounded by a moat, the Sujan Ganga. This dates from the eighteenth century when Bharatpur was a Rajput stronghold. An outer moat was built by the Rajputs to protect the town itself and much of the town remains inside this moat, although development has also spread beyond it. There are now some breaks in the outer moat and the sections that remain have reduced in size due to encroachment and infilling. Street patterns within the outer moat have not changed much over the years and this central part of the town still has relatively high population densities and a 'vernacular' feel. Housing densities outside the outer moat tend to be lower and there are areas of informal housing both within and outside the outer moat. Some of these are officially designated as 'slums', a term that is used in India for low-income areas that have been developed informally, usually on government land, and have subsequently been officially recognized by the government and given the right to receive basic services.

The Sujan Ganga and the outer moat were originally fed by clean water from outside the town but both are now heavily polluted with wastewater discharged from drains. Indeed, the channels that were originally built to bring clean water into the town are now used to drain dirty water out of it. Solid waste collection services do not reach all parts of the town, particularly lower-income settlements in urban fringe areas and disposal is to a 'dump site' rather than to a properly managed sanitary landfill. Bharatpur Municipal Council (BMC) has installed communal sanitation facilities in some low-income areas and has also provided individual twin-pit pour-flush latrines to some households, with funding from the Indian government's Integrated Low Cost Sanitation (ILCS) programme.

During the mid-1990s, the Water and

Sanitation Program – South Asia (WSP-SA), the regional arm of the WSP, wished to explore the practical application of the SSA. The UK government's Department for International Development (DFID) made funds available to support this work through its research budget and it was decided that one key aspect of the research would involve the implementation of a pilot strategic planning exercise in an Indian town.

Following discussions between WSP-SA and the Rajasthan State authorities in Jaipur, several potential locations were identified. Bharatpur was chosen from among these potential pilot project locations because BMC had expressed interest in the process and because the town presented a range of sanitation problems of the type that might be addressed through a strategic plan (WSP-SA 2000).

The planning process started in mid-1998 and continued through to the production of a strategic plan in early 2000. Jeremy Colin, one of the authors, acting as an external facilitator provided through WSP-SA, assisted the process. He was not based in Bharatpur on a full-time basis but provided inputs at key stages in the process, spending a total of about six months in Bharatpur over the two years of the pilot project.

Early activities

The facilitator's first task was to identify potential partners within the town. As he made contact with the various potential partners, he explained something of the background to the initiative, emphasizing that its objective was to develop a plan for the town in accordance with strategic principles that was agreed by a wide range of stakeholders. These stakeholders fell into two broad categories – government departments and non-government organizations.

Among government organizations, BMC had already expressed commitment to the pilot planning initiative. The other government organization with obvious potential interest in the process was the Public Health Engineering Department (PHED), which had prepared a plan to sewer the town some years previously, although this had not succeeded in attracting funding from the state government.

Among non-government organizations, one potential partner was the NGO Sulabh International,[1] which had installed some public latrines in the town and was also contracted by BMC to provide latrines under the ILCS programme. ACORD and Lupin, two NGOs with programmes in the surrounding rural areas, also emerged as potential partners in the course of the facilitator's initial contacts and discussions.

As the Bharatpur process developed, the various stakeholders were encouraged to think about current sanitation problems in the town, and to develop initial ideas on answers to the following questions.

○ Who is responsible for existing services?
○ What sanitation problems do we face?
○ What are the causes of those problems?
○ What resources do we have to solve them?

At this stage, the focus was on the need to gain a broad understanding of *how* services currently functioned in order to identify problems and gain an initial understanding of the causes of those problems. As part of this process, the two NGOs, ACORD and Lupin, carried out a consultation exercise with low- and middle-income communities in Bharatpur to assess perceptions of sanitation-related problems.

The first planning workshop

This initial process of contacting stakeholders and encouraging them to think about

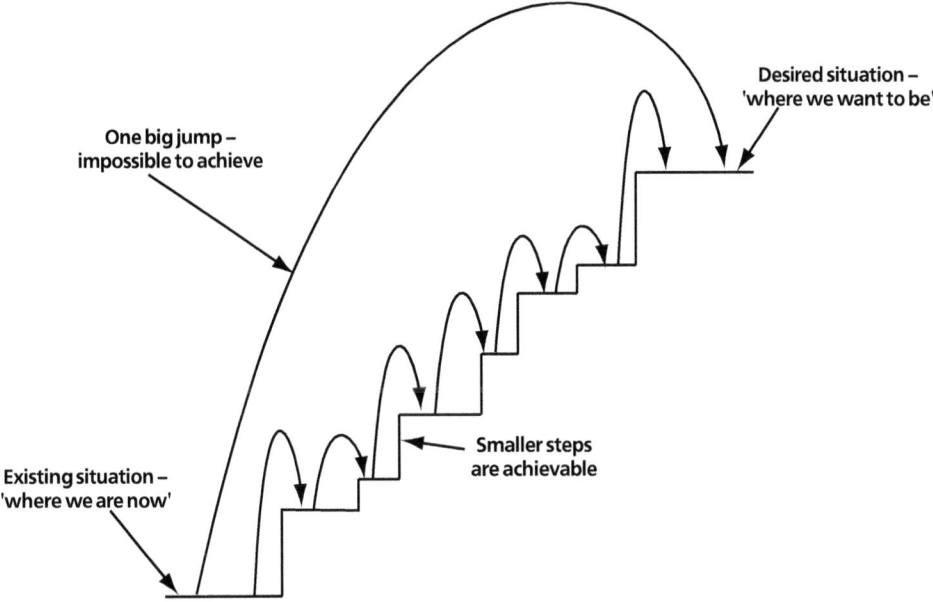

Figure 3.1 Small-steps approach towards achieving the desired situation

problems lasted about two months and culminated in a two-day planning workshop, which set the scene for much of what was to follow. The workshop objectives were to:

o reach agreement on current sanitation problems and their causes

o develop a framework for the production of a comprehensive sanitation plan

o allocate tasks and responsibilities for short-term action

o identify support requirements for developing the plan.

The first part of the workshop focused on problem analysis. Participants were invited to write cards on sanitation-related problems and these were then grouped to show how the problems were interrelated (Chapter 9 provides further information on preparing and using cards for participatory planning purposes). Following this, the two NGOs that had carried out consultation exercises presented their findings to the workshop. This helped to bring community concerns to the attention of workshop participants without increasing the number of participants to the point at which the workshop became unwieldy. The session ended with a plenary discussion structured around three questions.

o What do we need from the community?

o How do we get better community support?

o Which organizations should lead the various activities identified in response to the second question?

The first day concluded with a presentation on the need to take a strategic approach. This compared improving sanitation to climbing a flight of stairs, the analogy used for the small-steps approach described in Chapter 2. The facilitator stressed that the initial problem analysis had suggested that Bharatpur was near the bottom of the stairs (see Figure 3.1), with poor sanitation facilities and services. Clearly, everyone present would like to be at the top of the stairs, with the best facilities possible, but it would be impossible to arrive at this point in one leap. Just as with climbing a flight of stairs, it was necessary to proceed step by step. Some tasks would require more effort than others – represented by the height of the step, while others would take longer than others – indicated by the length of the step.

The second day started with a discussion of the strategic principles introduced on the previous day. One point to emerge from this discussion was the need to develop new mechanisms to provided links between the municipal authorities and the people that they were intended to serve. In theory councillors should have been providing this link but workshop participants thought that this mechanism was not working well.

The next session focused on the question of resources. To facilitate analysis, participants were asked to identify available resources in relation to a matrix which identified the various sectors to be considered in any plan along one axis and the tasks to be undertaken along the second axis. The techniques used are explored in more detail in Chapter 7.

Attention now turned to the way in which the planning process could be taken forward. First, an interim coordinating committee was set up to oversee activities during the next stage of the planning process. This was fairly small and included the Chairman, Medical Officer and Deputy Town Planner from BMC, the Superintending Engineer from the PHED and representatives of ACORD and Lupin. Next, a number of tasks, intended to prepare the way for the development of a full municipal strategic sanitation plan, were agreed and responsibilities for carrying out these tasks were assigned. The tasks identified are listed and briefly described in Box 3.1. A matrix system similar to that already used to identify resources was used to identify responsibilities for carrying out tasks.

Finally, a timetable for the completion of tasks was agreed and arrangements were made for a follow-up meeting to bring together the outputs from these tasks and finalize a strategic sanitation plan.

Follow-up to the planning workshop

Six months were allowed for the completion of the tasks identified in the planning workshop, following which it was agreed that there would be a follow-up workshop at which the overall structure and contents of the municipal plan itself would be agreed. In practice, some of the tasks took rather more than six months while others were not started.

The slow progress was partly due to the fact that some of the tasks proved to be more complex than had been realized during the workshop. For instance, it proved difficult to introduce an effective drain-cleaning programme. Drains that are prevented from flowing freely because of either a lack of fall or downstream obstructions tend to silt rapidly and therefore require high levels of maintenance. Bharatpur is a very flat town and, without information on drain levels, it was difficult to identify the causes of silting and decide where any increased maintenance effort could usefully be focused. Perhaps as a result of this, the municipality made little effort to develop a drain-cleaning programme in advance of the completion of the drainage survey and the information it would give on drain levels. Despite this, it should have been possible to identify areas with reasonable gradients in which improved arrangements for drain maintenance could usefully have been introduced.

A more general problem emerged during this period. Despite their exposure to strategic principles, government officials were unconvinced by the small-steps approach and

Box 3.1 Tasks identified during the Bharatpur workshop

Task 1 Drainage survey – covering the whole town and intended to provide the basis for understanding and, if necessary, redesigning its drainage system. Undertaken by consultants on behalf of the Municipal Council with assistance provided by WSP-SA.

Task 2 Drain cleaning – thorough cleansing of main drains in order to reduce flooding problems. Assigned to the Municipal Council with assistance again provided by WSP-SA. This task was scheduled to start immediately, rains permitting.

Task 3 Solid waste management – review of the existing solid waste management system in the town as a whole, with a special focus on one ward. Led by the NGO ACORD with funding provided from the research funds and routed through WSP-SA.

Task 4 Latrine survey – technical and social review of existing low-cost sanitation initiatives in one or more wards. Assigned to the Municipal Council in collaboration with Sulabh International and Lupin.

Task 5 Sanitation promotion – promotion of low-cost sanitation including hygiene education in the same ward/s as that in which Task 4 was carried out. Assigned to the Municipal Council in collaboration with Sulabh International. WSP-SA and UNICEF were identified as possible resources to provide training in basic sanitation and hygiene promotion for community workers.

Task 6 Social and technical mapping of town – to identify areas where sanitation needs were greatest. The lead agency was Lupin, with advice on methodology provided either by UNICEF or by the Indian Institute of Rural Development in Jaipur. Further details of social and technical mapping are given in Chapter 7.

Task 7 Community involvement – to develop proposals for community organizations to facilitate community involvement in a future comprehensive sanitation programme. Led by Lupin with advice from WSP-SA and other agencies as appropriate.

Task 8 Financial planning – focusing on collecting user contributions for the Integrated Low Cost Sanitation scheme, in accordance with state policy. The municipality and Sulabh International were to be the lead agencies with support provided by WSP-SA as required.

still tended to think that the only 'correct' planning option was the production of a comprehensive master plan. Perhaps as a consequence of this, many were more interested in building new facilities than improving the operation and maintenance of those that already existed. Not surprisingly, given its role as a planning and design agency, this was particularly true of the PHED.

Another problem related to the fact that municipal stakeholders did not always fully grasp aspects of the tasks that they had been asked to undertake. For instance, Lupin did not make much progress with the task of social and technical mapping, partly because they did not really understand its significance and were not clear on how to tackle it. In retrospect, it may have been better to delay this task and to carry it out in the context of the strategic plan itself. Similarly, limited progress was made with the financial planning task because BMC and Sulabh, which were responsible for this task, had not fully accepted the importance of recovering costs from users.

The NGOs proved adept at mobilizing communities but were then hampered by a lack of knowledge of the options for dealing with the problems of those communities. They also lacked experience in mediating between stakeholder groups with different viewpoints and concerns. For instance, efforts to improve solid waste management services on a pilot basis in one ward were resisted by the private sweepers working in the ward. It was clear that the NGOs and other actors in the process would need to develop new skills and techniques if they were to be effective in facilitating efforts to resolve differences.

The process was undoubtedly held back by the fact that there was no statutory requirement for the municipality to produce a strategic plan. Not surprisingly, municipalities with limited resources tend to focus on the activities that they have to undertake rather than those that are optional (Zaidi 1996).

Despite these problems, considerable progress was made during this stage of the planning process. The whole town was surveyed, maps were produced at a scale of 1:500 and an outline scheme for improving drainage was prepared. A pilot project to improve drainage and remove a large stagnant pond was identified in a low-income area. Options for improvements in the implementation of the ILCS were identified. The survey of existing solid waste management practices was completed and provided a good insight into existing services in the town and the possibilities for change.

A rather less tangible but equally important benefit was the fact that the various stakeholders became used to working together, increasing the likelihood that they would choose to collaborate further in the future.

The second workshop and the written plan

The activities described above culminated in a second workshop, during which the overall structure and content of the plan, together with responsibilities for producing and implementing it, were discussed and agreed. Work then continued on the development of the plan. This was a written document, covering a period of three years and containing detailed proposals for the actions required to address priority problems. The plan document was divided into two main sections and a number of annexes as follows.

Section 1 set out the overall framework for the plan, stating the overall vision and providing information on the principles underlying the plan, roles and responsibilities, arrangements for managing plan implementation, financial arrangements and responsibilities and an assessment of capacity-building needs.

Section 2 was divided into a number of chapters, each of which dealt with one of the plan components. For each component, information was given on the current situation, responsibility for implementation, the plan objectives and the strategy for achieving those objectives. Targets were given for the outputs to be achieved during the first year and at the end of the three year planning period. Information on additional resources required to implement the plan was also provided for each component.

The appendices covered the make-up and responsibilities of a Sanitation Coordination Committee, contact details for the various stakeholders, an inventory of capacity-building needs, an outline budget for items for which funding was not immediately available and an annual maintenance plan for drainage.

More detailed information on the structure and contents of a typical plan, based on that produced in Bharatpur is given in Boxes 3.3 and 3.4 later in this chapter.

Once complete, the draft plan was made available for comment by the various stakeholders. Following receipt of comments, it was amended and the amended version was formally adopted by BMC.

Stages in the development of a strategic plan

We now turn to the general lessons to be learnt from the Bharatpur experience, starting with what it tells us about the best way to structure a strategic planning exercise. Figure 3.2 shows, in broad outline, the stages in the development of a strategic plan at the municipal level. The essence of the Bharatpur process is represented by the three stages identified in the central box:

○ understand problems

○ develop solutions

○ plan city-wide.

Figure 3.2 also takes account of the need to prepare for any strategic planning exercise and to follow up on the plan to ensure that it is implemented.

The feedback loops illustrate the fact that analysis of completed activities can help to create a better understanding of problems and their causes and can thus influence the decisions made about later stages in the planning process. This suggests that planning should not be a one-off event. Rather, there is a need to develop solutions and amend plans in the light of experience

Bear in mind the fact that processes in the real world will always be more complex than can be represented by an idealized model. In particular, some activities can be started immediately and completed quickly while others may require a period of preparation and take longer to implement.

The process is compatible with the adaptive approach to strategic planning set out in Chapter 2. The initial emphasis on understanding problems helps to ensure that the planning process is firmly grounded in the existing situation. The developing solutions stage provides time for information to be gathered and objectives to be decided, allowing the process to proceed in a step-wise manner. The emphasis on taking account of lessons learnt from completed activities helps to ensure that the planning process is flexible and can be adapted in the light of changing circumstances and improved understanding of problems and possibilities.

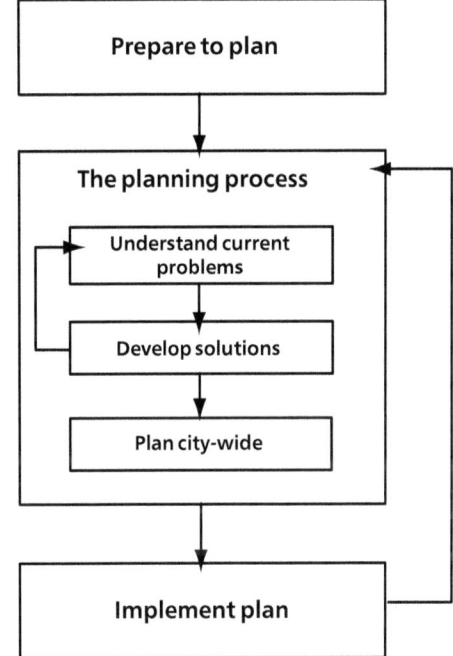

Figure 3.2 The strategic process at the municipal level

The approach adopted in Bharatpur has similarities to action planning approaches, which have been favoured by many development theorists and promoted by international agencies over the years.[2] Like these approaches, it involved an initial focus on understanding the existing situation, the establishment of an overall vision and a series of actions designed to lead towards the achievement of that vision. It differs from other action planning approaches in its emphasis on 'developing solutions'. The developing solutions stage provides time to:

○ extend and deepen the process of identifying the components of the final plan, thus overcoming what has been one of the major drawbacks of the traditional 'project cycle' – the identification of interventions on the basis of insufficient information

○ develop the commitment and capacity of the various stakeholders to implement the final plan.

Bearing these points in mind, we now consider each of the stages in the planning process in more detail, drawing on the lessons learnt from Bharatpur where appropriate.

Preparing to plan

The first priority when setting out to develop a strategic plan is to ensure that you have a remit to plan. Many municipal officials assume that they can only do what is specifically required by existing rules and regulations. They sometimes interpret these rules and regulations in a very conservative way, assuming that no aspect of currently accepted procedure can ever be changed. So, if there is no mention of strategic planning in the procedures, they believe that it cannot be considered. In fact, existing rules and regulations usually offer more flexibility than is commonly assumed (Cotton et al. 1998) and do not prevent committed individuals from seeking to act more strategically. Nevertheless, it is important to confirm that this is the case. Where approval from a higher level of government is necessary, obtaining this approval should be a priority.

Once it is established that a strategic plan is possible, preparations for planning can proceed. These preparations should seek to achieve the following.

○ Identify potential partners in the planning process. These are likely to include:

- municipalities and other government agencies with statutory responsibility for aspects of sanitation provision

- elected representatives, who may exercise some control over government development funds assigned to their constituencies

- NGOs, which may already be working closely with low-income communities and may possess skills in social investigation and analysis that are not available within government

- CBO leaders and other activists who, in some way, represent low-income communities.

○ Develop consensus on the need to plan. It will be easier to develop this consensus where government regulations require the production of a strategic plan and/or the plan can be used to attract government and/or external funding. Where this is not the case, it will be important to be able to demonstrate to stakeholders, and particularly key decision makers that the plan will make a difference and that they can influence the form that it will take if they engage in the planning process. One way of achieving this will be to arrange for local stakeholders to meet their counterparts in a municipality that has already carried out a successful strategic planning exercise.

○ Establish a core team to lead the process. It is unrealistic to assume that the planning process can be led by one person, or even by one organization. Efforts should therefore be made to identify those individuals and organizations with a possible interest in taking a leading role in the planning process.

The municipal authorities should always take a leading role in the process since it cannot proceed very far without their active participation. Where some other individual or organization instigates the process, its first priority should be to bring representatives of the municipality into the process and to ensure that they are prepared to become part of the core team.

Understanding current problems

Information requirements

The need at the understanding problems stage is not to collect large quantities of data. Rather, it is to answer the basic questions *how* do services function at present, *where* are problems and gaps in service provision found and *what*, in broad terms, are the reasons for those problems.

Answers to these questions do not need large quantities of data. Before collecting information, ask the question *'what am I going to do with this information?'* If you cannot answer this question, it is doubtful whether the information will be useful. Some ideas about the points to be considered in relation to the four basic questions posed in Bharatpur are given below.

Who is responsible for providing existing services?

Different government agencies will be responsible for different aspects of sanitation provision and there may be some duplication in their responsibilities and activities. However, government will rarely be the only provider of sanitation services and it will also be necessary to explore the activities of individuals, CBOs and NGOs. Look for any gaps in responsibilities for service delivery. For instance, there may be no agency with expertise in hygiene education, overall drainage planning or community mobilization.

What sanitation problems do we face?

The five types of sanitation deficiency identified in Chapter 1 are:

- an absolute lack of sanitation facilities
- sanitation facilities are inconvenient, unpleasant and/or unhygienic
- lack of access to sanitation facilities
- poor operation and maintenance of sanitation facilities
- environmental degradation caused by poor management of excreta disposal systems.

These should provide a useful framework for answering this question. It may be useful to divide the town into a number of zones, each exhibiting similar physical and social conditions, and to assess the sanitation-related problems in typical zones.

What are the causes of problems?

Answering this question will help you to understand why services are not working well and what can be done to improve their performance. The investigation should be promoted in a positive way, as the start of a process that will bring about change and improvement rather than as an opportunity for apportioning blame. Ask people how they think things could be done better in the future rather than focusing entirely on what was wrong in the past. This will reduce (although it may not eliminate) the risk that the management and staff of the various organizations providing services will feel threatened by the investigation and so refuse to engage with the planning process.

Consider what people's answers tell you about existing demand for improved sanitation, the extent to which this demand is informed and whether there is a need to promote improved hygienic practices. These initial investigations will give an indication of whether or not sanitation and hygiene promotion need to be included in the plan. (Chapter 6 provides further information on sanitation and hygiene promotion.)

What resources do we have?

In order to solve problems, you must have some idea of the ability of service users and/or providers to finance services and the availability of knowledge and skills. It is often assumed that problems stem mainly from a shortage of funds and can thus be solved by greater investment. While lack of funds can be an issue, it will rarely be the sole cause of problems. Some towns have a surplus of funds and many staff, but still suffer severe sanitation problems. This suggests that there are other constraints that must also be overcome if services are to improve. So, the investigation of available resources should ideally go beyond a simple listing of existing resources to an initial exploration of the factors that underlie any resource constraints.

Consultation with users will always be worthwhile, for the following reasons.

o Users know about their neighbourhood, the way in which municipal services operate there, and the sort of improvements that might work.

o It is only possible to find out about the services that people want and are willing to pay for by talking to them. This can help prevent money being wasted on services that people will not use.

o Users have responsibilities for the proper use and maintenance of sanitation infrastructure, particularly that which lies within their plot boundaries. However, it may be necessary to talk to them to agree and clarify these responsibilities.

Ideally, consulting with service users should become part of the routine of municipal service delivery and all municipal staff should be encouraged to consult in an informal way, as part of the routine of doing their jobs. It may be best to assign formal consultation exercises to a third party such as an NGO that is skilled in community liaison. Most municipal bodies lack skills in this area and it is probable that people will speak more freely if they are talking to a third party rather than to the service providers themselves.[3]

Some caution is needed here. Consultation raises public expectations. If the municipality is not serious about improving services, and no action follows the consultation, people may become frustrated and lose all confidence in the organization. So, you should always be clear about why you are consulting people and be able to tell them something about the planned follow-up action. Do not promise what you cannot deliver.

Further information on possible sources of information and methods to be used to collect and analyse information is given in Chapter 7.

Taking account of existing plans

Representatives of some organizations may be reluctant to join the planning process because they already have their own plans. For instance, the PHED representatives in Bharatpur saw little need to engage with the strategic planning process because they already had a sewerage plan for the town, albeit a plan that was over 20 years old and for which there was little prospect of obtaining funding. To overcome such resistance, stress that existing plans will be seen as resources, which will be taken into account when preparing the strategic plan. They will be reviewed in the course of the planning process but this review should be presented as a positive development that will increase the likelihood of relevant parts of the plans being implemented.

Reviews of existing plans should pay particular attention to the way in which existing plans deal with the need for operation and maintenance. Their contents should be checked against the principle that operation and maintenance costs should never be subsidized. This is a particularly important issue for sewerage. If sewerage plans do not include realistic consideration of operation and maintenance costs, together with workable proposals for cost recovery, they are unlikely to work.[4]

Developing solutions

While the information gathered during the initial understanding problems stage should provide a basic understanding of problems, it will rarely be sufficient to enable planners to move with confidence directly to the development of a sanitation plan. The developing solutions stage deals with this problem by providing time for the collection and analysis of more detailed information on specific problems and issues. At the same time, it provides an opportunity for the various stakeholders to become closely involved in the planning process.

Figure 3.3 is a diagrammatic representation of the developing solutions stage, based on the process followed in Bharatpur. Note the use of workshops to bring stakeholders together at the beginning of the process and then to review findings and develop the outline for the strategic plan. Further information on organizing and running a participatory planning workshop is given in Chapter 9. Each of the stages in the developing solutions stage is now discussed.

The first planning workshop

The first planning workshop provides an opportunity to:

○ Involve a wide range of stakeholders in problem analysis, thus bringing diverse experience and viewpoints to the analysis and helping to ensure that the outputs from the planning process will be widely owned.

○ Establish a structure for coordinated planning, along the lines of the Sanitation

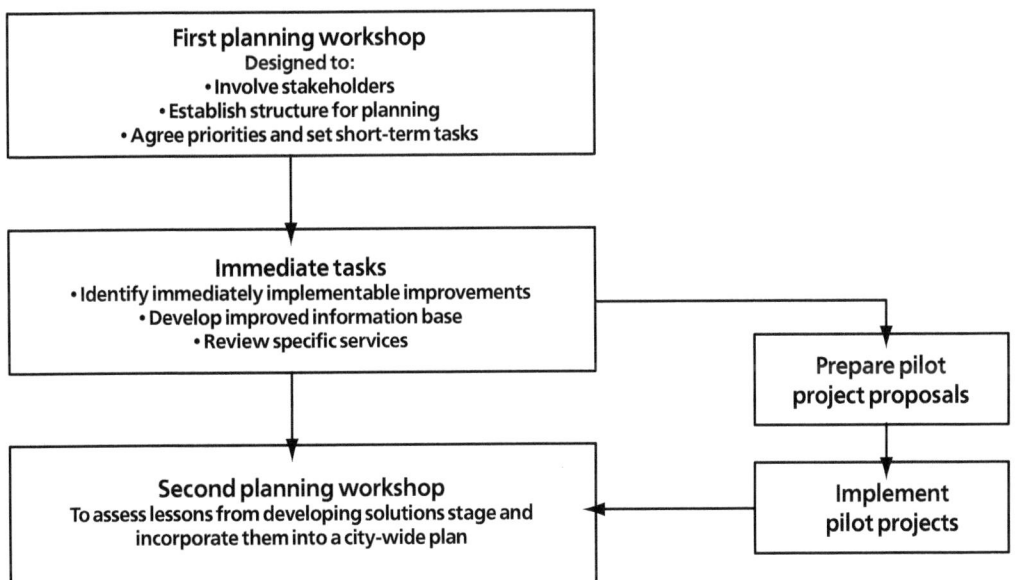

Figure 3.3 Steps in developing solutions

Coordination Committee established in Bharatpur. In order to ensure that the recommendations of the committee feed into the formal planning process and are officially recognized, senior municipal decision makers should be included on the committee. Any government regulations pertaining to the composition and activities of special committees should be observed.

o Agree priorities and assign short-term tasks, designed to provide the information required to move forward to the development of a full municipal plan. The aim should be to break problems down into their component parts and identify a series of clearly defined tasks, each of which tackles a specific problem and leads to a next step in developing better services. Hiring in specialist expertise for some of these tasks will be a worthwhile investment, provided that the tasks are well defined.

In accordance with our emphasis on informing demand, it will usually be desirable for the facilitators to emphasize some key points in the course of the workshop. Box 3.2 summarizes the points made in Bharatpur. These relate to the strategic principles outlined in Chapter 2 but are stated in a less formal way.

Analysis of the tasks identified in the Bharatpur workshop suggests that they can be divided into three categories relating to:

o improvements in working practices that can be implemented immediately

o improvements in the information base

o reviews of existing services and programmes.

It will also be worthwhile to start to investigate possible sources of funding at this stage.

As these tasks are implemented, some are likely to reveal the need for action to test out new concepts and approaches. The best way to meet this need will be through the implementation of pilot projects. Because of their time scale, the larger of these will often have to be incorporated into the strategic plan.

Action to develop solutions

Implement immediate improvements

The focus should be improvements that are relatively easy to implement but do not require a big injection of funds from outside. Many of these will relate to operation and maintenance. Efforts to improve routine maintenance tasks, for instance drain cleaning, may help to convince citizens that the municipality is serious about improving sanitation. It may be best to focus on selected areas in the first instance, later incorporating improved practices into municipal routines and budgets so that they become a standard feature of municipal operations in the future.

Small-scale physical improvements may also be possible. These should stand alone and be cheap and easy to implement. Some may relate to existing bad practice. For instance, in Bharatpur, ILCS leach pits were being lined with brickwork with closed joints so that water could not leach away from the sides of the pit. The use of open-jointed brickwork for all new leach pits was an obvious and immediately implementable improvement. In other cases, it may be relatively easy to introduce new responses to old problems. For instance, where good falls are available, the introduction of a programme to replace existing open drains with sewers may improve the local environment.

At this stage, it is important to *identify actions that have a chance of success*. Later, efforts can be made to deal with more intractable problems.

Figures 3.4 to 3.6 illustrate the point that local improvements may solve local problems at the expense of creating problems at

Box 3.2 Key points stressed during the Bharatpur workshop

1. *There is no maintenance-free option.* If the maintenance of existing facilities is neglected, the plan must consider how current practice can be improved. Responsibility for carrying out maintenance is unlikely to rest entirely with government and it is important that service providers and users agree on their respective duties and are willing to fulfil them.
2. *Sanitation problems are not only physical in nature.* Their root causes may relate to poor management, a lack of planning, and failure to generate enough revenue to provide a reasonable level of service. Sanitation services will only improve if these root causes are tackled.
3. *Sanitation problems are interconnected.* Excreta disposal, drainage and solid waste management are not isolated services, but are closely linked. Failure in one area can have damaging effects in another. One example is the dumping of uncollected solid waste in drains, which leads to blockages and flooding and allows insects to breed.
4. *Agencies need to plan together* both to coordinate their activities and to agree on action to fill any gaps in responsibilities, for instance the fact that there may be no agency with overall responsibility for hygiene promotion. Special attention needs to be paid to the interfaces between agency responsibilities and the role of non-government organizations should not be ignored.
5. *Low-income areas need special attention.* While problems with existing services may be acute, there may be some parts of the town, particularly informal low-income areas, where people have few if any sanitation services. If these areas remain outside municipal services and/or planning controls, sanitation in the town may never reach an acceptable standard.
6. *Sanitation is also about behaviour.* Sanitation services can do little to improve the local environment or protect health unless people use them responsibly and adopt basic standards of hygiene. For instance, it is easy to build toilets but there is no guarantee that people will use them or empty pits safely when they are full. Latrine construction should therefore be accompanied by efforts to promote latrine use and personal hygiene, and education in latrine maintenance.
7. *Sanitation services must be paid for.* Widespread use of subsidies to fund new sanitation facilities will take up financial resources and reduce the number of new facilities that can be provided. This may reduce the ability of sanitation programmes to make a real impact on sanitation deficiencies. Once provided, sanitation services are unlikely to continue to function satisfactorily unless someone, usually the user, pays for their operation and maintenance tasks, either directly or indirectly through a tariff.

the next level up in the service hierarchy. So, planners should be aware of the need to see such improvements as one stage in the improvement of services and not as an end in themselves.

Improvements in the information base

Efforts to improve the information base should aim to fill gaps that have emerged during the initial understanding problems stage. Examples of such gaps might include:

o the lack of an accurate map base

o a lack of information on facilities provided by individuals and organizations other than government (for instance toilet facilities, privately installed septic tanks and community built sewers)

38 URBAN SANITATION

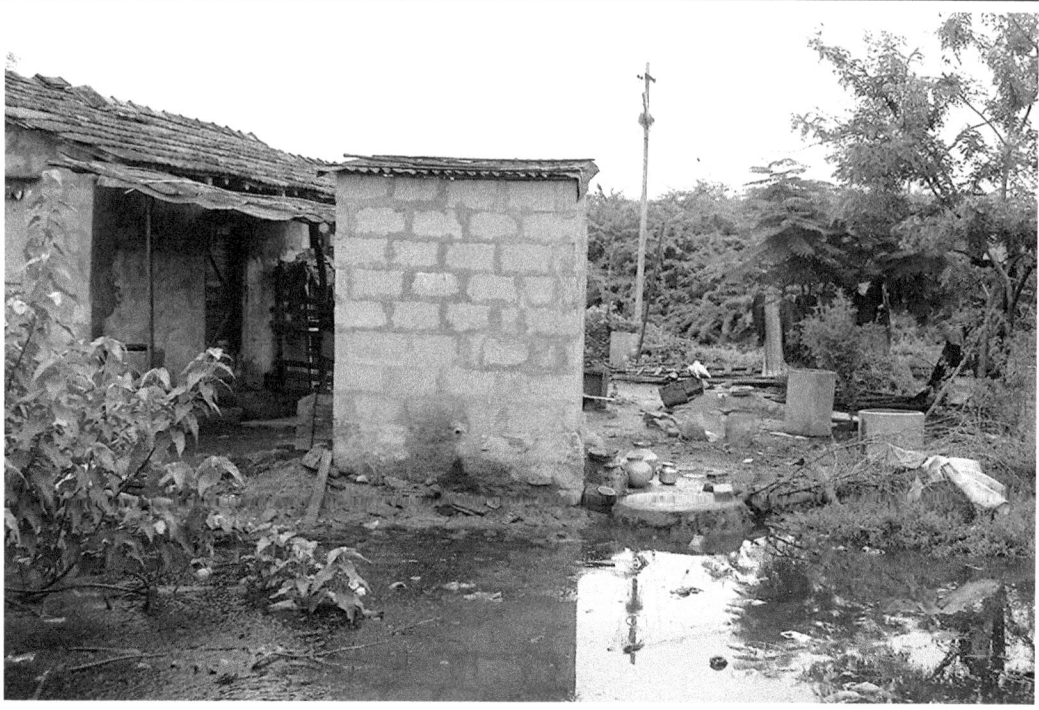

Figure 3.4 Problems caused by household level action
This latrine in Andhra Pradesh, India, has been built by the householder but it appears that wastewater is being discharged directly to the roadside drain, causing serious pollution.

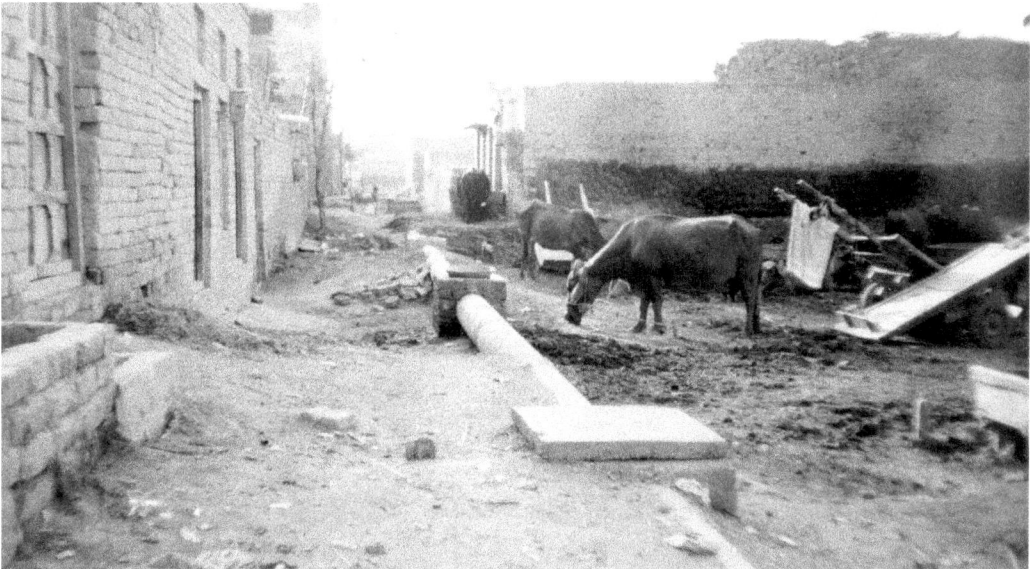

Figure 3.5 Problems caused by neighbourhood level improvements
This community-built sewer in Faisalabad, Pakistan, photographed before ground filling, certainly improved the local environment. However, untreated sewage was discharged to an adjacent field, causing friction with the farmer, until a secondary sewer was built.

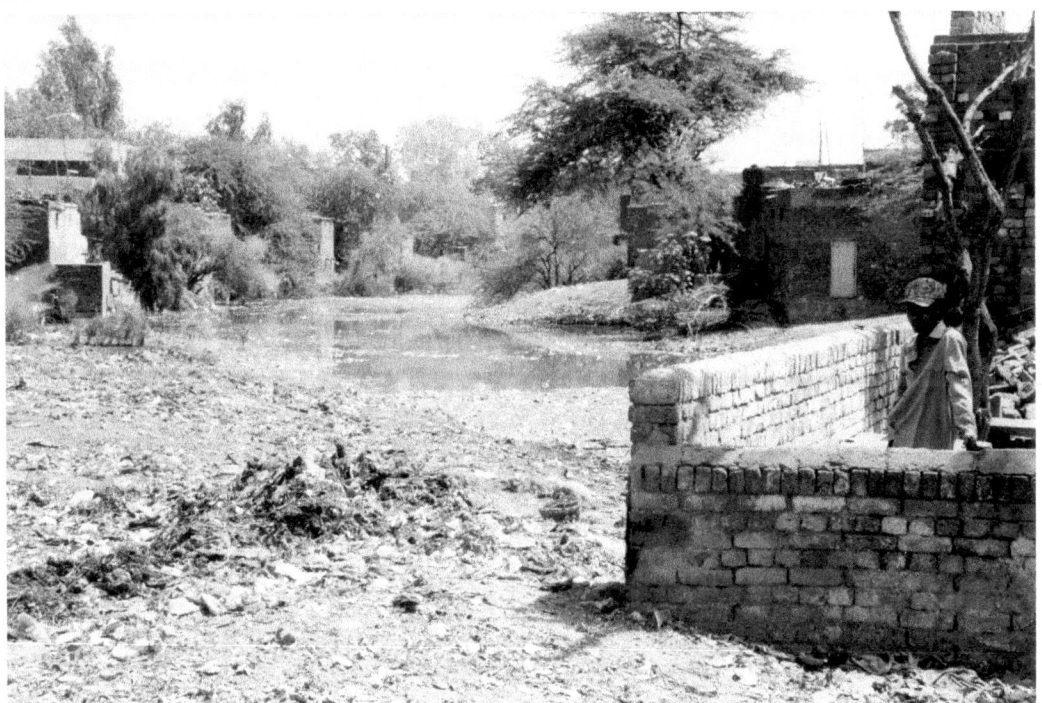

Figure 3.6 Problems with impacts at the municipal level
The Outer Moat in Bharatpur, Rajasthan, was once a clean water body but is now heavily polluted by discharges of municipal wastewater. Such problems can only be solved by action at the level of the town as a whole, including wastewater treatment where appropriate.

o lack of detailed information on municipal expenditure on and revenue from sanitation services so that it is impossible to tell whether services are affordable

o lack of accurate information on attitudes to sanitation and hygiene.

Obtaining detailed information for the town as a whole may be difficult and time consuming. There is much to be said for piloting information systems at a more local level, perhaps that of the ward. Information collection and analysis can be coordinated with reviews of existing services and efforts to bring about immediate improvements. This will help to ensure that information is used and will thus reduce the danger that improving the information base is seen as an end in itself.

It will often be useful to bring information from different sources together on a single map base, perhaps as the starting point for the development of a Geographic Information System (GIS) as described in Chapter 7.

Detailed reviews of specific services, programmes and schemes

While some improvements can be made immediately, there will be other cases in which the reasons for deficiencies and problems are not clear. For example, the workshop participants may identify the fact that garbage remains uncollected. However, further information is required before action can be taken. Is the problem caused by lack of staff, inadequately trained staff or poor supervision, access problems for collection vehicles, lack of cooperation from the public or some combination of these? A detailed review of specific services will often be needed before such questions can be answered and lasting improvements can be made.

A good way of reviewing a service is to investigate in detail how it operates in one ward or neighbourhood. This should reveal problems and bottlenecks that are typical of those affecting the whole town. Try to identify each step in delivering the service, from start to finish. For example, if there is a scheme to provide low-cost household toilets, what is the sequence of events, from first contact with households to completion of the superstructure? How effective is this process?

Any ongoing programmes and schemes should also be reviewed. In Bharatpur, for instance, study of the Integrated Low Cost Sanitation progamme revealed the lack of an adequate programme to educate users in the use of the latrines provided under the scheme. This resulted from a failure to budget for user education and hygiene promotion. Identifying the problem made it possible to investigate ways of solving it.

Assessing options through piloting

Efforts to carry out immediate improvements, improve the information base and review existing services will often create awareness of the need for changes and improvements in existing systems and perhaps of options for bringing about these changes and improvements. Where there is no local experience of a technology or approach, it will usually be wise to pilot test it on a relatively small scale before attempting to introduce it over the municipality as a whole. The design or model should be modified, as necessary, in the light of local conditions. If the outcome is successful, the model can then be recommended for wider use, perhaps in a modified form taking into account the lessons from the pilot.

Pilot projects may be used to:

- test new technologies or designs
- find the best way of organizing and delivering a service

and, on occasion, to do both.

Piloting should be seen as a learning process, enabling mistakes to be made and rectified at a manageable scale. It allows effective solutions to be developed in a systematic way and can prevent money being wasted on large-scale programmes that fail because they are based on insufficient information.

Before starting a pilot, its likely resource requirements, in particular the availability of land and management skills, should be assessed in relation to those that are available in the city as a whole (see Figure 3.7).

Pilots will sometimes involve attempts to use either composted solid waste or wastewater as a resource. From a city-wide perspective, the key questions to ask of these pilots are:

- Is the market for the waste likely to be sufficiently large to deal with a large proportion of the waste produced in the city?
- Is it feasible to either transport the waste to a central location or to find suitable locations for decentralized treatment/composting facilities?

If these questions cannot be answered satisfactorily, it does not mean that there is no place for composting within an overall solid waste strategy. For instance, it may be feasible to find suitable locations and markets for composting market wastes. It does mean that a city-wide strategy based only on composting and/or decentralized wastewater treatment is unlikely to work.

Pilots can vary in scale. As suggested in the discussion of options for immediate improvements, some will be small and immediately implementable, using municipal or

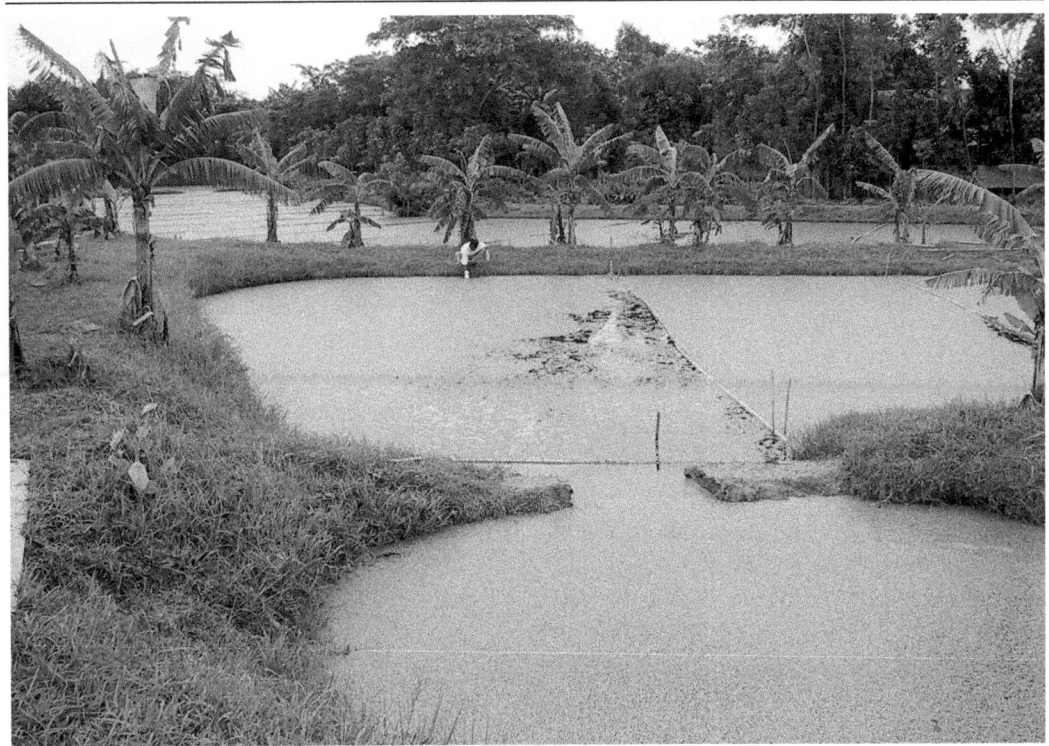

Figure 3.7 Considering resource requirements
This pilot wastewater management facility in Mirzapur, Bangladesh, produces duckweed for fish farming. The system has a high land take. The critical question to be asked when considering the suitability of the technology for inclusion in a city-wide strategy is whether sufficient land will be available at an affordable price to allow its widespread replication.

community resources. Others may be larger, perhaps covering one or two wards. Whatever their scale, pilot projects should relate to problems that are widespread and should be implemented in typical situations. To avoid delay and excessive expenditure, they should normally be carried out in locations where any higher-level services required for their operation are already in place.

Key institutional questions should be addressed as early as possible in the pilot project process. These questions include:

○ Which agencies will manage and deliver the service?

○ What will be the roles and responsibilities of the community, the service providers, and the municipality?

○ Who will pay for the service?

Time required for the developing solutions stage

The time required to develop solutions will vary, depending on local circumstances. The six-month period allowed in Bharatpur proved to be too short but there is a risk that stakeholders will lose interest if the developing solutions stage is too protracted. In general, the aim should be to move into the preparation of a strategic plan within one year of the start of the process.

Larger pilot projects may need more time that this. Rather than extending the developing solutions stage to accommodate them, they should be absorbed into the city-wide plan.

Developing the city-wide plan

The planning process

A good way to mark the transition from developing solutions to working on the city-wide plan is to hold a second planning workshop. This will serve to inform the various stakeholders of the results of the developing solutions stage and develop consensus around the broad contents of the plan, thus helping to ensure that the plan will be supported and followed by a wide range of agencies and organizations.

It is important to be clear about who is going to be responsible for the different components of the plan. Wherever possible, the organizations that are responsible for developing solutions and carrying out pilot projects should also take responsibility for the implementation of solutions and scaling up pilots to the level of the city as a whole.

Once the main components of the plan and responsibilities for those components have been agreed, time will be required to develop the plan document itself. It will be best if a small team is assigned to coordinate production of the first draft of the plan. However, it will be best if the sections of the plan that refer to specific actions are prepared by representatives of the organizations that will be responsible for carrying out those actions. The coordinating team should provide a basic template for how material should be presented (see Box 3.4, page 45).

Once the plan has been prepared in draft, it should be circulated for comment. The main points should also be presented at a follow-up meeting or workshop. Written comments, together with observations made in the course of the workshop can then be incorporated into a final version of the plan.

Structure and contents of the plan

The plan components identified in Bharatpur are represented diagrammatically in Figure 3.8. The main body of the plan, the overall framework and the chapters devoted to individual components should be fairly concise and supported by appendices as required. This will ensure that the plan is accessible to everyone while providing additional information for those who need it. For networked services such as sewerage and drainage, the annexes should include plans showing existing and proposed facilities. If possible, these should be at a sufficiently large scale to allow the location of existing and proposed facilities to be shown accurately.

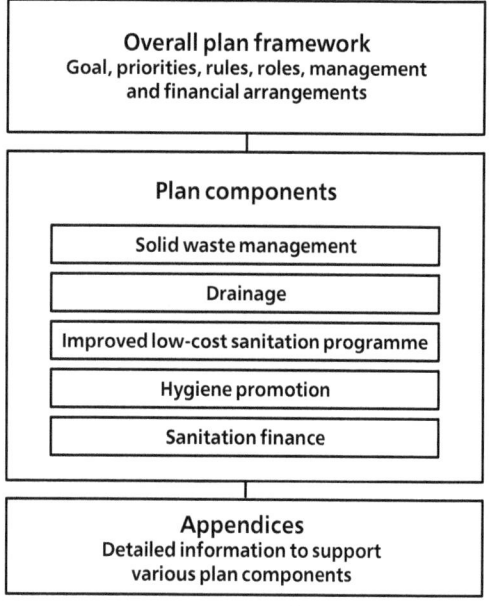

Figure 3.8 The typical structure of a municipal sanitation plan

The plan should *set priorities* for action and investment, and explain clearly how these priorities have been established. They should not just be about the provision of new facilities. For each component, options for improving management arrangements, particularly as these relate to operation and maintenance, should be included.

Individual plan components should include targets, which should be decided in the light of the availability of resources and the constraints presented by the existing situation, a reasonable understanding of which should have been obtained during the developing solutions stage. Particular attention should be paid to the targets for the first year. Achieving these targets will build confidence among all the parties involved. Conversely, if early targets are set at too high a level and consequently are not achieved, people will lose confidence in the plan and may ignore it.

Pay attention to the intermediate milestones that will have to be passed on the way to achieving each objective. For instance, a plan objective might be to improve solid waste disposal arrangements and this may require a new disposal site. Milestones on the way to opening a new disposal site might be the identification of a suitable site, the production of a costed scheme for the site and the securing of funding. Identifying intermediate targets or outputs in this way and assessing the time and resources required to achieve them will make it easier to estimate the time that is likely to be required to commission the new site.

The plan should be written as simply as possible, again with the aim of making it accessible to anyone who might be interested in its contents.

Further information on the contents of the framework section of the plan and a typical component, based on the Bharatpur plan, is given in Boxes 3.3 and 3.4.

Financing the plan

Many municipalities are dependent on funding provided from higher levels of government, the level of which cannot be guaranteed from year to year. Where this is the case, some flexibility should be allowed in the timing of components that depend on external funding. Do not assume, however, that government will be the only source of funding. The plan should be based on a realistic assessment of what intended users will pay for improved sanitation services and the resources that may be available through NGOs, local businesses and other non-government sources. Where appropriate, it should include some indication of action that might be taken to improve financial systems and the local financial base.

Funds will probably have been already earmarked for ongoing programmes and committed schemes. These funds represent another important resource and so linking the strategic planning process with existing schemes will help to ensure that resources are available to implement the plan. At the same time, the analysis and new thinking that has taken place during the development of the plan should help to improve the quality of existing schemes.

Ideally, the plan should allocate some funds to support the implementation of pilot and demonstration initiatives. Once an approach has been proved, it can be demonstrated on a wider scale, incorporated into mainstream practice and included in future plans.

Making the plan 'official'

Unless both municipal and state authorities formally endorse the plan it will be difficult or impossible to ensure that all concerned departments and agencies work within the framework it has established. Ideally, the plan should have an official status and should be designated as the framework for action by higher levels of government. You may have limited power to make this happen, but you should do everything that you can to have the plan accepted as the official sanitation plan for the town.

Box 3.3 Overall framework of the strategic plan

Overall goal
A brief statement should be provided, stating the purpose or purposes of the plan. This should set out its expected impact – a cleaner town? a healthy living environment?

Framework (rules, policy and principles underlying the plan)
This should explain how the municipality is going to tackle sanitation problems in the town. All agencies involved in sanitation should comply with this framework.
It should include information on:

1. *Priorities*

How will the municipality decide which activities or places to target first? How will priority areas be identified? Use social and technical mapping to identify the areas that suffer the worst sanitation problems (see Chapter 7).

2. *Roles and responsibilities*

What are the responsibilities of:
- communities, including those to both provide and pay for services
- the municipal authorities
- other government institutions, NGOs and the private sector?

3. *Communication and mobilization*
- How will community support for the plan be achieved?
- How will the municipality communicate with service users (e.g. via ward committees or via CBOs/NGOs)?

4. *Management and coordination*
- How will the inputs of different agencies (state and municipal agencies, NGOs, private contractors) be coordinated to achieve a common goal? If there is to be a Sanitation Coordination Committee, will it have formal status?
- What is the relationship between the plan and other formal plans and programmes, particularly those dealing with infrastructure and services for the poor?
- What will be the role of regulation and enforcement (e.g. to manage the private sector and control encroachments) and how will it be achieved?
- Supervision and monitoring of services: who, how, why (especially for services contracted out to NGOs or private contractors).

5. *Financial arrangements*
- What are the main sources of capital and recurrent funding? State the municipality's intentions regarding local taxes.
- Municipal policy on subsidies and cost recovery (e.g. for primary waste collection, household toilets, other services).

Box 3.4 The solid waste management component of the municipal plan

Current position
A summary of the current state of the solid waste management service, key issues and problems identified from recent investigations, and priorities for improvement (e.g. increasing the quantity of waste lifted by introducing a primary collection service). Make sure that this includes information on what is done formally and what is done informally.

Objectives
For example:
o To introduce a primary collection service in specified wards (eventually city-wide).
o To establish a properly managed disposal site.
o To extend secondary collection services to all areas currently unserved.

Potential constraints
Are there any constraints that might prevent the achievement of objectives? For instance, workers may be resistant to efforts to change working practices, particularly when they are gaining some unofficial benefits from the existing situation. How might such constraints be overcome?

Strategy
This section should identify the time frame for achieving each objective and set out how it will be achieved. For example:
o By piloting a primary collection service operating through small enterprises funded through direct payments from users, perhaps managed by a local NGO. To be harmonized with municipal secondary storage and collection.
o By purchasing land and developing a sanitary landfill operation under a competent manager.
o By piloting suitable technology and systems for collecting waste from informal settlements and other locations with access problems.

Targets (Year 1 and Year 3)
Clarify what is to be achieved, both in terms of quality and quantity.

Activities (Year 1)
List the main activities to be undertaken in the first year.

Implementing agencies
Set out the roles of municipal and state agencies, NGOs, CBOs and the community and indicate how their efforts will be coordinated.

Additional resource requirements
What financial, technical or other resources are needed to fulfil the tasks in addition to those already available?

Budget
Estimates of capital investment and operational costs making a clear distinction between activities that are and are not covered already by existing budgets or government schemes.

In particular, everything possible should be done to ensure that plan components are formally incorporated into the programmes and budgets produced by the various stakeholder organizations. This will help to lock these organizations into the planning process and reduce the probability that they will retreat from the commitments made in the plan.

Next steps

The process does not end with the production of the plan. Indeed, any plan is only as good as the action that flows from it. We will return to the subject of implementation in Chapter 10. However, one key point is worth making here. No plan will ever be perfect, certainly not at the first attempt, and thinking may change as a result of the experience of implementing the plan. So, the production of the plan is not the last step in the planning process but rather a point of departure. Although the Bharatpur plan had a city-wide focus, it covered a limited time period and certainly did not represent the last word in planning for the town. In accordance with the philosophy presented throughout this book, the achievements of the plan should be reviewed at the end of the planning period and used in the development of a new plan covering the next three to five-year period.

Key points in this chapter

1. Planning should always start with efforts to understand existing problems and the options that might be available to tackle them.
2. A developing solutions stage will often be necessary to prepare the ground for a plan covering the town or city as a whole.
3. This will often involve action to explore possibilities and test new approaches at a local level, perhaps that of a ward or a specific low-income settlement.
4. To be effective, planning processes must involve all the stakeholders, including elected representatives. A planning committee including representatives of all those with an interest in sanitation can provide a useful focus for planning activities.
5. Plans should not be only about new facilities. You should be equally concerned with the operation and maintenance of those facilities that already exist.
6. The plan itself should include a statement of its overall goal and the principles that underpin it. Priorities should be identified together with an indication of the roles and responsibilities of the different organizations that will be involved in implementing the plan. Special attention should be paid to the arrangements for coordination.
7. The plan should also contain detailed guidance on the action to be taken in relation to a number of key issues. For each of these components, the aim should be to set out an action plan to be implemented over a limited period, typically 3–5 years. Particular attention should be paid to the targets to be achieved in the plan's first year.
8. Plans should take account of available financial, human and institutional resources.
9. It is important that the plan is locally 'owned', that it has an official status and that the plan components are incorporated into the programmes and budgets of the various stakeholder organizations.

Chapter 3 endnotes

1 Pathak (1999) provides a profile of Sulabh International.
2 The concept of action planning was first introduced by Patrick Geddes in India in the early twentieth century, but the first formal presentation of the concept was by Koenigsberger (1964). A more recent and more detailed outline of an action planning approach is provided by Hamdi and Goethert (1997).
3 Some Indian cities have formalized consultation with users on the quality of services through a 'report card' system (see Paul 1996).
4 The issue of operation and maintenance is particularly important. For further information on assessing the current operation and maintenance status, see IRC (1997).

CHAPTER 4
Developing a supportive context

ONE OF THE important lessons from the Bharatpur pilot project was that strategic planning initiatives are likely to be constrained by the lack of a supportive context – the attitudes, assumptions, policies, rules and procedures within which planning efforts take place. This chapter is concerned with the action that might be taken to develop this supportive context. Following a brief exploration of the links between the overall policy context, municipal level activities and local initiatives, it identifies a number of barriers to the widespread adoption of a strategic approach to sanitation planning. The actions required to overcome these barriers are then examined. The initial focus is on options for changing attitudes to sanitation itself and the role of strategic planning in sanitation service provision. Attention then turns to the critical need to develop a policy context that is supportive to improved sanitation provision in general and strategic planning issues in particular. Finally, options for overcoming resource constraints and increasing capacity to plan strategically and respond to sanitation needs are considered.

Municipal planning in context

Some government officials in Bharatpur were not convinced of the step-by-step approach to sanitation planning promoted in the planning workshop. They saw it as a poor substitute for comprehensive plans, despite the fact that the latter were rarely implemented as intended and sometimes were not implemented at all. This notional commitment to comprehensive planning contrasted strongly with the reality that most officials worked in a reactive rather than a proactive way, responding to directives from higher levels of government and/or pressure from elected representatives. This situation appears to be widespread, whether or not there have been formal moves towards decentralization of powers and responsibilities.[1]

Two important points emerge from the Bharatpur experience.

○ Prevailing attitudes and assumptions, sometimes described as mental models,[2] may place constraints on the possibilities for action. Attempts to increase the priority given to sanitation and to introduce strategic planning will often have to start with efforts to change the mental models of both sanitation users and sanitation providers.

○ The policy environment – current policies and the rules and regulations that support them – is likely to influence the approach to planning taken by municipal officials. In Bharatpur, there was a strong emphasis on following the rules and procedures set by the Rajasthan State Government. Indeed, experience elsewhere suggests that municipal officials are often reluctant to diverge from existing rules and procedures in any way. It is usually safer for an official to follow the rules, even those that do not appear to make sense, than to take initiatives that may be rewarded with disciplinary action if they fail.

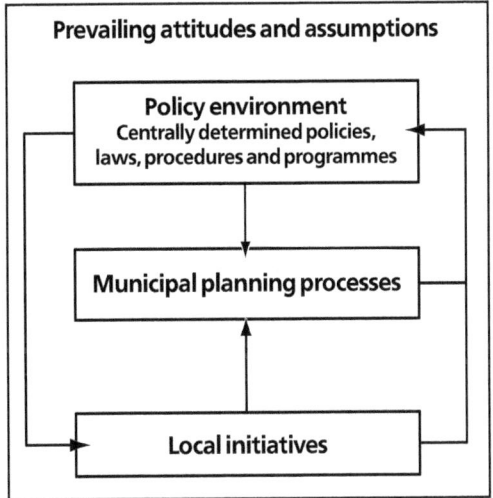

Figure 4.1 Municipal planning in context

Figure 4.1 provides a diagrammatic illustration of the relationships between prevailing attitudes and assumptions, the policy environment and action at the municipal and local levels. The outer box shows that all sanitation-related decisions, activities and processes take place within the context provided by prevailing attitudes and assumptions. The links from the policy environment box indicate the important point that planning processes at the municipal and local levels are likely to be strongly influenced by the policy environment.

Of course, attitudes and assumptions are likely to vary between individuals and groups. Without such variation, there would be few prospects for change and development since there would be no voices other than those supporting the generally accepted status quo. Indeed, it can be argued that, at its most basic, development is all about changes in attitudes and assumptions.

If this is accepted, the key question becomes 'where might beneficial changes be initiated?' The feedback loops directed upwards from the local and municipal levels in Figure 4.1 suggest two possible answers to this question:

○ Champions of change, including both politicians and senior officials, may emerge from within the 'official' system.

○ NGOs and other civil society groups may develop ways of thinking about sanitation and related problems that are very different from the 'received wisdom' found among senior politicians and government officials. Over time, the initiatives taken by these organizations and groups can have a profound impact upon the approach taken to sanitation problems. We will see in Chapter 5 that such initiatives can incorporate strategic characteristics and can thus provide an entry point for the development of a strategic approach to planning.

External organizations and agencies can play an important role in introducing new ideas and supporting the efforts of internal champions of change. However, the role of external stakeholders is to assist rather than to lead the process of development. In the end, new ways of thinking and acting are unlikely to be sustained and replicated unless they are reflected in changes in the policy environment that are initiated and carried forward by national stakeholders.

Four barriers to improved sanitation

We now turn to the options for developing an improved context for strategic sanitation planning. We start by identifying four barriers to improved sanitation, as shown in Figure 4.2.

The first two barriers relate to existing attitudes and assumptions. The third is explicitly related to the policy environment and in particular to the need to encourage those responsible for municipal sanitation planning to think and act more strategically. Even when decision makers and planners are well informed and motivated to provide

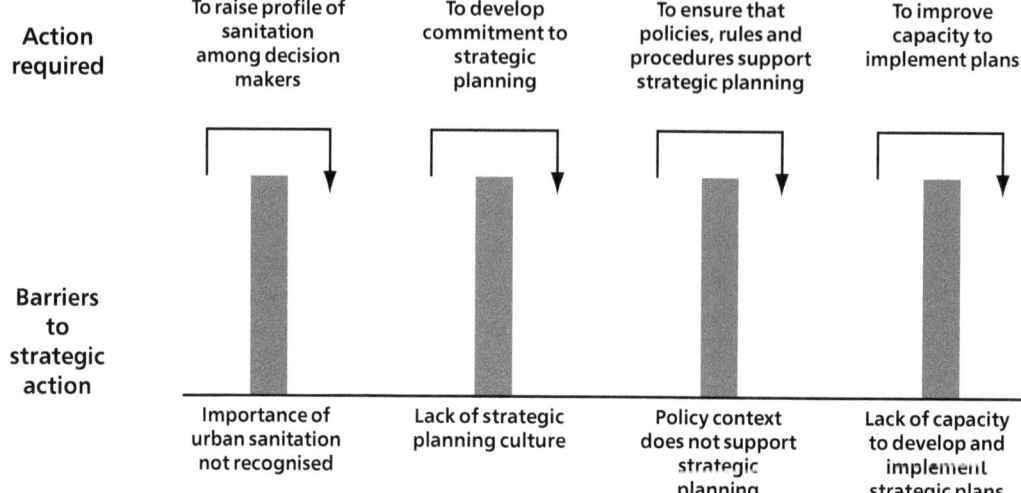

Figure 4.2 Requirements for widespread adoption of strategic planning

better sanitation services and are working in a supportive policy context, they will make little impact unless they know what to do and have the capacity to do it. So, the fourth barrier identified in Figure 4.2 is lack of capacity to develop and implement strategic sanitation plans.

Committed leaders at the municipal level can take action to overcome these barriers, at least temporarily, within their own towns and cities. Nevertheless, as we have already indicated, it is unlikely that strategic approaches to sanitation planning will be widely adopted unless action is taken at the 'centre' to promote and support them.

Figure 4.2 involves a simplification of reality, insofar as it ignores the interactions between actions taken to overcome the four barriers. For instance, appropriate policies and rules handed down from higher levels of government can have some impact upon the attitudes and assumptions of those working at the local level. Bear this in mind when reading the remainder of this chapter and be aware that it will sometimes be necessary to take action to deal with more than one barrier at the same time.

Raising the profile of sanitation

General recognition of the importance of good sanitation, particularly among those who are responsible for making policy decisions, is required if sanitation services are to improve. Where this recognition does not exist, there will be a need for efforts to raise the profile of sanitation. There are two issues here – the arguments to be used and the responsibility for putting forward these arguments.

A range of arguments for improved sanitation has already been given in the section entitled 'why improve sanitation' in Chapter 1. These arguments go beyond the traditional concerns with health and the environment to include the potential economic and social benefits of improved sanitation. When exploring options for raising awareness of sanitation, it will be important to consider the full range of these arguments and to tailor arguments to the interests and concerns of those you are trying to convince. So, for instance, when talking to economists, the main focus of the argument might be on the links between sanitation, health and a more productive economy. In contrast, the best approach to local politicians will often be to focus on the link between improved environmental sanitation conditions and voter satisfaction.

Efforts to raise the profile of sanitation are more likely to be effective if they involve a wide range of stakeholders and are not restricted to either one target group or one set of arguments. Possible roles for different groups include the following.

- *Senior officials and politicians* should aim to increase awareness of the importance of sanitation among their peers. Those working within central and state/provincial government can use their influence in committees and think tanks, where possible facilitating action to gather the information required to support the case for improved sanitation. Strong leaders at the municipal level can act as advocates for improved sanitation in the towns and cities for which they are responsible.

- *External agencies and NGOs* can promote greater awareness of the importance of sanitation through reports and publications,[3] advocacy campaigns,[4] high-level workshops, sponsorship of short training courses and emphasizing the importance of effective sanitation during the development of project and programme proposals.

- *Local non-government organizations* can play a role by demonstrating effective sanitation approaches at the local level, advocating the widespread adoption of such approaches and drawing attention to the needs of the urban poor.

Developing a commitment to strategic planning

Even where the importance of good sanitation is recognized, there will still be a need to develop commitment to a strategic approach that:

- is grounded in appropriately detailed information about the existing situation
- recognizes the need for a step-by-step approach to sanitation planning
- recognizes the importance of strategic principles.

The options for developing commitment to strategic planning are limited by the fact that, almost by definition, many of those who might otherwise act as advocates for more strategic approaches to sanitation planning are firmly entrenched in the prevailing non-strategic culture. Champions of change may exist at various levels of government. However, they will usually have to battle against an unresponsive institutional culture, which seeks always to return to the status quo and provides no support for attempts to bring about change.[5]

There is no easy solution to this problem. However, efforts to bring about change are more likely to be successful if they receive support from 'external agents', which may include international and bilateral development agencies, international and national NGOs and the consultants who work for them. These external agents can act as catalysts for change, providing ideas and technical assistance and working with local stakeholders to ensure that financial assistance is linked to efforts to promote the adoption of strategic principles.

Workshops and think tanks (groups of concerned individuals who meet regularly to discuss key issues) offer a possible starting point for efforts to raise awareness of the importance of strategic planning. For instance, WSP-SA holds regular workshops in India, which are attended by senior politicians and officials with an interest in change. During and after the Bharatpur pilot project, some of these workshops were devoted to strategic planning. Such workshops are most likely to have an impact if they:

o impart relatively simple messages – in the first instance that planning is important, that it should be information based and that it should be responsive to improved knowledge and changing circumstances

o provide concrete suggestions as to the ways in which participants might follow up with more strategic action in their local situations.

In order to have a lasting effect, workshops and think tanks must form part of a wider programme of change. External agencies and internal 'champions' of change can contribute to this wider programme by promoting strategic planning at a pilot scale at the municipal and local levels. When doing so, they should look for ways to:

o integrate pilot initiatives into existing systems and procedures

o disseminate positive lessons to individuals, groups and organizations that might be in a position to act upon them.

External agencies will achieve a greater impact if they work together to seek ways of integrating their activities and maximizing their effect. There is much to be said for bilateral agencies encouraging the adoption of strategic approaches on a pilot scale. This relatively small-scale action can pave the way for the development banks to support more ambitious programmes, which will have more chance of success once capacity and willingness to plan have been developed.

External agencies should avoid undermining the development of a strategic planning culture by promoting solutions to development problems that ignore basic strategic principles. An example would be implementing a project that subsidizes forms of sanitation that are unaffordable to poor households. They should also seek to integrate their initiatives into national programmes and planning systems so that they become part of a process that is owned by national stakeholders rather than one-off initiatives, which are unlikely to have a long-term impact. To do this, they may need to balance their concern with what they see as fundamental principles with recognition of the constraints imposed by the situation in the country in which they are intervening.

Developing a supportive policy context

A strategic approach to policy development

The experience in Bharatpur and elsewhere suggests that strategic planning is unlikely to take root at the municipal and local levels unless there is a supportive policy context. As with other aspects of developing a strategic approach, the development of an improved policy context will require answers to the three basic questions.

1. What is the present situation or *where are we now?*

2. What are the characteristics of a comprehensive, equitable and institutionally sustainable approach to sanitation provision or *where do we want to go?*

3. *How do we get from here to there?*

Figure 4.3 shows the way in which the various stages in the development and implementation of policy might be linked to these questions.

Figure 4.3 illustrates the following important points:

1. Policy should be informed by experience, including that from initiatives at the local and municipal levels.

DEVELOPING A SUPPORTIVE CONTEXT 53

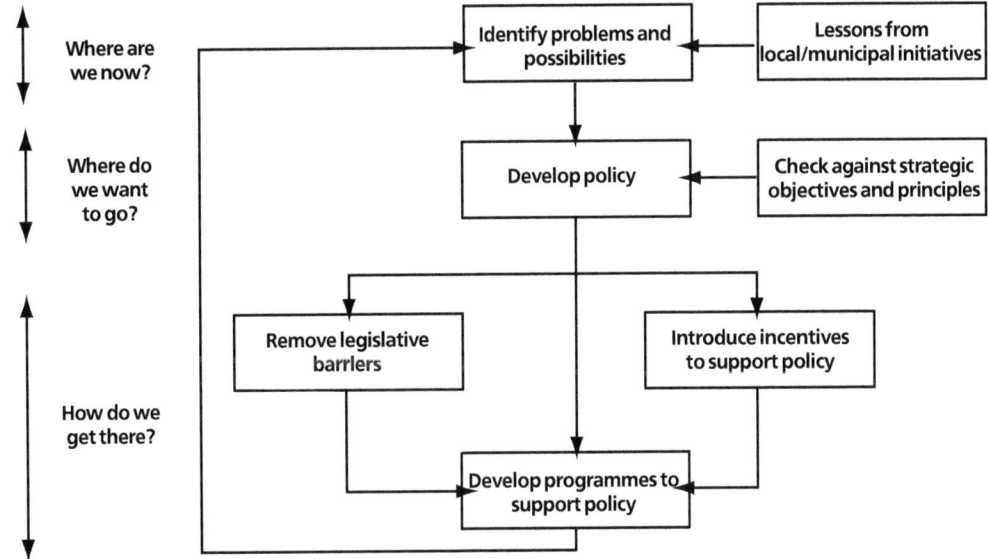

Figure 4.3 Stages in developing and implementing policy

2. Policy should be informed by the strategic objectives and principles set out in Chapter 2.

3. Policy should be supported by a range of actions designed to ensure that it is implemented. These may include action to change laws and accepted practices in order to both remove barriers to the implementation of policy and provide incentives for action that will help to achieve policy objectives.

4. Centrally funded programmes can be a significant source of funding for municipal sanitation programmes and should be designed to support key policy objectives.

Who should be involved in developing policy?

Policies are likely to be more effective in responding to needs if they draw upon the insights and experience of all those who are working to develop improved sanitation services. Their development should not be seen as the sole preserve of government.

Officials of multi-lateral and bilateral agencies and the consultants who work for those agencies have an important role to play in promoting discussion of key strategic concepts and facilitating knowledge transfer between different countries and regions. They should aim to influence policy where appropriate but never to force policies on partner governments. International NGOs and those who work for them may also possess knowledge of sanitation initiatives incorporating strategic principles in other countries and regions.

National NGOs may be able to provide information on existing initiatives in the non-government sector that incorporate some aspects of a strategic approach. They also have an important role to play in ensuring that those responsible for policy receive information from the 'grass roots'.

Within government, efforts should be made to draw upon the knowledge and experience of those who are involved in implementing projects and programmes in the field. This will help to ensure that policies are realistic and address real problems and needs.

What practical steps can be taken to involve the various stakeholder groups in policy development? One step will be to ensure that they are represented on any working group that is set up to consider policy. By its very nature, the working group will be fairly small and there will be a need to develop ways of consulting more widely. This might be done through a series of workshops to discuss the key issues to be addressed when considering changes in policy. Later, it should be possible to prepare and circulate discussion documents on key policy issues and to ask for comments on these documents. Further workshops, at which proposals are presented and discussed, will provide opportunities to obtain feedback on policy proposals.

Assessing the existing situation

Policies should always be based on a realistic assessment of the existing situation, which should be structured around the following broad questions.

○ *What is the nature and scale of existing problems?* The five types of sanitation deficiency identified in Chapter 1 may provide a useful framework for answering this question.

○ *How do existing policies and programmes impact upon existing problems?* Where an existing policy or programme appears to be ineffective or problematic, it may be useful to commission a study to explore its deficiencies and the reasons for those deficiencies.

○ *What resources are available?* The aim here should be to obtain an overview of the available financial, human and institutional resources.

○ *How do existing systems work in practice?* This is an important question. It is all too easy to assume that the systems for delivering and managing services operate as intended by existing legislation and procedures. In practice, they are also influenced by the way in which institutions are structured and the resources that are available to them (see Box 4.1).

○ *What constrains progress towards better sanitation services?* It may be that existing legislation, institutional structures and procedures are limiting the scope for change. Institutional and human resource constraints may also inhibit change and development.

Box 4.1 The influence of limited resource availability on operational systems

Indonesia has recently gone through a process of decentralization. It now requires that all municipalities produce a range of planning documents, which together should in theory provide an integrated planning system. In practice, because the previous system was so centralized, few of those working at the municipal level have good planning experience. As a result, many municipalities struggle to produce realistic plans.

In Bharatpur, efforts to introduce a more systematic approach to drain maintenance were hampered by the lack of accurate plans of the system. This problem is common in India.

Even where good plans exist, they are often held at the 'centre'. For instance, most towns in the Indian state of Andhra Pradesh have been mapped using aerial photographs but the maps are kept in Hyderabad and are not available in the towns themselves. So, current hierarchical systems contribute to the lack of resources at the municipal level.

Existing information may provide a starting point for answering these questions, particularly when this relates to previous pilot projects and case studies. Any existing initiatives that embody at least some of the strategic principles described in earlier chapters should be assessed. We will see in Chapter 5 that these do not necessarily have to be formal initiatives supported by government.

Where initial assessment of existing information sources reveals that there are gaps in knowledge, it will be necessary to commission additional studies to obtain the information needed to develop policy. These studies have a similar role to that played by the activities undertaken in the developing solutions stage of the planning process at the municipal level. Information requirements for policy development are discussed further in Chapter 7.

Developing the policy

A dictionary definition of policy is 'a plan of action adopted by a person, organization or government'. The policy is normally produced in the form of a written document, setting out the aims and ideals of the organization that produced it. It may take the form of a general vision statement, setting out qualitative rather than quantitative objectives. To provide justification for overall aims and visions, most policies also provide a brief review of the existing situation and some indication of the route that is to be followed to achieve the overall vision. There are clear similarities here with strategic plans developed at the municipal level with the main differences relating to the focus of policies, which normally relates to a country, state or province as a whole rather than an individual town or city.

If the policy is to support the approach to strategic planning set out in earlier chapters, it should include reference to the following.

○ The focus of efforts to improve sanitation services – in particular the way in which they address the needs of the poor and the balance to be struck between new provision and operation and maintenance. Is there a need to address the specific needs of particular groups, including women, old people and the young?

○ The overall approach to sanitation provision – focusing in particular on the need for adaptive information-based processes that allow for wide stakeholder involvement.

○ The need for a demand-based approach – which provides the services that users want and for which they are willing to pay.

○ The options for providing and managing sanitation facilities – including those for involving stakeholders other than government in providing and managing sanitation services. The policy should refer to the options for involving both private sector and civil society organizations in aspects of sanitation provision (Hardoy and Schusterman, 1999; Solo, 1999). The need for improved coordination should also be addressed and this suggests that the policy should address the need to reduce duplication of responsibilities and, where possible, streamline and simplify administrative systems.

○ The adoption of appropriate sanitation technologies – recognizing that the technologies adopted have to be affordable to users and that different technologies may be appropriate for use in different areas.

○ Capacity-building priorities and approaches – with particular emphasis on developing capacity to prepare and implement strategic plans.

Care should be taken to ensure that policy statements are not too prescriptive, particularly when they deal with situations that are characterized by uncertainty and lack of information. For instance, while there should certainly be reference to the desirability of involving a range of stakeholders in sanitation planning and provision, it will normally be best if the policy avoids specifying exactly how this should be done. In particular, do not assume that technologies and arrangements for the division of management responsibilities that work in one country will necessarily be transferable to another country with quite different social and physical conditions.

Communicating the policy

The policy will only be implemented and so have a real impact upon sanitation conditions if key stakeholders:

○ are aware of the policy

○ understand its implications

○ are willing and able to implement it.

The chances of achieving these conditions will be increased if representatives of the various stakeholder groups are involved in the development of the policy. However, the number of people directly involved in policy development is bound to be small and there will always be a need to communicate policies to stakeholders and to make sure that those policies are widely understood and accepted.

An essential starting point for communicating policy will be to make sure that the written policy document is widely circulated. Ideally, the policy itself should be supported by written guidance on its implications and how to implement it.

Workshops can be a useful tool for communicating policy. In order to develop consensus, those presenting the policy decisions should ideally include representatives of groups other than central government, in particular municipal officials and representatives of NGOs.

Demonstration projects can be used to show the implications of policy decisions, particularly where these have physical implications and/or involve cooperation between different organizations and groups. For instance, a demonstration scheme involving facilities provided by community groups and including facilities constructed to appropriate standards may be used to make the point that it is possible to involve stakeholders other than government in sanitation provision. Information on demonstration projects can be communicated by arranging visits to the projects themselves and circulating information on their achievements. Videos may provide a good mechanism for circulating information. The impact of site visits and videos will be greater if the users of the facilities, those who are responsible for managing them and those who have been involved in their provision are involved in presenting the scheme.

Government training institutions can provide training on policies and their implications. However, this training should not consist only of lectures since more lasting results are likely to be achieved if trainees engage in training sessions as active participants rather than passive recipients. Where possible, formal classroom sessions should be combined with site visits so that trainees can see what the ideas that they are absorbing mean in practice. In many countries, this 'learner-centred' approach to training will require big changes in the way in which training institutes deliver training and this needs to be taken into account when developing the policy communication strategy.

Amendments to legislation and procedures

Amendments in legislation and procedures will often be needed to remove barriers to the implementation of policy. The precise details of these amendments will, of course, depend on the existing situation but changes are likely to relate to the following.

- *Recognition of informal areas.* Some governments still view most informal settlements as illegal and pursue policies that focus on removing rather than improving them. For instance, in Zimbabwe, the Harare City Council was reported to have plans to destroy over 145 000 backyard structures, making around 500 000 people homeless.[6] Where existing legislation and procedures do not recognize the existence of informal development, it may be impossible to include the needs and concerns of the poor people who live in them in strategic plans.

- *Demand.* The focus here should normally be on amending rules and procedures to ensure that at least part of the cost of new sanitation facilities is recovered from users. While there should be some flexibility to allow for differences in local circumstances, everyone should be required to follow a broadly similar approach to charging and cost recovery. For instance, a policy statement that users should pay a 'realistic' connection charge for connection to sewers will be undermined if some government programmes and/or elected representatives continue to provide facilities free of charge.

- *Roles and responsibilities.* Changes in legislation will often be required to allow different organizations to take responsibility for sanitation provision in different areas and at different levels within hierarchical service provision systems. Where facilities managed by one organization are linked to facilities managed by another, it will be necessary to provide clear guidelines on the way in which revenues and financial responsibilities are to be shared between the parties. It will usually be necessary to develop procedures to resolve disagreements. Consideration also needs to be given to the options for promoting better coordination. There may also be a need to legislate for the changes needed to clarify and simplify the division of responsibilities between government departments.

- *Sound finances.* In recent years, there has been a strong emphasis on the need to devolve responsibility for aspects of service provision from higher levels of government to municipalities. This emphasis on devolution of responsibilities is certainly compatible with the need to involve stakeholders in appropriate ways. However, real devolution will only be possible if municipalities know what finances are available to them. Ideally, revenue raising powers should be devolved to the local level. Where this is not possible, there must be clear guidelines on the allocation of funds between municipalities (and, where appropriate, other local stakeholders) and the mechanisms used to distribute the funds.

- *Technologies and standards.* Existing standards based on conventional 'western' approaches to sanitation can seriously constrain opportunities for developing appropriate sanitation technologies, strategies and programmes. For instance, current legislation in Zimbabwe compels local authorities to provide water-borne sewerage in urban areas. Even where a standard relates to an apparently appropriate technology, it may be unrealistic. Again Zimbabwe provides an example. Even in the limited areas in which pit latrines are acceptable as an option for urban sanitation, they must be of the relatively expensive ventilated improved pit design (See Appendix 2). This contrasts with the

> **Box 4.2 Principles for the development of appropriate standards and specifications**
>
> When deciding what constitutes an appropriate standard, the following basic principles should be kept in mind.
>
> 1. *Standards should relate to the function that a facility is intended to perform.* For example, a manhole on a sewer with a depth of more than about 1.5 m must be large enough for a man to gain access and work with drainage rods and other sewer maintenance equipment. A chamber on a shallow sewer can be smaller because it is intended to be accessed from the surface and so does not have to be big enough to allow a man access.
> 2. *Standards must be framed in the light of local conditions.* For example, a sewer laid in a main road carrying heavy trucks needs to be laid at a greater depth than one laid in a narrow lane carrying nothing heavier than handcarts.
> 3. *Specifications should relate to the performance required of a component or facility.* For example, when considering the jointing arrangements for sewer pipes, the most important concern should be to avoid the possibility of a poor fit between the two pipes, which might create an obstruction on which sewage solids can become caught and thus cause an obstruction to the flow in the sewer.

situation in neighbouring Mozambique described in Box 4.3 (see page 60).

Box 4.2 suggests principles for the development of appropriate standards and specifications. Where there is disagreement on what constitute acceptable standards and specifications, the best way forward will normally be to develop a programme to test a range of possible standards and/or specifications and demonstrate the viability of those that are found to be satisfactory (see Figure 4.4). Ideally, the testing programme should be discussed and agreed with both government technical advisers and those with practical knowledge of the standards and specifications used in the non-government sector.

Testing programmes can be developed at the level of a single town or city. However, their impact will be greater if they are sanctioned by higher levels of government so that their results can be used as the basis for either developing or amending 'official' standards and specifications.

It may take time to achieve changes in legislation. To avoid long delays, efforts to develop changes in legislation should be started as soon as the need for those changes has been identified. Even then, do not assume that the new legislation will be in place in a matter of weeks or even months. It will usually be useful to gather support for the required changes at an early stage and look for 'champions' who will take the lead in promoting them.

Incentives as a support to policy

Appropriately targeted incentives can provide a powerful means of ensuring that local stakeholders follow policy recommendations. In particular, incentives can encourage municipal and local stakeholders to take a more strategic approach. These incentives might involve the following.

Rewards for good performance. In particular, additional funds might be awarded to those organizations, whether governmental or non-governmental, which have been effective in delivering good quality sanitation services in accordance with strategic sanit-

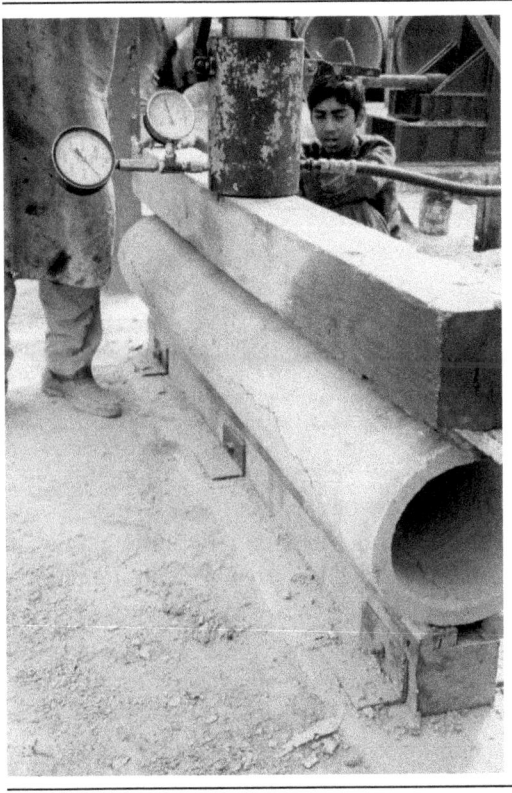

Figure 4.4 The place of testing in developing appropriate standards

In the course of the DFID-funded Faisalabad Area Upgrading Project, pipes from officially approved and 'informal' pipe casting yards were tested in order to establish their relative strengths. The testing proved that the quality of both officially approved pipes and those used by local community organizations left a lot to be desired. The results were used to develop recommended standards for pipes used for community-built sewers (Parkinson and Alam 2002).

[Photo Paul Dean].

ation principles. To avoid a tendency for funding to gravitate towards those organizations that perform well, leaving other organizations further and further behind, rewards for good performance must be linked with efforts to provide support to and build capacity in poorly performing municipalities and government departments.

Encouragement for strategic planning. As a first step in rewarding good performance, higher levels of government might require that all municipalities produce a strategic sanitation plan. As with providing rewards for good performance, this approach will only be successful if the requirement that a plan is produced is linked with assistance to enable the municipality to produce the plan. Involving a wide range of stakeholders in the planning process will help to reduce the likelihood that municipalities will produce plans purely for the sake of receiving funding. Plans are more likely to be followed if projects developed in the context of an overall strategic plan are given priority when considering applications for funding through national and state/provincial government programmes.

Increased municipal accountability. Ideally, municipalities should be responsible for repaying any loans and/or repayable transfers of funds that they receive from either higher levels of government or development banks. This will provide an incentive for them to spend money wisely and will thus help to ensure that their finances are sound. In many cases, there will be a need to move towards this overall goal in manageable steps that match increased financial responsibility to increased capacity to plan and budget. As a first step, consider whether there is scope for applying any existing rules and procedures that are currently ignored.

> **Box 4.3 Provision of materials as an incentive for investing in sanitation**
>
> The national programme for low-cost sanitation in Mozambique (PNSBC) has been based for many years on a simple pit latrine design, incorporating a simple domed slab. The slab is unreinforced and can be produced by workers with basic skills. The implementation strategy of PNSBC is based on the establishment of a relatively large number of production units for these slabs in peri-urban settlements. The programme has been very successful. Between 1985 and 1998, the programme sold and installed 230 646 improved latrines and slab production capacity grew to about 25 000 units per annum. No subsidy was provided on the cost of the slabs but they proved popular with users because they were readily available and could be easily transported. (Saywell and Hunt, 1999)

The role of centrally initiated programmes in supporting policy

Programmes designed and funded by higher levels of government but implemented through local stakeholders provide a means of introducing appropriate incentives and channelling resources. These programmes are likely to include both:

○ *targeted programmes*, which often promote a specific low-cost technology and which are likely to have a poverty focus. Examples include the Indian Integrated Low Cost Sanitation (ILCS) programme and the Mozambique Government's National Program for Low Cost Sanitation (PNSBC).

○ *general infrastructure financing programmes*, which will typically take the form of an 'annual development programme' designed to provide finance for larger infrastructure development projects, for instance new collector and trunk sewers.

Existing programmes should be assessed to determine the extent to which they already comply with strategic sanitation principles as embodied in the policy. Action can then be taken to bring the programmes into line with policy.

Centrally initiated programmes may provide one or more of the following.

Finance. In this case they should require that sanitation providers pay increased attention to demand. This may take the form of a requirement that users pay part of the cost directly and/or that tariffs are increased to cover capital and recurrent costs. Avoid schemes that require that users pay a small proportion of the cost of facilities directly, since the cost of administration of such schemes will often exceed the amount collected through them. Either ask users to pay a higher percentage of the cost or look at indirect cost recovery options, such as increased tariffs.

Materials. In some cases, the provision of essential materials may be a better incentive than providing finance for latrine construction. An example of what this might mean in practice is given in Box 4.3.

Technical guidance. The aim should be to ensure that a range of technologies, suitable for use in the range of conditions that is likely to be encountered, is available. When developing new programmes, the options for improving the technologies that people are already using should always be explored. The assumption that 'one technology fits all' should be avoided. Technical guidance programmes should also provide funds to support experimentation and innovation.

Support to human resource development. This important requirement for improved sanitation provision is often neglected. There is a need for greater emphasis on providing support to human resource development (HRD) programmes that are responsive to organizational needs and provide sound advice on strategic planning principles.

Support to strategic planning. It may be appropriate to develop a programme with the specific objective of supporting strategic planning. This might provide:

- modest funding for both workshops and activities carried out to develop solutions
- technical support, covering the provision of trained facilitators for workshops, advice and guidance and training in strategic processes.

The process might be implemented in pilot municipalities. Following this, the achievements of the pilot projects would be disseminated through workshops, publications, videos and exchange visits as appropriate. At the same time, a start should be made on the changes in legislation and procedures required to allow general replication of the process. These activities will lead into the introduction of strategic planning processes on a national or state-wide scale.

This process requires that higher levels of government are committed to the concept of strategic planning but uses a step-wise approach to changes in legislation and procedures, based on the lessons learnt from practical field experience. Box 4.4 provides an example of how such a process might operate in practice.

Integrating externally funded initiatives with government programmes

Government officials and representatives of funding agencies often treat externally funded projects as separate entities from the government's own ongoing programmes. There is a need for greater emphasis on the links between the two and the ways in which externally supported projects can be integrated into government and other local programmes. Ideally, the development of an overall sanitation policy based on strategic principles should lead to the development of a programme into which externally supported projects can be integrated. External funding can be used to test out ideas and theories, but it is important to consider the ways in which any lessons learnt can be integrated into mainstream procedures.

Increasing capacity to produce and implement strategic plans

In many countries, resource constraints are likely to seriously limit the ability of local government and other local organizations to produce and implement strategic plans. Given the limited financial resources of many municipalities, it may be necessary for higher levels of government to make finance available to support strategic planning activities, at least until action to introduce better municipal financial systems has been introduced. It will normally also be necessary to either develop or reinforce local capacity, looking at the options for human resource development and the possible roles of the private sector in delivering sanitation services.

Human resource development

Human resource development is achieved through formal education and subsequent practical experience and technical training. We will focus on training rather than formal education, although some of the points made will also apply to university and college courses.

The most obvious focus for efforts to improve capacity for strategic planning will

Box 4.4 WASPOLA – a project approach to policy development[7]

The Water Supply and Sanitation Policy Formulation and Action Planning Project (WASPOLA) aims to develop a partnership approach to policy development for the water supply and sanitation sector in Indonesia. It began in 1998, with a five-year implementation period, and focuses on those services that require input from both formal institutions and the communities that will benefit from the services. It is led by the Indonesian government through a multi-agency Central Project Committee with day-to-day activities undertaken by a working group of the participating agencies, led by BAPPENAS, the national planning agency. This, in turn, is supported by a small project secretariat, which receives technical support from the World Bank through the Water and Sanitation Program for East Asia and the Pacific (WSP-EAP) and financial assistance from the Australian government and the World Bank.

The project's overall objective is to enhance the Indonesian government's capacity to develop and adopt policies for water supply and sanitation that encourage demand-driven and participatory initiatives. It also seeks to test policy-related options in selected provinces and to establish and develop capacity in Indonesia to collect and analyse data on the water supply and sanitation sector.

The approach is strategic, not only in its emphasis on developing an inclusive information-based approach to policy formulation but also in its step-wise approach to the development of policy and the strong emphasis on obtaining feedback from field studies and tests. Steps in the process include:

- Reviews of existing case studies in order to identify key policy issues. (Answering the question 'where are we now?')
- New case studies, focusing on key policy issues, action to improve information systems and further analysis of available information.
- Development of a Draft Preliminary Policy Framework.
- Field trials to test policy-related service improvement initiatives. (This stage of the project fits well with the concept of developing solutions.)
- Revision of the Draft Preliminary Policy Framework, incorporating the results of field trials.
- Trial activities in selected provinces to explore the implementation of the policy.
- Dissemination of the findings of the project and support to implementation at the district level. These activities will also feed back into the revision process.

be on courses designed to provide knowledge and skills that are directly relevant to the strategic planning process. These should cover:

- the strategic approach itself, with particular reference to the need to see planning as an information-based process and to follow basic strategic principles
- the skills required to facilitate strategic processes and the involvement of the various stakeholders in those processes.

This training should ideally be linked to strategic planning activities in the field so that the trainees can see how strategic principles and processes might apply in concrete situations.

Important as training is, it should be seen as just one aspect of an integrated approach to capacity building. In order to understand why this is so, problems relating to demand for training and the supply of training are listed below.

Demand-side problems include the following:

o The low priority given to training and human resource development by many government departments.

o Wider organizational problems, which inhibit the use of the knowledge and skills acquired through training.

o Personnel policies which award promotion on the basis of seniority and length of service rather than performance and achievement, which mean that there are few incentives for staff members to undertake training.

Supply-side problems include the following:

o The poor quality and lack of relevance of many training courses, many of which rely largely on 'standard' materials with little attempt being made to tailor training to the situations encountered by trainees in their working environment.

o The lack of provision for amendment in the light of feedback from trainees. This clearly contributes to the lack of relevance.

o A lack of trained trainers. It is common for trainers to be professionals, who may know their jobs but have had no exposure to training methods. The result is a preponderance of top-down training methods that provide little opportunity for feedback from students.

The overall result of these deficiencies is that many officials working at the municipal level often have limited technical skills. So, even if a strategic planning process is completed successfully, there is no guarantee that the elements of the strategic plan will be implemented satisfactorily.

This situation can only be addressed by taking coordinated action to both:

o increase demand for training

o ensure that the training that is available is relevant and well delivered.

As with other aspects of strategic processes, it will be important to first identify the exact nature of current problems and then take action to deal with those problems.

On the demand side, an increased emphasis on the need to produce good quality strategic plans will help to focus attention on the need to build capacity to produce and implement those plans. Ideally, this should be accompanied by changes in personnel policies to encourage merit-based promotion although this may be easier to promote than to achieve.

On the supply side, the starting point for improving the quality of training will often be to give training institutions more autonomy and allow them to develop their own courses and materials to suit demand. Allied to this, they should be given more control over staff appointments. As far as is possible, training must be delivered by trained trainers who are committed to their training role and do not regard involvement in training as some form of 'punishment posting'.

Training materials should place greater emphasis on the way in which particular tasks fit into the overall planning and implementation process. This will help to ensure that trainees know not only how to carry out a particular task but when and why it is required. The present focus on how tasks should be done rather than when they are required militates against efforts to ensure that training is more relevant to trainees' work situations.

In many countries, these changes will

require both a fundamental shift in attitude towards training and major efforts to improve the quality of training. Options for helping to bring about these changes include the following.

o Ensure that policies refer to the actions required to build capacity.

o Develop some training institutions as centres of excellence and provide support for those institutions to facilitate the production of improved training material and methods.

o Place greater emphasis on training of trainers.

o Include an allowance for training in the funding provided for projects and to support strategic planning processes.

These options are not alternatives but rather should be considered together as part of an integrated approach to developing a more effective context for capacity building. International agencies will often have an important part to play in providing funding for such efforts.

The possible role of the private sector in increasing capacity

The approach to building capacity outlined above will not achieve results overnight and should not be pursued to the exclusion of other options for increasing capacity. One of these options is to involve the private sector in sanitation provision. Indeed, the concept of unbundling was originally used by World Bank economists in the context of their strong belief in the benefits of private sector involvement in infrastructure delivery (World Bank 1994).

Involving the private sector may provide access to capital and skills that are not available in the public sector. In practice, it seems that the skills that are relevant to sanitation provision are currently more likely to be available in the informal private sector than through formal private companies. Nevertheless, the possibilities for developing roles for these companies should not be ignored. For instance, in relation to training, it may be that expertise in training of trainers is available in the private sector.

Where government departments are bound by rigid rules, regulations and ways of thinking, as is often the case, the greater flexibility of the private sector may offer significant cost savings. Indeed, figures provided by municipal officials in Andhra Pradesh, India, suggest that the introduction of privately operated solid waste collection and water tanker services has reduced costs to less than a third of those previously incurred by the public sector in providing the same services. On the other hand, there is a real danger that poorly monitored private sector operations may provide poor quality services and it should not be assumed that the private sector will automatically be more efficient and effective than the public sector.

Most efforts to involve the private sector in infrastructure provision focus on large contracts that cover whole cities. The size of these contracts means that they are usually let to large multi-national companies based in industrialized countries. Some international agencies appear to assume that this comprehensive approach to private sector involvement is the only worthwhile approach to private sector involvement. They dismiss the fragmented and small-scale ways in which the private sector is already involved in infrastructure provision as being irrelevant since they will not contribute to fundamental reforms in government systems.

Most of these informal and small-scale initiatives are less than perfect. It can be argued that reliance on them enables decision makers to put off hard decisions on much-needed reforms. There are no obvious ways of regulating them so that there is an obvious danger that they will tend to perpetuate inefficient and even corrupt practices. All these points have some validity. However, there are equally persuasive counter arguments. In particular:

o Small-scale forms of private sector involvement provide opportunities for local companies and thus help to develop in-country capacity. In contrast, the comprehensive approaches to private sector involvement favoured by many international banks and agencies only provide opportunities for large international organizations, which are invariably based in the 'North'.

o Where the government 'culture' is unsympathetic to the idea of wholesale reform, efforts by eternal agencies to introduce such reform are likely to be subverted by the attitudes and assumptions of key stakeholders within government. More limited approaches to private sector involvement provide opportunities for ideas to be absorbed and allow time for attitudes to change. Far from being barriers to necessary reform, these more limited approaches represent necessary steps on the way to that reform.

o Comprehensive regulatory systems are not required for small-scale forms of private sector participation. Rather, the need is for clear contracts, ideally backed up by some form of monitoring by service users. Where existing arrangements for contract supervision leave much to be desired, as is often the case, the need is to explore options for improving those arrangements rather than to introduce high-level regulatory systems. The latter will certainly represent a very unwieldy approach to monitoring local initiatives and are likely to suffer from many of the same problems as existing monitoring systems.

The arguments in favour of small-scale private sector provision are sufficiently compelling to suggest that policy makers should look for ways of encouraging municipalities to engage with the private sector. This encouragement might take the form of guidelines, standard contract documents, circulation of information on examples of good practice and, where necessary, changes in legislation and procedures to remove any barriers to participation that might exist. However, you should beware of assuming that private sector involvement provides a panacea for all the problems associated with municipal infrastructure provision.

Key points in this chapter

1. The lack of a strategic planning 'culture' often constrains efforts to introduce a more strategic approach to sanitation planning.

2. Strategic planning is unlikely to take root at the municipal and local levels unless the policy context supports it. The term 'policy context' refers not only to policies themselves but also to the laws, regulations and procedures that help to ensure that they are implemented.

3. These efforts to improve the context for strategic planning require action at the 'centre'. This suggests that efforts to introduce strategic planning cannot be confined to individual municipalities.

4. Policies should start from a sound understanding of the existing situation, based on accurate and relevant information. They should reflect the ideas, concerns

and experience of all stakeholders and not just a small group at the centre.

5. Limited resources may affect the way in which policies are implemented in practice.

6. Appropriate incentives, enshrined in legislation, can play an important role in encouraging a strategic approach to urban sanitation planning.

7. Programmes, developed at the centre but implemented through local stakeholders, can serve to introduce appropriate incentives and channel resources.

8. There is a need to develop capacity to prepare and implement strategic plans. This will often require coordinated action both to create increased demand for training and to build capacity to deliver relevant training in a learner-centred way.

9. The private sector may provide additional capacity for sanitation provision and sanitation service management. This does not necessarily mean bringing in large contractors on long-term contracts and should include efforts to develop a role for local companies.

Chapter 4 endnotes

1 India illustrates this point very well. Under the 73rd and 74th Amendments to the Indian Constitution, enacted in the early 1990s, a considerable degree of devolution of power and responsibility to local levels of government was to have taken place. Despite this, most responsibilities for infrastructure planning and implementation continue to lie with state level agencies and departments.

2 Senge (1990, p.8) defines mental models as 'the deeply ingrained assumptions, generalisations, or even pictures or images that influence how we understand the world and how we take action'.

3 See, for example, UNICEF (2000), WSSCC (2000),

4 An example is the 'Water Matters' campaign in 2002, which focused on the need to ensure that everyone has access to safe water and adequate sanitation. The aim of the campaign was to ensure that the issue of sanitation was given prominence in the World Summit on Sustainable Development held in that year. (WaterAid and TearFund 2002).

5 Carley et al. (2001) suggest that the term 'institutions' should be used in two ways. Institutions are not just 'organizational forms' but are also defined by the mental models that underpin those organizational forms and the ways in which organizations operate.

6 Information provided by Gift Manase, when a research student at Southampton University.

7 The information contained in Box 4.4 is based on a note on WASPOLA produced by the WSP-EA on behalf of the WASPOLA Project Office. The stages in the project process are our interpretation of the process described in the note.

CHAPTER 5
Developing a strategic process from the local level

As indicated in Chapter 4, there will be situations in which official attitudes and assumptions preclude the immediate adoption of a strategic approach at the municipal level. Nevertheless, stakeholders working to improve conditions in particular local areas can think and act more strategically and, in doing so, provide an entry point for strategic thinking at the municipal level. This chapter provides guidance on how they might do this.

The first part of the chapter provides examples of planning initiatives that either operate or have been initiated at the local level. In particular, the case of Pakistan is used to illustrate the way in which action initiated outside government, in the first instance to address local problems, can have a profound effect on official thinking. Following this, a structure is suggested for a local strategic planning process and guidance is then provided on the various stages of the process. Finally, the options for moving beyond the local level are briefly reviewed.

Three approaches to planning at the local level

It is possible to discern three broad approaches to planning at the local level. These are:

○ Government or NGO initiated local plans that deal with specific, usually low-income, areas. Such plans are usually multi-sectoral but sanitation services often figure prominently in them.

○ Plans produced by local stakeholders, usually with the help of an NGO, often in response to the lack of government action in their areas. Many take an incremental approach to problem solving, focusing first on the problems that affect small groups of households and only moving on to consider action at a higher level if local action does not solve those problems.

○ Local plans initiated by government but intended to feed into a hierarchical systems of plans designed to provide a planning framework for the municipality, or indeed the state or province, as a whole.

This chapter is concerned mainly with the first two, although it draws on experience with the third. The ways in which local planning initiatives could provide the starting point for more comprehensive approaches to planning are briefly examined at the end of the chapter.

Local plans initiated by government

The micro-planning approach adopted during the Million Houses Program (MHP) in Sri Lanka is a good example of a local planning approach initiated by government. The MHP began in 1984 and included both rural and urban components. The MHP was a government project, located within the National Housing Development Authority and managed by committed individuals within that organization. However, its underlying philosophy was based on the assumption that the state should participate in the people's processes rather than the other way round (Fernando et al. 1987). While both rural and urban components provided support to people who wanted to improve their own houses, the urban component also had a strong emphasis on local infrastructure provision.

An important feature of the MHP, as implemented in urban areas, was its use of a participatory micro-planning process to facilitate the identification and prioritization of community needs (Hamdi and Goethert, 1988). As the term 'micro-plan' suggests, the approach was small scale and very local in nature.

Micro-planning activities were normally confined to specific low-income settlements and implemented through community development councils (CDCs), organizations representing groups of around 50 families. For larger settlements, a number of CDCs were formed and were then encouraged to come together to form a 'CDC federation'.

This approach is not without problems. There can be problems in sustaining local community-level organizations, particularly when they have no clear official status. From the perspective of this book, it is questionable whether micro-plans can really be considered as strategic since they have no city-wide or even district perspective. Nevertheless, the micro-planning approach provides some useful lessons on *how* to facilitate participatory planning processes at the local level and we will draw on its experience when providing planning guidelines later in this chapter.

Incremental community-based initiatives

In Chapter 1, we noted the existence of three basic approaches to sanitation provision, the third of which was described as the 'local collective action' model. Much of the activity that currently takes place in informal areas, those developed outside official government rules and procedures, falls into this category. Local people come together to solve problems as and when they occur, either acting directly or putting pressure on elected representatives and government officials to solve the problems for them.

Given the importance of informal settlements as places where many poor people live and work, any strategic approach that is serious about the need for equity and hence for a clear poverty focus must take account of these activities. Furthermore, as we have indicated in Chapter 4, where the prevailing attitudes and assumptions of official decision makers are not conducive to change, it is quite possible that local initiatives may provide the best entry point for attempts to introduce a more strategic approach to sanitation planning.

As an example of how this might happen in practice, we now will now briefly summarize the situation in Pakistan, focusing on the role of the Orangi Pilot Project (OPP) as a catalyst of change.

Community initiated sanitation – the case of Pakistan

In Pakistan, there is long tradition of local groups coming together to solve the sanitation problems that government departments are either unwilling or unable to tackle. Most groups are concerned only with their immediate environment and their activities typically involve the construction of a sewer along a road or lane to connect to the nearest open drain or government sewer. Such local actions clearly cannot be considered to be strategic. However, there are examples of more ambitious schemes, which require a degree of planning and which, perhaps unconsciously, follow some of the strategic principles outlined in Chapter 2. Box 5.1 provides an example of such a scheme.

Box 5.1 Saifabad 2, Faisalabad – an area-based scheme

Saifabad 2 is an informally developed housing area on the south-western fringe of Faisalabad, which is Pakistan's third largest city. It lies just outside the municipal limits and the 'developer' provided no services to the 400 or so plots in the scheme. When faced with drainage problems, the residents formed a society to explore the options for sewering the area. Initial investigations revealed that they could expect little help from the Faisalabad Water and Sanitation Agency (FWASA), the official sewerage provider, because they were outside the municipal limits. In any case, it seemed that the area could not be connected to FWASA sewers without pumping. So, they developed their own self-contained scheme, a system of branch and collector sewers discharging to a local pond. A local NGO, Community Action Programme (CAP) encouraged the society in its endeavours and arranged for a topographical survey to be carried out. The total investment was estimated to be about 2.8 million Pakistani rupees, (1998 prices), the equivalent of about US$60 000.

Once the scheme was operational, it became clear that seepage from the pond was insufficient to match the inflow of wastewater. The society responded by purchasing a diesel-powered pump, which was used to pump the wastewater from the pond to a wide verge alongside a nearby main road out of the city. For three days, for a few hours every evening, the wastewater was directed along the verge in one direction. The direction of discharge was then reversed and wastewater drained in the other direction. Residents paid a regular monthly fee to the society to cover the costs of operating the pump and any maintenance work required. The community recognized that this arrangement was not satisfactory and investigated other options, including the possibility of using the wastewater for irrigation in fields owned by an agricultural institute close to their current disposal point and that of pumping their sewage back to the FWASA sewer. However, to date these efforts have been unsuccessful.

How do such schemes measure up against the strategic principles set out in Chapter 2? Answers to this question are suggested below. They are clearly demand-based in that residents plan, finance and manage all aspects of the scheme themselves. The example of Saifabad 2 shows that the level of investment can be high and that, in the short to medium term at least, the finances of such schemes can be reasonably sound. Saifabad 2 residents paid for construction of the scheme and also make monthly payments to the society to cover the cost of pumping so that the scheme is self-supporting and has sound finances.

The Saifabad scheme developed in a series of steps, the first involving the construction of sewers and the second the purchase of the pump to provide a rather ad hoc solution to the problem of wastewater disposal. Residents then talked to official stakeholders, including FWASA, in an effort to identify a more permanent and acceptable solution to the problem of wastewater disposal.

However, local schemes can be unsatisfactory in other respects. Because of the flat topography, many sewers are laid to fairly flat gradients and the standard chamber details are often poor. One result of this is that chamber covers are often broken or removed, allowing solid waste to enter the sewer. This has serious implications for maintenance and for the long-term viability of sewerage. In Saifabad 2, the most serious deficiency lay in the arrangements made for wastewater disposal. It seems that some local schemes will prove to be unsatisfactory unless it is possible to link them to higher-order facilities installed by official service providers.

The Orangi Pilot Project – a model for a locally based strategic approach?

The Karachi-based NGO, the Orangi Pilot Project (OPP) has gone some way towards tackling the issues raised above. It started work in Orangi, a large informal settlement on the outskirts of Karachi, in the early 1980s and, on the basis of initial observation and discussions with local residents, identified sanitation and drainage as being the most serious problems facing residents (Hasan 1997). Taking its lead from local residents, it decided that sewerage provided the best option for improving sanitation and drainage. It also recognized that government was unlikely to provide improved services and encouraged local people to take responsibility for financing, building and managing their own sewers.

The initial focus was on tertiary sewers, serving a single street or lane. This was possible because Orangi is a hilly area, cut by many natural drainage channels or 'nullahs' so that it was often possible to build a sewer to the nearest nullah. There were, however, many situations in which there was no obvious outlet for a sewer serving a single lane. OPP responded by encouraging larger groups of residents to come together to plan, finance and construct the secondary sewers required to collect flows from a number of tertiary sewers.

By the early 1990s, much of Orangi was served by secondary and tertiary sewers although there was still a need to provide trunk sewers to remove flows from the major nullahs and to treat sewage before discharge to the Lyari River. OPP responded by:

○ producing an overall sewerage plan for Orangi Township

○ lobbying government authorities and international agencies to develop an integrated approach to sewage disposal services in the area, building on what it had already achieved.

It also provided advice and encouragement to NGOs in other cities in Pakistan with an interest in adopting its approach to sanitation provision, encouraged government authorities and international agencies to adopt its approach to sewerage provision and provided advice to a number of externally funded projects (see Boxes 5.2, 5.3 and 5.6).

OPP's work is internationally recognized.[1] Its approach is, in many ways, consonant with the strategic principles introduced in Chapter 2. In common with other examples of local collective action in Pakistan, it is clearly demand-based in that the users of sanitation facilities are responsible for providing and paying for those facilities (Zaidi, 2001). In order to ensure sound finances, it has placed considerable emphasis on overcoming what it calls the economic barrier, the fact that the *'conventional cost of building an underground sanitation system is unaffordable to users'* (Hasan 1997).

It has done this by:

○ developing appropriate standards and designs, for instance small concrete inspection chambers for community-built sewers

○ encouraging community groups to manage schemes themselves, thus cutting out what it sees as the excessive profit made by contractors on government schemes.

In both cases, it has clearly been concerned to inform demand.

The idea of unbundling is enshrined in

Box 5.2 The CKAIP in Hyderabad and the consequences of failing to take a wide view

The Collaborative Katchi Abadi Improvement Programme in Hyderabad was a pilot project, supported by the World Bank and the Swiss Development Corporation, and intended to test and demonstrate an unbundled approach to upgrading services in low-income areas in Pakistan. It involved collaboration between the Sind Katchi Abadi Authority (SKAA), the Hyderabad Municipal Corporation (HMC) and OPP, which acted as technical adviser. The ultimate aim was to cover a range of services, including roads, water supply and streetlights but, following the standard OPP model, the initial emphasis was on sanitation. It was clear from the start that on-site sewers could not be built before the installation of off-site sewerage facilities. The Hyderabad Water and Sanitation Agency prepared a design for off-site sewerage involving pumping. OPP, quite rightly, argued that a pumped scheme was likely to be problematic and produced an alternative design involving gravity sewers laid to very flat gradients and discharging to the nearest collector drain. These sewers were built but the project progressed very little further. OPP blames government for the situation and there is little doubt that government failings were a contributory factor. However, inspection of one of the project sites suggests that there were other factors. A combination of the extremely flat sewer gradient adopted, the channelling of wastewater from open drains through the sewer and the lack of a solid waste collection service in the project area had resulted in blockage of the sewer and it was clear that it would be very difficult to unblock it and reclaim the situation. A wide view of sanitation would have identified the need to tackle the problem of solid waste collection either before or at the same time as efforts to provide sewerage. It would also have identified the need to remove solid waste and silt from flows entering the collector sewer before construction of tertiary sewers and to provide interceptor tanks on house connections while building those sewers.

OPP's concept of 'internal' and 'external' facilities. Internal facilities are those that people can provide and manage themselves. They include household and tertiary facilities, together with those secondary facilities that serve clearly defined neighbourhoods. All other facilities are considered to be external. OPP argues that local communities should take full responsibility for financing, providing and managing internal services, leaving government to concentrate its limited resources on what it should theoretically do best – plan, provide and manage the more complex external facilities and services.

OPP's whole philosophy is founded on the idea of moving forward in achievable steps. Its approach in the early years in Orangi was not dissimilar from the understand problems – develop solutions – plan city-wide sequence described in Chapter 3. To understand problems and possibilities, it looked at what was already happening in Orangi and talked to local residents. It then developed and tested an approach to local sewerage improvement before moving on to consider the needs of Orangi Township as a whole. Its stepwise approach to sanitation problems is illustrated by a quote from its founder, Dr. Akhtar Hamid Khan, *'Nearly two years ago, we began to organise the lanes. Gradually, after much fumbling, a viable pattern emerged, which is now popular. In the last six months, we tried tentatively to climb from the lane level to the mohalla and circle levels* (Khan 1985, p. 262).

(The terms *mohalla* and *circle* refer to a local neighbourhood and a councillor's ward respectively.)

The OPP approach has had a wide influence within Pakistan. NGOs such as Anjuman Samaji Behbood (ASB) in Faisalabad (Alimuddin et al. 2000) and Youth Commission for Human Rights (YCHR) in Lahore, CBOs throughout the country and some government projects have adopted its concepts and techniques in whole or in part (see Figure 5.1).

However, the OPP model is not without its problems. It is arguable that, in stressing the need to identify the people's main problem and solve that before moving on to solve other problems, it takes a rather narrow view of sanitation. This, together with its tendency to assume that the first priority will always be sewerage, can lead to problems, as illustrated by the example described in Box 5.2. However, perhaps the greatest problems relate to coordination with government and other 'official' sanitation providers. OPP has had limited success in persuading government agencies and departments of the validity of its view of what constitute appropriate standards. Problems also remain with the arrangements made for sharing operation and maintenance costs. Orangi itself has good falls and sewers can therefore be laid to self-cleansing falls without resorting to pumping but this is not the case in some other parts of Karachi and in many other cities in Pakistan. Box 5.3 illustrates the problems that can arise when the arrangements made to deal with operational costs, particularly those associated with pumping, prove to be inadequate.

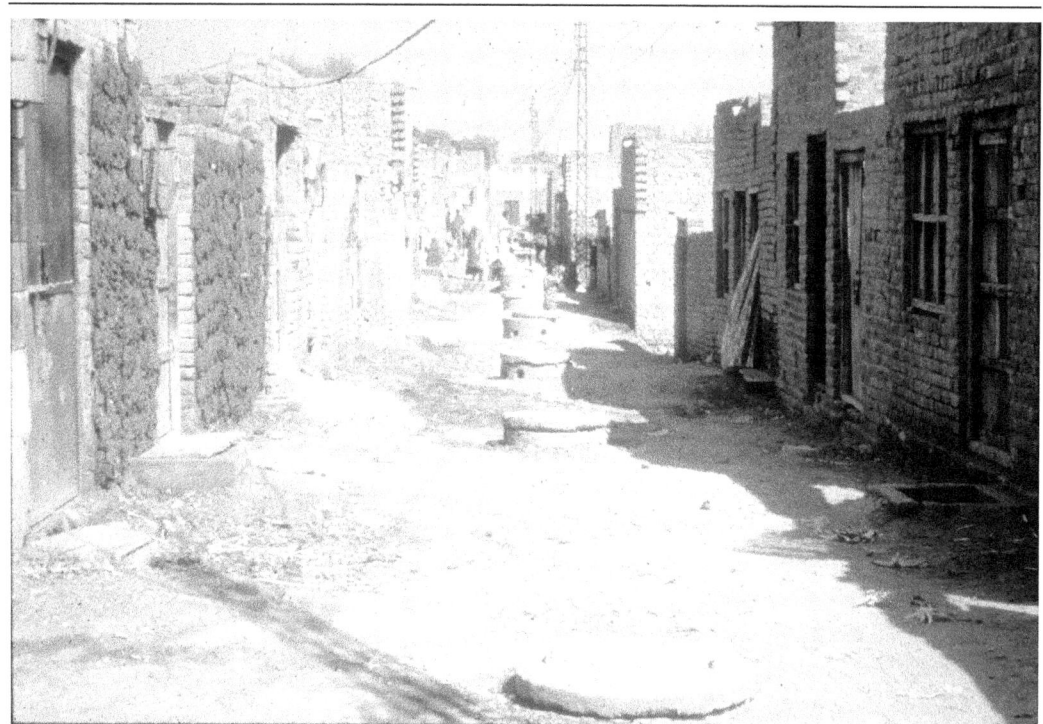

Figure 5.1 Orangi Pilot Project (RTI) access chamber under construction
An OPP-style access chamber under construction. The sewer is being constructed by the DFID-funded Faisalabad Area Upgrading Project. The design for access chambers is based on that developed by OPP.

Box 5.3 Sukkur, Pakistan – an example of failure to deal with operating costs

The Urban Basic Services Program (UBSP) in the town of Sukkur, Pakistan involved efforts to improve sanitation and drainage in and around an area called Gole Takri. The houses to be served were located in low lying excavated land and any drainage scheme for the area must involve pumping. Before the UBSP scheme, open drains discharged to a large wastewater pond in the centre of Gole Takri.

Community members were required to pay the full cost of lane sewers. Government and UNICEF paid the capital cost of collector sewers, a pumping station to lift sewage and a rising main to convey it to the Indus River. In effect, there was a generous subsidy on the higher order 'external' facilities while people paid the full cost of local facilities themselves. This division of responsibilities was based on the approach advocated by the OPP, which acted as adviser for the scheme. After only six months, the Sukkur Municipal Corporation (SMC) stopped operating the pumping station, at least partly because it was receiving no revenue from users to pay for its running costs. It seems that insufficient attention had been paid at the planning stage to the question of who would pay for this critical ongoing cost. Without the pumping station, the scheme started to fail. The pond in the centre of Gore Takri reappeared, sewers were surcharged so that they could not run freely and there were frequent problems with sewer blockages. As a result, some residents abandoned their sewers and reverted to the use of open drains.

OPP has since made efforts to revive the scheme but with the sewer users themselves taking financial responsibility for the operation of the pumping station.

A process for planning at the local level

The brief review of activities in Pakistan shows that:

- it is possible for concerned individuals, groups and organizations to take action at the local level, even where the government authorities with official responsibility for sanitation provision have little interest in an area
- these initiatives can incorporate many of the strategic features that have already been identified in this book
- there will often be problems in convincing municipal stakeholders to officially agree to the connection of local community-initiated sewers into their own systems.

Bearing these points in mind, we now explore a possible process for planning at the local level. In doing so, we recognize that many of the points made in Chapter 3 apply, with some minor modifications, at the local level. In particular, the basic sequence of understanding problems and developing solutions before going on to plan for an area as a whole should still be followed unless the area covered by the plan is small and the actions identified at the first planning workshop are simple and self-contained. Figure 5.2 shows the process diagrammatically. Like both the Sri Lankan micro-planning process and the Bharatpur pilot planning process, it is built around one or more planning workshops, which allows the various stakeholders to identify problems and to develop proposals for moving towards solutions.

74 URBAN SANITATION

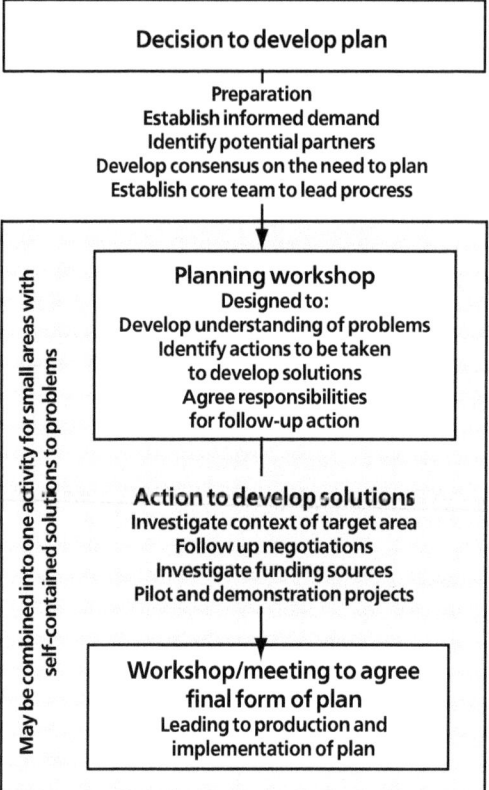

Figure 5.2 The planning process at local level

The suggested process is rather more formal than that used by OPP. There are two reasons for this:

o providing a formal structure will help to reduce the tendency for local initiatives to degenerate into isolated ad hoc actions; and

o the planning workshop provides a forum to which all stakeholders, including official sanitation providers, can be asked to contribute, thus helping to build bridges and provide a starting point for later cooperation and the institutionalization of strategic planning processes.

Figure 5.2 indicates the need for a period of preparation, during which demand for sanitation improvements can be established and informed and the various stakeholders can be convinced of the need for a strategic approach to planning. However, much of the detailed assessment required to develop an initial understanding of problems and possibilities can be carried out in the workshop itself.

A period is then allowed in which action can be taken to develop solutions. Figure 5.2 indicates that this period can be attenuated or even left out altogether when the area to be planned is small and the proposed actions are relatively simple and self-contained. For larger areas, a final workshop or meeting will be required to agree the final form of the plan.

The planning process does not have to relate to sanitation alone. Indeed, there is much to be said for taking an integrated approach to service provision at the local level, covering water supply, street paving and social services as well as the disposal of liquid and solid wastes. Where appropriate, efforts should then be made to have outputs relating to the different services incorporated into the plans and programmes of the agencies with overall responsibility for the provision of these services.

Bearing these general points in mind, we now move on to examine each stage of the process in more detail. The focus is on sanitation-related issues rather than services as a whole, but much of what is said will also apply to other services.[2]

Preparation stage

First steps

When the drive to improve sanitation comes from outside the 'target area', there will be an initial need to make contact with recognized local leaders and activists within the target community. Without the blessing of these recognized leaders, local people may be hesitant to work with outsiders.

Once it has been established that local leaders will not oppose the planning process, it is possible to move on to identify potential partners. These might, of course, include the local leaders themselves and we have already noted in Chapter 3 that elected representatives often play a role in promoting action to improve services in the areas that they represent. Even where these leaders do not wish to play an active role in the planning process, they should be asked to endorse the process and perhaps accept an honorary role in the management team.

Other potential partners include those who are already involved in attempts to improve conditions within the target area, in particular CBOs and community activists.

Investigating demand

There is no point in producing plans for improved sanitation if demand for sanitation is either absent or uninformed. So, efforts to identify potential partners in the planning process should be accompanied by investigation of demand. This investigation should normally take the form of a rapid appraisal of existing practices and attitudes to sanitation based on observation of facilities and services and conversations with local people. It will be good to involve local people in this rapid appraisal, both to ensure that the appraisal takes account of local knowledge and to encourage them to take an interest in the planning process. Women should be involved in this process since their perspectives and priorities may differ from those of men.

Even where government has a duty to provide services, it will rarely have the resources to provide those services to everyone without charge. Despite this, it may still be necessary to challenge the assumption that government should provide services free of cost. Encourage community members to think about who should be responsible for paying for both the capital and recurrent costs of service provision. Point out that all sanitation services have to be paid for and that the greater the level of subsidy, the more difficult it will be to ensure that everyone will receive subsidized services. In this way, you can raise awareness of the importance of paying for services and this should help to inform the debate about developing solutions.

Where initial investigations reveal that there is clearly a limited demand for sanitation, existing demand is poorly informed and/or existing practices are unhygienic, there will be a need to include sanitation and/or hygiene promotion in the plan. An introduction to sanitation promotion is given in Chapter 6.

Developing consensus on the need to plan

Where efforts to improve sanitation already exist, the initial aim should be to convince stakeholders that these efforts could benefit from efforts to develop a more integrated and strategic approach to sanitation planning. The immediate need may be to overcome the tendencies:

○ to react to problems on an ad hoc case by case basis

○ for politicians and CBOs to focus on what they can do for people rather than working *with* local people to bring about improvements in service provision, either directly or by putting pressure on government departments to provide improved services.

Tackle the first obstacle by making local stakeholders aware of the advantages of planning. Emphasize that efforts taken to improve local conditions are more likely to be successful if people work together and pool their resources within the framework provided by a shared plan. Point out that planning is nothing more than thinking ahead to ensure that the best use is made of available resources and that everyone plans in some way, even though they may not commit their plans to paper. The issue is not whether or not to plan but rather what form the plan should take and how it should be prepared and presented. If people cooperate they will also be in a stronger position to negotiate with the municipal authorities to play their part in providing better services.

Efforts should also be made to convince local politicians to work with local people rather than providing political favours and political patronage in return for votes. Use the argument that planning enables limited resources to go further, bringing about improvements that would otherwise be impossible to achieve. If this is not sufficient incentive in itself, point out that local people will welcome the improvements that can be brought about by a rational planned approach and should then be more inclined to vote for the politician at the next election.

Developing a core team

Once there is at least the beginning of a consensus on the need to plan, it will be possible to start thinking about the planning process itself. As with planning at the municipal level, it will be necessary to develop a core team to promote and manage the planning process. This should certainly include any local activists and/or representatives of CBOs who show an interest in the idea of strategic planning. People with specialist skills, for instance masons with knowledge of constructing sanitation systems, health workers and those with experience of managing small projects can also be valuable members of the team. As far as is possible, they should be from the community or at least known to it although there may also be a need to bring in outsiders to provide specialist skills and knowledge. Make sure that women are represented *and* listened to. Do not assume that they should only be concerned with 'soft' subjects such as hygiene education. Women, children and old people stand to gain the most from sanitation improvements and their views should be heard on *all* subjects.

Deciding the area to be covered by the plan

Physical and social boundaries will help to determine the area to be covered by the plan.

Physical boundaries might include major roads, canals, railway lines, hills and rivers, whereas social boundaries relate to:

○ the boundaries between different housing areas, particularly where the characters of the two housing areas is very different

○ boundaries between clearly distinct social or religious groups.

Where possible, encourage different communities to work together – after all neither floodwater nor wastes recognize religious and ethnic boundaries.

Regardless of this, the causes of problems will often lie beyond the boundaries of the immediate target area for the plan so that the scope of the plan will have to be extended, at least when addressing these problems. Situations may also arise in which a low-income area can benefit from being considered in conjunction with its higher-income neighbour. For instance, it may be relatively easy to extend the sewers, drains and solid waste collection services planned for a higher-income area to cover an adjacent low-income area.

Obtaining basic information

In Chapter 3, we noted how NGOs may undertake investigations into the views and concerns of primary stakeholders and feed this information back to the planning workshop. For more local workshops, it may be appropriate for a similar exercise to be carried out to obtain information on the views and plans of the municipal authorities and other government stakeholders. Particular attention should be paid to any funding from government and other sources that might be available to support improvements in local sanitation facilities.

The planning workshop

Workshop participants, objectives and process

A planning workshop provides a focal point, which can bring the various stakeholders together and ensure that the various stakeholders are aware of the planning process. The participants in the workshop should include:

- *community members* – if the area is small, everyone can be invited. For larger areas, you may have to ask local people to select representatives, at least one man and one woman from every street, lane or cluster of houses within the area. Community members with specialist knowledge, for instance masons and health workers should also be asked to participate.

- *representatives of adjacent communities* – those might be affected by the activities to be included in the plan.

- *selected specialists* – those from outside the community who provide or could be called upon to provide services to the community.

The workshop will normally last two days, with the first day devoted to problem identification and analysis and the second to the development of proposals for follow-up actions. See Chapter 9 for further information on preparing for and conducting a planning workshop.

The key objectives for the workshop relating to the stages of identifying problems, problem analysis, and developing solutions are considered in detail below.

Understanding problems

A good way to identify problems will be to divide the workshop participants into groups and ask them to walk around the area to be planned in order to assess the situation with regard to excreta disposal, wastewater and stormwater disposal and solid waste management. Suggest that, while identifying problems, participants should also note examples of good practice.

The groups should ideally comprise four to six people. They should be briefed on what they have to do and where they have to go before being sent out. There are two broad possibilities for organizing the groups:

- Divide participants in terms of their roles, so that one group might consist of men from the community, one of women from the community, one of government employees and so on.

- Ensure that each group includes people from a range of backgrounds.

A basic version of the first approach was used for the micro-planning workshops held in Sri Lanka. Three groups were formed, one technical group, one health and social group and one community group.

The advantage of the first approach is that it helps to ensure that the voices of groups that might otherwise be marginalized, for instance women and tenants, will be heard. In doing so, it should also help to counter the possible tendency of professionals and politicians to try to dominate the workshop on the basis that they know what is good for the people. It should also bring out differences in perceptions about what the problems are, how they should be tackled and, indeed, what the objectives of the plan should be.

The advantage of the second approach is that it ensures that various viewpoints are brought to bear on problems and possibilities when the participants are in the field.

As a general rule, use the first approach for areas that are relatively small, so that everyone looks at the same area and, by implication, the same problems and possibilities. Where the area to be planned is larger so that it is not possible for one group to cover the whole of the area, mixed groups have the advantage that all areas will be looked at by people with different roles, knowledge and experience so that there is less chance that problems and possibilities will be missed.

Problem analysis

It is not sufficient simply to identify problems. It will also be important to agree on which problems are important and to analyse those problems in order to establish their causes. Only then will it be possible to develop a plan of action to address them.

The approach to prioritizing problems used in the Sri Lankan micro-planning process is briefly described in Box 5.4.

Although the details vary, most recognized workshop procedures use a similar approach to reaching agreement on priority problems. Many use cards, on which each group writes the problems that it has identified, one problem per card. The advantage of this approach is that it is flexible. Cards can be moved around, duplicates can be discarded and new cards can be written to capture important ideas that emerge in the course of discussion. Further details are provided in Chapter 9.

Some key points to be considered during the problem analysis are introduced and discussed below.

Hygiene

Workshop participants should be encouraged to assess the current situation with regard to current hygiene practices. The two key questions are:

○ Are people aware of what constitutes good hygiene and its role in ensuring that the full benefits are derived from improvements in sanitation provision?

Box 5.4 Problem analysis in the Sri Lankan micro-planning process

Each of the three groups formed to investigate problems was asked to prepare a chart with three columns, the first listing the problems identified, the second the reason why they were problems and the third to whom they were problems. The workshop leaders then listed the problems identified into three categories:

○ those on which all three groups agreed
○ those on which two groups agreed
○ those identified by only one group.

Those problems that were agreed by two or three groups were automatically accepted as being worthy of further analysis and action. Where only one group had identified a problem, that group was asked to convince other workshop participants of its importance. If they could do so, it was carried forward to the next stage of the analysis.

○ To what extent do current conditions prevent good hygiene? For instance, it may be that regular hand-washing is not possible because water is not always available at existing public toilets.

It will often be useful to aid the discussion by arranging for information on current hygiene practices, gathered before the workshop by a small team, including community members, to be presented to the workshop participants. (See Chapter 6 for further information on participatory hygiene assessment).

Location of the causes of problems

When considering the problems identified in the course of fieldwork, encourage workshop participants to consider the extent to which:

○ problems originate outside the project area, as would be the case where flooding is caused by storm flows from other areas

○ deficiencies in off-site or 'external' facilities affect the performance of local services. For instance, local sewers may not function effectively because an off-site pumping station is not operating so that collector sewers are full and the local sewers cannot flow freely.

If such problems and deficiencies are not tackled, they will undermine efforts to improve local services. This may even lead to a final situation that is worse than that at the start (See Box 5.3). This will certainly discourage local people from continuing to engage with the strategic planning process. So, it will be important to consider the extent to which problems either originate outside the area of immediate concern or are affected by facilities and services outside that area.

Figure 5.3 suggests a conceptual approach to assessing problems and their causes and so deciding the area to be included in the plan.

If it is clear that problems either originate or require action outside the project area, the following questions can be used to guide problem analysis.

○ Which organizations have responsibility for dealing with externally generated problems?

○ Will they be prepared to take action to deal with those problems?

○ If so, will it be feasible to extend the scope of the planning exercise so that it includes action to deal with these off-site problems directly?

○ What arrangements will be needed to manage this wider planning exercise, bearing in mind the fact that it will almost certainly involve external stakeholders?

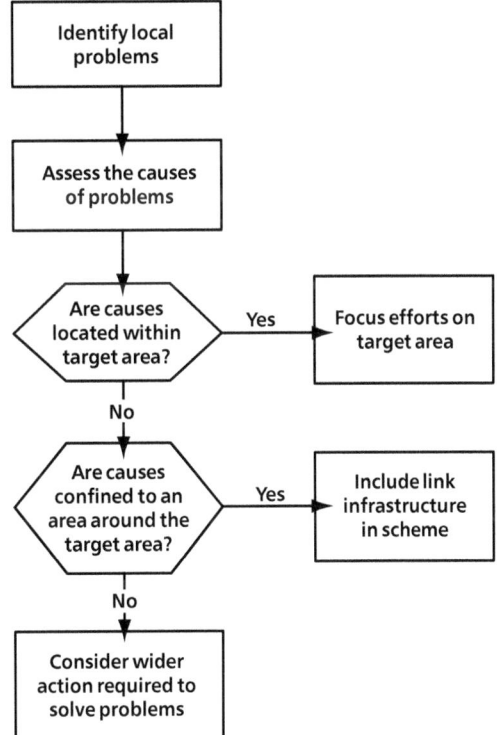

Figure 5.3 Procedure for assessing appropriate responses to local sanitation problems

It may be difficult to answer some or all of these questions directly. Where this is the case, one of the objectives of the workshop should be to reach agreement on the subsequent actions to be taken to answer them. These subsequent activities will form part of the developing solutions stage of the planning process.

Available resources
Available resources include both:

○ internal resources – the funds that community members can raise themselves, together with the commitment, knowledge and skills that are available within the community

○ external resources – the funds and support that might be provided by government, NGOs and other external stakeholders.

In order to prepare the ground for discussion of available resources, encourage workshop participants to look for examples of attempts to address sanitation problems during their field visits on the first day. It may be good to give them examples of the form that such efforts might take (local solid waste collection services, the construction of drains and sewers, etc.) and ask them to look for similar examples of people using their own resources to solve sanitation problems. They should also look for any evidence of government initiatives in the area.

The following questions may be used as a structure for discussing available resources.

○ What services and facilities should people reasonably be expected to provide from their own resources?

○ Where free services have been provided in the past, perhaps by local elected representatives, is this the best use of limited resources? Would it have been better if community members contributed some of their own resources and worked with the ward councillor to develop a more comprehensive response to drainage problems?

○ Are there problems which clearly cannot be solved locally and if so where might the resources required to solve these problems be found? Can these resources be accessed and can they be relied on?

Deciding on the way forward

The last part of the workshop should be devoted to deciding the steps to be taken to carry the planning process forward. Tasks designed to address priority problems should be identified and responsibility for carrying out those tasks should be allocated in the light of existing responsibilities and available resources. As we will see shortly, it is likely that some at least of these tasks will be dedicated to developing solutions to problems in preparation for the production of an overall plan for the area.

Responsibilities for coordinating and carrying out follow-up activities and reporting back to the community must also be agreed. It may be appropriate to appoint a small team to follow up on progress and report back to the community. Arrangements for liaising between the community and external organizations need to be agreed. A date for a follow-up event, at which progress will be reported, should also be agreed.

Developing solutions

Given the relatively small size of local planning initiatives, it might be assumed that there will be no need for the planning process to incorporate a specific developing solutions stage. Indeed, most existing models for local participatory planning processes proceed directly from problem identification into action plan proposals.

However, there will be many situations in which the way forward is not immediately clear. It may be that:

o it is not clear how local facilities can be integrated with city-wide systems

o it is proposed to use technologies and approaches that are not familiar to the majority of community members

o the causes of some problems, particularly those relating to drainage, are not clear.

In all these cases, it will be advisable to spend some time developing solutions before finalizing an overall plan for the area. For those working at the local level, developing solutions is likely to involve some or all of the following.

o Follow-up negotiations with outside stakeholders such as government departments, first to determine the extent to which they can be relied on to support the plan outputs and then to agree on responsibilities and outputs.

o Investigations of sources of funding that might be used to supplement the resources available through the community itself.

o Pilot and demonstration initiatives to test new approaches and/or convince people of their benefits.

The time allowed for developing solutions can generally be shorter for local plans than for municipal plans and ideally should not exceed about three months.

It may be that initial investigations have revealed that action to solve off-site problems will require massive expenditure, for which no funds will be available in the short term. Where this is the case, look for immediately implementable actions that will ameliorate problems while seeking support for the longer-term development of comprehensive solutions to those problems. For instance, flooding may be a general problem for which no immediate solution is available. Possible short-term responses to this problem include improving drainage systems to reduce the duration of flooding, and raising the floor levels of pit latrines to a level above normal flood levels in order to reduce the possibility that flood water becomes contaminated with faeces.

Another possible scenario is that the authorities responsible for higher order facilities are unwilling or unable to engage with the planning exercise and/or cannot be realistically relied upon to provide external services. The developing solutions stage provides an opportunity to explore options that are less dependent on external stakeholders. These options might include the discharge of WC wastes to leach pits rather than sewers and the development of local disposal arrangements for solid waste. However, in many cases, there will be no alternative but to negotiate with external 'authorities' on the provision of off-site facilities and services. Indeed, this may be an important step in developing a more strategic approach to sanitation planning in the town or city as a whole. Box 5.5 provides basic guidance on preparing for and conducting follow-up negotiations.

Pilot and demonstration initiatives

It may be that some of the possible solutions identified in the course of the planning process are unproved and/or unfamiliar to local people. Where this is the case, it will be advisable to pilot the solutions on a small scale before introducing them more widely. As far as is possible, pilot initiatives at the local level should be kept fairly small and self-contained so that they can be implemented reasonably quickly and assessed in good time for the development of the final

> **Box 5.5 Points to bear in mind when conducting follow-up negotiations**
>
> 1. Make sure that you know who has the power to make decisions on behalf of government departments and other external organizations and work out the best way to reach them.
> 2. Be clear about who is to represent the community in meetings and negotiations and ensure that they continue to do so throughout the process of negotiation.
> 3. Be clear about what you want from those with whom you are negotiating and present what you want simply and unambiguously.
> 4. Ask one of your representatives to write down what is said in the meeting, focusing especially on any verbal agreements and promises.
> 5. Send a record of your understanding of the agreements reached in each meeting to the other participants in the meeting as soon as possible after the meeting. This should set out what each group, including your own, has agreed to do.
> 6. If possible, conclude negotiations with a written agreement or memorandum of understanding setting out what has to be done to implement and manage sanitation improvements and defining the roles of the various parties to the agreement.

plan. The situation addressed by the pilot should be representative of the situations found in the area as a whole. Where the pilot is likely to be relatively large and/or complex, it will be best to incorporate it into the early stages of the main plan.

The pilot may also serve as a demonstration of any ideas that are new to the community. Alternatively, it may be desirable to implement projects and initiatives purely for demonstration purposes, using an approach that has already been developed and proved under similar conditions elsewhere. In both cases, an early small-scale initiative can help to ensure that people understand what is on offer to them. It is all too easy for external professionals to assume that they have explained the basic features of a sanitation option, only to discover once the option is in place that community members thought they were being offered something different altogether.

Demonstration projects must be 'visible' to those whom they are intended to influence. This can sometimes be achieved by ensuring that they are located in a public place. (For example, demonstration latrines have sometimes been located in a school or health centre). Where demonstration facilities are located on-site, make sure that the owners of these facilities are aware that people will want to look at the facilities once they have been completed.

Once a project is complete and has been operational for some time, you should aim to:

○ evaluate its performance and identify any changes that may be necessary before introducing the approach more widely

○ ensure that findings are communicated in a way that encourages other people to adopt the approach (assuming that it has produced good results). Community members are more likely to listen to and understand people like themselves than outsiders, who may literally or metaphorically speak a different language. So the best way to convince people that an initiative really works may be to ask those who have benefited from it to tell others about it. Other options for communicating findings are to prepare posters and videos on pilot and demonstration initiatives and their results. Whichever communication method is used, the focus should be on the most important findings. Extraneous detail should be avoided. Further information on sharing information is given in Chapter 10.

The sanitation plan

Developing the draft plan

Once negotiations have been completed, pilot and demonstration projects have been initiated and funding options have been agreed, the plan can be finalized. Start by holding a general meeting or workshop and use it to establish consensus on the overall structure and contents of the plan. Those who have been responsible for negotiating responsibilities, exploring funding options and managing pilot and demonstration projects should briefly report on their activities. They should present material as simply as possible, bearing in mind that not all people in the community will be literate. It may be appropriate to walk round the area included in the plan with community members and to talk about individual plan components at the locations where they are to be implemented.

Once agreement has been reached on the outline plan, a smaller group should be charged with producing a first draft. This group should include representatives of the community, including but not limited to those who have been active in investigating and developing solutions. Ideally, the group should also include representatives of government agencies and other external stakeholders with responsibility for the area. This will increase the likelihood that the plan will be taken into account by government service providers and others who might help to implement plan components.

Form and content of the plan

The draft plan should be a simple written document, backed up by plans, drawings, activity schedules and the like, as required to present a clear picture of the activities to be undertaken. As with the municipal plan, it should include a general section, setting out the overall framework of the plan and sections devoted to the various components to be included in the plan should follow. These are likely to relate to some or all of the following.

o *Physical improvements*, including new sanitation and drainage facilities and improvements to existing facilities.
o *Changes in behaviour*, for instance handwashing after defecation and ensuring that children use latrines.
o *Improvements in the way that services are organized*, for instance increased community involvement in the management of local sewer systems.
o *New services*, for instance solid waste collection services.

Use the information on the structure and contents of the municipal plan given in Chapter 3 as a general guide for the preparation of a local plan, focusing particularly on the need to define first-year targets. However, local plans will normally be much shorter and simpler than municipal plans. Think of the intended audience and be realistic about what they will and will not read.

Arrangements for managing and funding services

This is an important issue that should not be neglected in the plan. Two issues are likely to need particular attention:

o the extent to which it will be possible and desirable for community members to take responsibility for the management of their own facilities

- the allocation of responsibilities and duties when local facilities and services are dependent on higher-order facilities and services.

The plan should pay particular attention to the options for funding the various proposed activities. Households should normally pay for on-site facilities. If an exception is made to this general rule, for instance to cater for the needs of low-income households in rented accommodation, the plan must be very clear about how any subsidies are to be funded. In any case, it will usually be wise to ensure that the household pays some part of the cost of the facilities.

Avoid loans for sanitation facilities since they are difficult to recover. Where people cannot meet the full cost of improvements in one payment, it may be worthwhile to encourage them to start a savings scheme to put aside money to pay for their share of the proposed improvements.

Whatever arrangements are made to cover the capital cost of improved sanitation facilities, the users of those facilities must pay their operational costs, either directly or through a service charge. The experience from Sukkur described in Box 5.3 illustrates the problems that can arise if one or more of the parties involved in the planning process ignores this principle. Every effort should be made to write financial responsibilities into the plan so that there can be no subsequent argument about who is responsible for meeting what expenses.

Publicizing the plan

Once the plan has been completed in draft form, it should be presented to the various stakeholders, including the people living in the area that is the subject of the plan. Options for presenting the plan to the community include the following:

- hold a community meeting at which the key points in the plan are explained
- produce a map or even a model, showing the location of proposed activities and display this in a prominent location such as a community centre or school
- talk to groups of people about the plan activities that will affect them directly and/or in which they will be involved.

Copies of the plan should be given to external stakeholders, including government departments and potential funding organizations. Representatives of these organizations are more likely to take account of the plan and its contents if someone talks to them about it. So, every effort should be made to present the key points contained in the plan to these external stakeholders at the time that the plan is given to them.

Provide opportunities for people to comment on the plan. The various stakeholders are more likely to take the plan seriously if you respond to any comments and suggestions that they make and so you should be prepared to modify the plan in the light of the feedback that you receive.

Moving beyond the local level

The planning approach outlined above can be used solely to deal with the problems of a specific area. While valuable, this approach falls short of being fully strategic in that it does not have a city-wide perspective. The challenge for those who have successfully planned for improved sanitation at the local level is to explore ways in which their experience can be communicated to other people so that they can replicate and/or build on it. There are two options for moving beyond the area in which the local approach is initially implemented:

- encourage other local organizations to adopt the approach

○ work for the acceptance and adoption of the approach by government and other formal sector stakeholders.

These options should be viewed as complementary rather than as alternatives.

The starting point for promoting interest in your initiative will be to share your experience with other stakeholders. Pay particular attention to those people and organizations that might act as 'champions' of your approach. These might include senior government officials at the municipal, state/provincial and national levels. It will also be worthwhile to gain the support of international agencies, which may be more aware of the value of locally initiated action than government. Further information on sharing experience is given in Chapter 10.

Regardless of where efforts to garner support for the replication of local planning efforts start, the ultimate aim must be to ensure that government planners and decision-makers accept the viability of the planning process and incorporate it into mainstream practice. There are two ways in which this might happen.

○ Municipal decision makers accept the basic model developed at the local level and adapt it for use at the municipal level (see Box 5.6).

○ Local plans are seen as a resource that can be incorporated into an overall planning process at the municipal level and perhaps beyond (thus moving towards the third approach identified at the beginning of this chapter).

The first is likely to be more appropriate for small to medium-sized towns, those with populations up to around 100 000 but perhaps rather less in Africa where towns tend to be smaller and more spread out.

There are various examples of planning approaches that incorporate local plans into larger municipal plans. Most of these initiatives are initiated by government and start with a city-wide perspective. The main purpose of local planning processes in such initiatives is to provide an input to the development of higher-level plans, ensuring that the latter are based on local concerns and priorities. Examples of the approach include the Kerala People's Planning Campaign (KPPC) in India (Isaac 1999) and the participatory budgeting approach adopted in Porto Alegre (Abers 1997). Both are multi-sectoral initiatives, which do not restrict themselves to either sanitation or low-income areas.

Their significance within the context of this chapter is that they both grew out of situations in which there was a background of neighbourhood-level organization, together with political support for the idea of participatory planning.

In Porto Alegre, neighbourhood leaders had already cooperated to form 'regional' level organizations. Many of these were supporters of the left wing political party that introduced the participatory budgeting process. The KPPC was developed in the light of the support for decentralization and participation contained in the 73rd and 74th Amendments to the Indian Constitution, passed in 1993, and the 1994 Kerala Municipality Act.

One last point is worth making, again drawing on the experience of Porto Alegre. Local groups did not have to take part in the process. Their incentive to do so was the fact that their participation made it more likely that their needs would be considered in the overall planning and budgeting process. Abers (1997, p. 50) states that her qualitative research indicated that *'the first neighbourhoods to receive investments through the policy were for the most part those*

> **Box 5.6 The Lodhran Project – adapting a local model to the municipal level[3]**
>
> Lodhran is a small town (population about 65 000) located in the south of Pakistan's Punjab Province. Sewerage was provided in the centre of the town in the mid 1960s and expanded in a haphazard manner over the years. However, by the late 1990s, the system was in a poor state of repair and did not cover many parts of the town.
>
> The Lodhran Pilot Project (LPP) was set up through the UNDP-LIFE programme. OPP was designated as the Chief Technical Adviser for the project. LPP itself is an NGO with a mandate to implement an urban sewerage and sanitation project in line with OPP principles and in direct partnership with the municipal council. It develops the basic OPP model in a number of ways, in particular its focus on the town as a whole, the partnership with municipal government and its concern with wastewater disposal and treatment issues. However, it is firmly based in OPP's basic paradigm, emphasizing the need for sanitation users to take responsibility for internal facilities while the municipal authorities are responsible for main drains, pumping stations and sewage treatment plant. The first task undertaken through the project was to produce a map showing all the streets and lanes in the town, together with existing sewerage facilities. An overall sewerage plan, based on this map, was prepared. This provided the main management tool for planning for both new external development work and the operation of completed facilities.
>
> Other activities undertaken through the project include:
>
> o Rehabilitation of non-functioning sewers. The municipality carried out this work with support from LPP.
>
> o Construction of new lane sewers. This work is financed and managed by local communities, through their appointed lane managers in accordance with the basic OPP model.
>
> o Collaboration with the Rural Sanitation Cell of the National Rural Support Programme to provide sewers, using the same basic model, in 13 peripheral villages.
>
> The efforts of LPP are not intended to substitute for those of government service providers. Rather, the aim is to strengthen the capacity of local government organizations.
>
> The LPP clearly has a town-wide focus although it is perhaps too early to judge its medium- to long-term success. Interestingly, sanitation options other than sewerage do not appear to have been considered.

known historically for their strong organisational capacity. Over time, as others saw infrastructure being built and became convinced that participating in the program could potentially bring such infrastructure to their neighbourhoods, whole new groups of people began to mobilise.' The lesson is that it is best to be flexible when attempting to bring together local initiatives to inform a municipal-level plan. People should be given time to 'grow' into a more comprehensive approach to planning.

Key points in this chapter

1. Government is not the only provider of sanitation services. Indeed, individual households and informal groups of residents are the main providers of sanitation services in many areas.

2. While many of these activities are ad hoc and uncoordinated, some show a degree of planning and hence have the potential to be starting points for developing a more strategic approach to sanitation provision.

3. Some NGOs have developed approaches to local sanitation provision that build on these initiatives and which follow some of the strategic principles outlined in Chapter 2.

4. Efforts to develop formal plans at the local level should be preceded by action to ensure that there is genuine demand for sanitation and to draw the various stakeholders into the planning process.

5. Local problems do not always have local causes. In order to take account of this, there will often be a need for negotiation with government stakeholders to ensure that any off-site actions required for the success of the plan are carried out.

6. Where off-site problems are too large to be dealt with immediately, the focus may have to be on managing rather than eliminating problems. Where government action on off-site facilities cannot be guaranteed, on-site solutions to problems should be explored.

7. As with planning at the municipal level, local plans should make allowance for developing solutions although the time allowed for this should not normally exceed about three months.

8. The plan itself should be a simple written document. The key points contained in the plan should be publicized in ways that are accessible to people living in the plan area.

9. Local planning initiatives can provide a starting point for efforts to plan more strategically for towns and cities as a whole.

Chapter 5 endnotes

1 For instance, it was quoted as a UNCHS Best Practices Initiative of the Habitat II Conference 1996. Orangi Pilot Project – Research and Training Institute (OPP-RTI) also received the World Habitat Award 2000 for its Low Cost Sanitation and Housing Programme.

2 For more information on planning for service provision at the local level, see Section 3 of Cotton and Tayler (2000).

3 Information on the LPP is taken from the case study produced by UNDP-LIFE in March 2002.

CHAPTER 6
The role of sanitation and hygiene promotion in developing and informing demand

THIS IS THE first of four chapters that focus in more detail on critical aspects of the strategic planning process. In this chapter, we are concerned with sanitation and hygiene promotion, both of which may be required to create and inform demand for better sanitation and improved hygiene practices. The main focus is on sanitation and hygiene promotion at the municipal level although much of what is said here will also apply at other levels.

The need to ground both sanitation and hygiene promotion in realistic assessment of the existing situation is emphasized. Following this, we consider the steps required to identify promotion options, decide messages, develop materials and carry out the promotion campaign itself, linking these steps to the basic understand problems – develop solutions – produce an overall plan model. The chapter closes with brief notes on the action necessary to create an enabling environment and provide funding for sanitation and hygiene promotion. Further information on the links between sanitation and health is given in Appendix 1.

Sanitation and hygiene promotion and the links between them

It is not uncommon to find projects that promote latrine construction without promoting hygienic behaviour. There is a real danger that such projects will result in under-used or misused facilities that quickly fall into disrepair. On the other hand, it will often be hard to achieve good hygiene in a slum. Without improvements in water and sanitation services, people may not be able to respond to hygiene education messages. For instance, there is little point in telling people to wash their hands after defecating if there is no source of water close to the point at which they defecate, as would be the case where either the water supply to a communal sanitation block is unreliable or lack of sanitation facilities forces people to practise open defecation some distance from their houses. So, it will normally be desirable to develop a combined hygiene and sanitation promotion programme, as indicated by Figure 6.1, rather than to consider the two separately.

Figure 6.1 indicates the need for initial assessment of the existing situation in order to answer the question 'where we are now?' and determine where the focus of sanitation and hygiene promotion efforts should lie. It also suggests the need for initial assessment of sanitation needs to consider not only whether there is a demand for improved sanitation but also whether that demand is informed. At the municipal and local levels, this initial assessment should be part of the process of understanding problems.

The results of this initial assessment will influence the objectives of the promotion effort.

○ Where there is limited demand for improved sanitation, it will be necessary to promote the construction of latrines and their effective operation and maintenance.

THE ROLE OF SANITATION AND HYGIENE PROMOTION IN DEVELOPING DEMAND

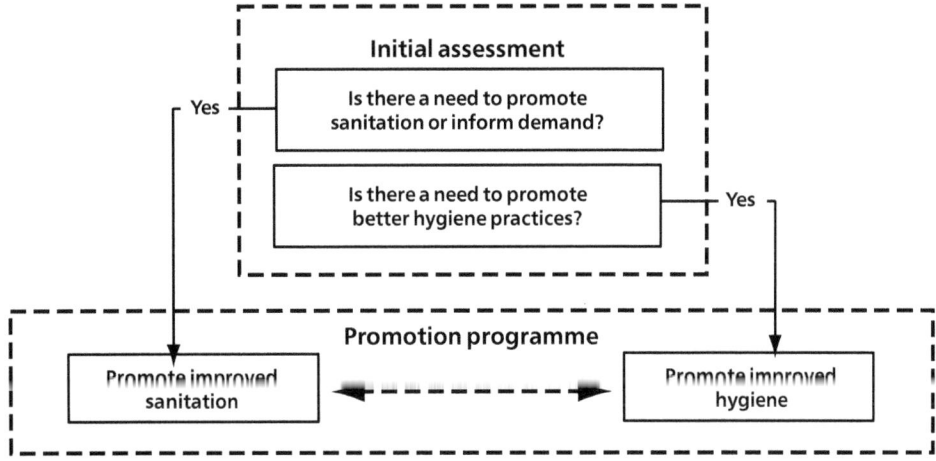

Figure 6.1 An integrated approach to sanitation and hygiene promotion

○ Where demand exists but it is for unhygienic, environmentally damaging or inappropriate forms of sanitation, the need will be to inform demand. This will require efforts to identify and promote sanitation technologies that are suitable for use in the local situation, while discouraging the use of inappropriate technologies.

○ Where existing facilities are poorly maintained, informing demand may also require an emphasis on the need for maintenance and the possible health implications of poor maintenance.

○ Even where there is a demand for appropriate forms of sanitation, there may be a lack of awareness of good hygiene and hence a need to promote better hygiene practices.

Bearing in mind these general points, we now turn to the various stages in developing and implementing a sanitation and hygiene promotion programme, linking these steps to the main stages in the strategic planning process.

Where are we now? Assessing current sanitation and hygiene practice

Some basic questions

Asking the right questions will help in the assessment of the current situation. The three basic questions are:

○ Is there a demand for improved sanitation?
○ Is that demand informed?
○ What action needs to be taken to improve hygiene practices?

The first two relate to sanitation promotion and the last to hygiene promotion. These questions are rather broad and it will normally be helpful to develop supplementary questions around them.

Supplementary questions that will help to establish the situation with regard to demand for sanitation include:

○ How do people dispose of excreta and wastewater at present?

○ Is there any evidence that they have tried or are trying to improve their sanitary conditions, for instance by building latrines, constructing drains or lobbying elected representatives to provide facilities?

○ Are people willing to pay for improved services?

Supplementary questions relating to hygiene promotion include:

○ What are the likely risk practices? An example would be failing to wash hands after defecation.

○ Who carries out those practices? Think, for instance, about the groups within the family and society whose members are least likely to wash hands after defecation.

Questions that might throw light on the approach to be taken to promote improved sanitation and better hygiene include:

○ How do people communicate? The answer to this will influence the approach taken to sanitation and hygiene promotion.

○ What prevents change? There are two possibilities:

- people cannot practise improved hygiene because of the lack of basic water supply and sanitation services
- people's beliefs and attitudes may be barriers to change.

Bear these questions in mind when identifying problems and possible solutions to those problems.

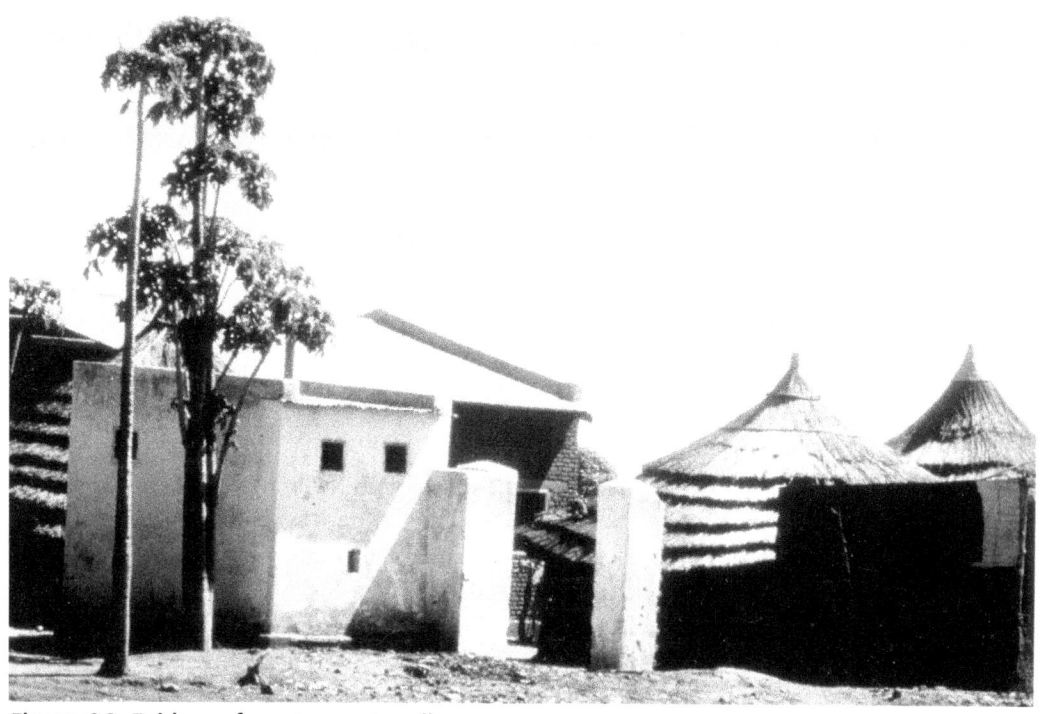

Figure 6.2 Evidence from transect walks

A plot in Juba, Southern Sudan. The ventilation pipe, small high windows and opening in the wall suggest that the structure in the foreground is a latrine. The opening in the wall is provided to allow a suction pipe to be passed from a desludging tanker into the latrine.

Initial identification of problems

During the understanding problems stage of the planning process, transect walks and conversations with community members, government officials and representatives of NGOs and CBOs can be used to provide a basic understanding of existing attitudes to sanitation and hygiene. For local workshops, it will normally be better for participants to look for evidence themselves during field visits. Guidance should be given by people with experience of good sanitation and hygiene.

In the course of transect walks, look for evidence that people have built or are trying to build new or improved sanitation facilities. Vent pipes, septic tanks and pipe connections to drains may all provide evidence that householders are using some form of on-site sanitation (see Figure 6.2). Walking through the land on the outskirts of a housing area will quickly reveal whether or not open defecation is taking place. Conversations with community members can provide initial information on activities and initiatives that might not be obvious through casual observation in the street.

Developing solutions

If initial investigations reveal the need for sanitation and/or hygiene promotion, follow-up investigations will be required to develop understanding of sanitation and hygiene practices and identify actions that can be taken to improve them. These investigations should be included in the developing solutions stage of the planning process. They will normally focus on representative localities and communities and involve:

○ more detailed investigation of problems

○ identification of options for dealing with those problems.

Responsibilities for carrying out these tasks should be allocated during the first planning workshop, bearing in mind the probability that the organization that is responsible for the investigations is likely to take a leading role in implementing any subsequent sanitation and hygiene promotion programme. If possible, use an organization that has already been involved in aspects of either hygiene or sanitation promotion. The next best option will be to use an organization that has strong communication skills and experience of working with communities, possibly an NGO and possibly a community development section located within a municipality. Make sure that the organization commissioned to do the work has women fieldworkers and is committed to talking to women, young people and old people about their perceptions regarding problems. It may be necessary to provide training and this should be discussed during the planning workshop. It may be that the first step in developing solutions for sanitation and hygiene promotion will be to identify a suitable support organization to provide training and back-up. If so, the options for financing its inputs must be explored.

Assessing needs in a participatory way

Promotion works best when it allows people to present their own views and discover the benefits of improved sanitation, rather than being told what is good for them. It is also more likely to succeed when some community members are already concerned about the effects of poor sanitation. This suggests that detailed investigation of sanitation and hygiene conditions should ideally be carried out as a participatory needs assessment. Participatory assessment involves mobilizing community members and working with them to first establish the facts about the existing situation and then discuss the nature of their problems, concerns and aspirations. Which homes have a toilet already?

Why are others without one? What drainage facilities are available? What arrangements are made for solid waste disposal? While exploring the existing situation, needs and options can be explored in a structured way.

Table 6.1 indicates the range of participatory methods used to investigate hygiene behaviour in low-income communities in three towns in Andhra Pradesh, India.[1]

Where initial assessment suggests that people have little interest in using toilets, the early focus should be on generating demand for latrines. Efforts to generate demand should start from the reasons why people are not currently interested in investing in toilets. In the Andhra Pradesh example from which the information in Table 6.1 was taken, the great majority of latrines installed under the ILCS were unused. The reasons given by respondents for this situation included the following:

- lack of water
- men prefer open defecation
- lack of knowledge of operation and maintenance requirements
- too close to water point – fear of groundwater contamination
- incomplete construction
- fear of pits (3 ft depth) filling fast (for this reason, some were kept for occasional use, and for the aged and infirm)
- fear of bad smells if used heavily and close to house.

The fact that men preferred open defecation suggests a need for promotion messages that focus on the potential health dangers of

Table 6.1 Participatory investigations used in the APUSP[1]

No.	Activity	Explanation
1	Health walk (in essence a health-focused transect walk)	Direct observation of existing water and sanitation facilities and associated practices. Includes discussion with focus group.
2	Resource mapping	Residents (male and female) produce a map of the slum showing key features relevant to the study (housing, water points, defecation areas, garbage dumping points, etc.)
3	Timeline	Respondent group outlines history of the slum including key events such as disease outbreaks, floods, installation of piped water supply, etc.
4	Health ranking	Respondents identify most common types of sickness in the community.
5	Women's issues	Discussion with all-female group on women's health issues including water supply and sanitation needs and aspirations.
6	Seasonality analysis	Discussion to identify seasonal variations in community activities, water resources, water quality and other relevant factors.
7	Hygiene behaviours (pocket chart exercise)	Using picture cards provided by facilitator, respondent group identifies 'good' and 'bad' hygiene-related behaviour practised in their community, and discusses potential for change.
8	Sanitation ladder	Respondent group discusses current excreta disposal arrangements and their adequacy, and identifies the type of facilities or services they would like.

(For further information on participatory methods, see Appendix 3).

open defecation, not the least of which is the fact that people are unlikely to wash their hands after defecating in an open space some way from their homes.

The answers relating to the lack of knowledge of operation and maintenance requirements and the fears relating to groundwater contamination, pits filling rapidly and bad smells suggest the need for action to inform demand. This does not just mean convincing people that their fears are groundless. Rather, the aim should be to develop a shared understanding of the present situation and the options that are available for improving it. Box 6.1 provides an example of what this might mean in practice.

The answers relating to incomplete construction and the lack of water indicate a need for improvements in physical facilities, suggesting that it will be best to link sanitation and hygiene promotion to a programme of physical improvement.

Adopting a participatory approach does not remove the need for inputs by those with knowledge of what constitutes good sanitation and hygiene practice. The Andhra Pradesh survey provides an example of a situation in which such inputs are needed. In two of the three towns covered by the survey, mothers did not appear to encourage small children to use toilets, even when these were available. Children's faeces were swept into drains, thrown on to open ground or diluted with water prior to sweeping the area in which they were deposited. In the first instance, it may be necessary to bring in people with specialist hygiene knowledge from outside but the medium-term aim should be to train local people to recognize and promote good sanitation and hygiene practices. We will return to this shortly.

The various insights gained during the participatory needs assessment can be brought together to provide a summary of high-risk behaviours. The Andhra Pradesh study identified the need for behaviour change interventions relating to the following practices and issues:

o open defecation (especially by males)

o inadequate latrine operation and maintenance

o children's defecation practices and the disposal of children's faeces

o handwashing practices

o food hygiene (domestic and commercial)

o hygiene at school

o the disposal of wastewater (it appeared that soakpits were a viable option in many locations)

Box 6.1 Developing solutions on the basis of pooled knowledge

Initial investigations suggested that the fears expressed in Andhra Pradesh about the pits filling too quickly were not justified. The standard pit depth for ILCS latrines is 0.9 m, which should be sufficient to provide about two years sludge storage for a family of six. However, further investigation revealed that masons sometimes built latrines with the inlet pipes entering the pit at a low level so that the effective storage volume was considerably reduced. Possible responses to this situation include:

o increase the depth of the pits by perhaps 0.3 m
o ensure that masons are trained to plan installations to minimize pipe runs
o raise the floor of the latrine to ensure that the inlet pipe enters each pit at the highest possible level.

o water collection and storage practices.

Some of these high-risk practices are likely to be fairly widespread while others will be specific to the local situation. An example of the latter might be the need to encourage people to wear shoes in areas where hookworm is prevalent.

Planning a promotion campaign

If the participatory needs assessment reveals the need to promote sanitation and/or improved hygiene, a promotion campaign should be included in the strategic plan. In most cases, this will involve an integrated approach that both emphasizes the need for changes in behaviour and provides the physical improvements that allow people to make those changes in behaviour. Points to be considered when planning a promotion campaign are discussed below.

Deciding the target area and time frame

The size of the area to be covered by the programme will clearly influence the resources needed for implementation and may have an impact on the overall approach adopted. If a municipal plan is to have a city-wide impact, the long-term aim must be to cover all areas of the city in which sanitation and hygiene promotion are required (although the message to be transmitted may be different in different areas). However, it will usually be best to test the approach in a more limited area. Ideally, the area chosen for the initial participatory assessment should be used to pilot the programme and the first year objective of the plan might be to complete promotion activities and initiate follow-up action to improve sanitation in this area. The plan might then include allowance for the phased expansion of the programme, at a pace that can be managed with available resources.

Do not underestimate the time required for campaigns. Behavioural change is usually a slow process. Short-term campaigns, involving high-profile public events, can be useful in launching or publicizing a project but are unlikely on their own to have any lasting effect on people's behaviour. The repeated delivery of a small number of appropriate messages to a defined audience is needed and it may take a long time for significant change to happen. It is essential to recognize this when designing sanitation projects. Do not be governed purely by the speed at which hardware can be installed but leave time for meaningful hygiene promotion activity.

Who should be responsible for sanitation and hygiene promotion?

It will be best if the organization that has been responsible for investigating sanitation and hygiene-related problems and issues also plays a part in sanitation and hygiene promotion. For large cities, it may be desirable to develop the capacity of several organizations to carry out promotion activities in different areas, providing training as required. Whichever organizations carry out the work on the ground, the municipality or some other government agency will normally continue to have a role in overseeing the programme.

The number of people required for promotion will depend on local circumstances but a typical neighbourhood-level programme serving a few thousand people might require a team leader and four or five fieldworkers. It may be possible to train community members as fieldworkers, taking advantage of their local knowledge and the fact that they should be better placed to communicate with residents than outsiders. Do not assume that community members will work free of charge. Unless they are paid, it is likely that the time and energy they devote to the programme will be limited, particularly if it lasts for many months.

Children can be effective promoters of behavioural change. They have energy and enthusiasm and are likely to be less bound than adults by traditional assumptions and long-held beliefs and less inhibited about 'mentioning the unmentionable'. Older children often care for younger children and can influence them to change their habits and beliefs. One possibility is to use child-to-child methods for encouraging improved hygiene practices. However, do not assume that these will provide a panacea. Child-to-child approaches require effective training for teachers and follow-up support. If you wish to consider using child-to-child methods, take advice from those who have had practical experience of implementing such methods, make realistic estimates of costs and ensure that there is a mechanism available for meeting those costs. If necessary, develop child-to-child methods specifically aimed at behavioural change for sanitation.

Another mechanism for promoting improved hygiene and sanitation among children is the formation of school health clubs in which pupils are trained and progress through various stages, as in organizations like the Scouts. This approach has been successfully used in Zimbabwe as described in Box 6.2.

Providing training

Good quality training for fieldworkers is important if the promotional work is to be effective. This training should cover:

- sanitation and hygiene promotion methods
- key points about the technologies that might be appropriate in the local situation.

The latter is often overlooked. If hygiene education staff have insufficient technical knowledge, they may give people poor advice. For instance, the team responsible for providing ILCS latrines in Bharatpur were convinced that the brickwork lining the latrine pits should not have open joints. As a result, no seepage from the sides of pits was possible, a violation of the basic principle on which they are intended to operate.

Training relating to promotion methods and technologies should be integrated so that fieldworkers develop a holistic approach to promotion. Those who are responsible for developing and implement-

---

Box 6.2 School health clubs in Zimbabwe[2]

The first step in the Zimbabwe campaign was to ask pupils to collect small pieces of soap that their mothers could no longer use for washing clothes and bring them to school, where they were combined into larger blocks. This was done at the beginning of a new term and produced enough soap to ensure that soap was available for hand washing every day during a whole school term.

The health clubs also provided practical demonstrations of the benefits of good hygiene practice. For instance, a group of children was divided into two sub-groups, each of which was lined up behind a bucket of water. Each of the two groups washed their hands in one of the buckets, the first with and the second without soap. At the end of the exercise, the children could see that the bucket in which hands had been washed without soap remained relatively clear, indicating that the dirt had stayed on their hands rather than being washed off.

ing training are likely to be health or community development specialists. They should work closely with their technical colleagues to ensure that the messages imparted through the training are technically sound. One way to do this will be to form a combined team to work on the development of training materials, based on shared experience in representative field conditions. In this way, it should be possible to develop training messages that synthesize the views and insights of community members, promotion specialists and technical specialists.

Deciding the message

The message to be promoted should relate to changes that are achievable within the constraints imposed by the local situation. Some key points relating to this overall principle are introduced and briefly discussed below.

Avoid promoting latrines in a vague and general way. Where people have limited knowledge of available and appropriate technologies, a general message may encourage them to build a latrine that is inappropriate to the local situation or poorly constructed. When it fails, producing bad smells, blocking up, overflowing or even collapsing, the whole promotional drive will be undermined. Sanitation promotion should start with explanation of the practical implications of basic choices (see Chapter 8). It should then focus on a limited number of specific designs that have been tested locally and found to be affordable, effective and (potentially at least) acceptable to local users.

Concentrate on high-risk practices, at least in the first instance. Washing hands after defecation and safe stool disposal should always be stressed, but other more location-specific high-risk practices may have emerged in the course of the participatory appraisal. For instance:

○ There may be danger of hookworm transmission where many people do not wear shoes and it is common to either irrigate fields with sewage or defecate in fields.

○ Eating uncooked or partially cooked meat may lead to infection with tapeworms when animals graze on grass irrigated with untreated wastewater.

○ Dumping solid waste in open drains may lead to local flooding and create ideal breeding grounds for culex mosquitoes, which may transmit filiarasis.

Recognize the reality of current constraints, for instance the fact that there may be no reliable source of water close to people's houses. In such situations, the initial focus will usually have to be on improving services although hygiene messages might help to inform demand and persuade people that they should be willing to pay for improved services.

Do not make messages too technical. You may know about pathogens and how they are transmitted but do not assume that local people understand disease and its transmission in the same way.

Where sanitation facilities already exist but are unsatisfactory, it may be best to focus sanitation promotion messages on what can be done to correct their faults and deficiencies. Training local artisans in construction may be an important part of the promotional campaign.

The operation and maintenance requirements of each sanitation technology should be explained at an early stage in the promotion process. There are many examples of sanitation facilities that have failed because their intended users were unaware of the need to carry out essential tasks. For example, many (perhaps most) users of double pit latrines are unaware of the need to use the pits alternately and to empty each pit once the other is almost full.

The willingness and ability of potential users to adopt any particular sanitation option will be influenced by its price. Users should therefore be provided with information on the capital and operation and maintenance costs of different sanitation options (or the amount they need to pay where costs are to be subsidized). In accordance with the principles set out in Chapter 2, users should normally pay operation and maintenance costs in full, either directly or through user charges.

Deciding on appropriate media for promotion

Hygiene messages must be communicated to the people for whom they are intended. This can be done:

- one-to-one, which can be very effective but might also be expensive
- to groups at meetings, video showings and other special events
- through mass media such as radio and television.

In general, the more personal the promotion medium, the higher will be the chance that the listener will heed the message that is being promoted. Indeed, there will be very few cases in which messages communicated through mass media alone will bring about changes in attitudes and behaviour.

When considering a city-level programme, it may be appropriate to use the mass media to spread information on the programme, to raise its profile and perhaps to provide information on 'hardware' (for instance pit latrine slabs) and where to obtain it. However, mass media outlets should be seen as supplementing rather than replacing one-to-one and group work carried out in the field.

People working on small, community-based projects are unlikely to have access to mass media outlets and so their sole emphasis will normally be on one-on-one and group options.

Methods based on 'popular' culture can be useful in promoting behaviour change. Options include short plays and sketches, songs and dance. For instance, a short play might be written and performed with the objective of showing that a person with diarrhoea can pass the disease on to other people if they do not wash their hands after defecation. Where possible, encourage local people to develop their own stories to illustrate specific points since these are more likely to convince their peers than stories developed by professionals. Some external specialist input to this process will be necessary to ensure that the main promotion messages are transmitted.

One potentially effective promotional tool will be to take people to see sanitation improvements that have been successfully implemented by people like themselves (see Box 6.3). When considering a sanitation option that requires communal effort, it will be better if a group of people visits the community with the improved facilities. This group can then present what they have seen to the wider community when they return.

Some points on promotion materials

Promotion materials will be required to illustrate the messages to be promoted. These might include some or all of the following:

- Simple written handouts providing information on the reasons why improved sanitation is important.
- Diagrams and pictures illustrating:
  - possible technologies and the ways in which they might be used

- examples of good and bad practice
- options for improving existing facilities.

When using plans and drawings to illustrate technical points, you should check that people understand them before using them widely in a promotional campaign.

○ Videos, which might be used both to draw attention to the problems associated with poor sanitation and to show the available technologies and the ways in which they might be used. These should be accompanied by a commentary and ideally by guidance on the key questions that people need to ask themselves in order to make decisions on what they should do in their own situation.

Written materials present a potential problem in that some of the target group for sanitation and hygiene promotion may be illiterate. The use of diagrams and pictures can help to overcome this problem but these will only be understandable to illiterate people if they do not contain text and captions.

Do not assume that other people will draw the same conclusions as you from a particular diagram, picture or video image.[3] In particular, be wary of the use of:

○ abstract approaches to physical phenomena – for instance the use of lines behind an object to suggest fast movement

○ extraneous detail, which can be a major source of confusion.

Before using a series of images to show change over time, be sure that people see that they represent a sequence of events rather than a series of unconnected situations.

Implementing the programme

The points made above indicate a need to pilot promotion methods and materials in one or more typical areas before introducing them more widely. During this piloting stage, and indeed afterwards, hygiene promotion staff should be required to keep simple records of their activities so that it is possible to monitor progress, identify which areas have been covered and determine whether any particular problems have arisen. Early experience can be used to check whether your initial assumptions about the rate of progress and cost of the programme were justified, providing a basis for amending the follow-up programme where these initial assumptions prove to be unjustified.

As the programme expands and develops, activities will start in new areas. Arrange meetings with the community leaders in these areas before promotion activities commence. It will usually be worthwhile to arrange for people from areas that have

---

Box 6.3 Exchange visits in Ouagadougou, Burkina Faso

In the Strategic Sanitation Project in Ouagadougou, Burkina Faso, implemented in the early 1990s, arrangements were made for people without adequate sanitation to visit households that had already installed on-site facilities. These potential participants in the project were able to find out more about the facilities, including their cost, repayment schedules, operational requirements and allay their concerns about perceived problems such as lack of space and smells from the latrine. All of the 100 prospective participants in the project who were involved in these exchange visits subsequently went on to invest in the programme.

Saidi-Sharouze (1994)

already been covered to attend these meetings and talk about their experience and the ways in which the promotion campaign has affected their lives. It may also be possible to use local media to provide information on the programme and let people know what is happening.

Regular team meetings should be held in order to discuss progress and address any problems that may have arisen in the course of fieldwork. Encourage promotion staff to talk about any problems and share their experiences with their fellow workers.

Do not assume that people will change their behaviour just because they have new theoretical knowledge. They may not relate this knowledge to their daily lives. This will be particularly true if they are constrained by lack of money or time from changing their routines and practices. There will be a need for follow up to determine whether people are changing their behaviour in the light of hygiene promotion messages. There are two aspects to this.

o Do people remember hygiene promotion messages?

o Do they respond to them by changing behaviour?

A monitoring programme may be developed to assess the impact of the promotion programme over time, using the same tools and techniques used at the needs assessment stage. This should not be seen as an end in itself but as a tool for improving the programme. If your investigations show that people do not remember messages, there is a need to review the approach to sanitation promotion. If people do remember messages but have not changed their behaviour, you need to explore the reasons. It may be that there are barriers to change that are not obvious to outsiders. Where this is the case, there is a need to consider what parallel action can be taken to remove those barriers.

A general point on monitoring and evaluation is that it is often difficult to detect and measure the impacts of hygiene education directly. The use of proxy indicators of hygienic behaviour can help to overcome this problem. Such indicators might include the presence of a functioning latrine, whether it is used, whether it is kept clean, whether soap and water are kept by the latrine and so on.

Creating an enabling environment

Sanitation promotion needs to be underpinned by a supportive government environment. This might involve action in a number of areas, for example:

o Policy. Extending basic service provision to established informal settlements; allowing low-cost designs and technologies; decentralizing the planning of sanitation services to municipal and ward level and incorporating community consultation; promoting collaborative approaches that draw on the resources of NGOs and the private sector.

o Funding. Providing sufficient funding to allow sanitation and hygiene promotion programmes and campaigns, together with any related action to provide improved sanitation facilities and services, to be implemented and sustained.

o Institutional arrangements. Assigning clear roles and responsibilities for the promotion, installation, operation and maintenance of sanitation infrastructure and services; strengthening and capacity building of key government agencies.

Where an adequate enabling environment does not exist, advocates for sanitation promotion have a vital role to play, by convincing decision makers of the need to give sanitation the priority it deserves.

International agencies and NGOs often take the lead here. However, as we have already noted in Chapter 4, change and development will only come about if it has strong internal support, particularly from key decision makers within government.

Funding options for sanitation and hygiene promotion

Failure to identify large-scale funding for sanitation promotion is a major drawback in many countries, and responsibilities for funding are often ill-defined. Possible sources of funding include:

o External agencies (including multi-lateral and bi-lateral agencies and international NGOs). External resources can be useful for testing approaches and providing a demonstration of the benefits of sanitation promotion. However, they are not sustainable in the long term and must eventually be replaced by internal sources of funding.

o Central or state/provincial government. To ensure continuity, leading to sustainable systems and results, state funding must be guaranteed over a reasonably long period.

o The agency with responsibility for sanitation provision at the municipal level (this may be a state or provincial level agency). The agency does not have to carry out the sanitation promotion work itself but should ideally set aside some of its funds for sanitation promotion and user education.

o A national NGO. There are examples of NGOs using their own funds to support sanitation promotion efforts but the more common situation is that they rely on funding from government or some other source (often an international agency or NGO).

o Community-based organizations (CBOs). For smaller initiatives, CBOs may be able to develop capacity for sanitation promotion, for instance by training people from the community as hygiene and sanitation promoters. A key question is whether these people should be paid and if so, at what rate. Will it be possible to raise the money from within the community or will you need to seek external funding?

The funding options available to you will depend on the local situation and the scale at which you intend to work. As the programme expands, it may be necessary to identify new sources of funding.

Key points made in this chapter

1. The provision of improved sanitation facilities will not reduce the incidence of faecal-oral disease unless it is accompanied by good hygiene, which in turn will often require hygiene promotion.

2. Adults are not clean slates upon which educators can write new ideas. Rather, their response to sanitation and hygiene promotion efforts will depend on their existing understanding of the issues surrounding sanitation. So, sanitation and hygiene promotion must start from an understanding of existing beliefs and practices.

3. Hygiene promotion messages should relate to the reality of the situation in which people find themselves and the possibilities that are open to them. This will usually mean that hygiene promotion efforts must be linked to efforts to bring about the physical improvements required to make improved hygiene possible.

4. The use of participatory approaches to needs assessment can ensure that the knowledge of both local people and

outside specialists is used to inform sanitation and hygiene promotion exercises.

5. Hygiene promotion messages should focus on a limited number of high-risk practices.

6. NGOs and other organizations with experience of working with communities may be the best option for delivering promotion programmes but will need training and support if they do not have previous sanitation and hygiene experience.

7. Promotion methods should be piloted, assessed and, where necessary, modified before being introduced more generally.

8. Sanitation and hygiene promotion have costs and it will be important to plan any proposed programme in the light of the finances that are likely to be available.

9. In general, one-to-one and group promotion methods will have a larger impact than those that use mass media such as television and radio. The latter may have a place but normally as a supplement to rather than a replacement for more personal methods.

10. It will often be necessary to create an enabling environment for sanitation and hygiene promotion. This will normally require action at higher levels of government, as indicated in Chapter 4.

Chapter 6 endnotes

1 This work was carried out as part of the DFID-funded Andhra Pradesh Urban Services for the Poor (APUSP) project.

2 Source: contribution by Brian Matthew to email conference on hygiene education. The proceedings of the conference are available at http://www.jiscmail.ac.uk/lists/HYGIENE-BEHAVIOUR.html.

3 See Dudley (1993) Chapter 5 for more information on this.

CHAPTER 7
Gathering and using information for strategic planning

THROUGHOUT THE BOOK, we have stressed the need for planning decisions to be information-based. In this chapter, we suggest a phased approach to information collection and analysis, linked to the planning processes that have been described in earlier chapters. The first part of this chapter provides an introduction to the types of information that sanitation planners are likely to require, the forms which that information may take, the level of detail that is likely to be required and how you might decide whether information is suitable for your purposes. Attention then turns to the specific information needs of those working at the municipal level. The main focus is on information to understand problems and develop solutions but the need to develop improved information systems is also stressed. The last part of the chapter provides an introduction to information requirements for policy development.

Information and planning processes

Information is required to:

○ inform decisions

○ monitor the progress of plans and activities

○ assess the effect of those plans and activities.

The first relates to planning and the second to the implementation of plans and their components. The third is required after a plan or a plan component has been completed to determine how successful it has been and inform follow-up activities and plans. We use the term 'assess' rather than the more commonly used term 'evaluate' because the latter tends to be seen, both by those who evaluate and those who are evaluated, as being primarily about judging performance rather than informing future action.

Monitoring can relate to:

○ the progress made towards the completion of a particular activity or output, for instance whether a strategic planning workshop has been held and whether the actions agreed at the workshop have been implemented

○ the quality of that process – in the case of the strategic planning workshop, which groups were represented at the meeting, who spoke, how the strategic principles were explained and so on.

Assessment can relate to:

○ the outcome of a particular initiative, for instance whether a particular latrine construction programme has achieved its target in terms of the number of latrines constructed

○ the impacts of that initiative – in the case of the latrine construction programme, whether people are using the latrines and the resultant health benefits for individuals and the community.

The main focus of this chapter is on the use of information for planning purposes.

Chapter 10 contains additional information on monitoring and assessment.

Types of information

Information will normally fall into one of the following four categories.

Spatial information. This provides an indication of the location of facilities, people and events and is best recorded on maps and plans. The routes of sewers and the extent of areas subject to regular flooding are examples of spatial information.

Quantitative information. This provides details of numbers and/or percentages, for instance the number or percentage of households that have on-site sanitation facilities.

Qualitative information. This relates to the quality of a process or service but does not define it in numerical terms. An example would be the information that municipal sweepers do not remove all the solid waste from local waste collection points. Photographs and videos are a particular form of qualitative information. They have the advantages that they are fairly easy to use and are easily accessible to community members.

Definitive information. We use this term to denote information that defines a particular facility or detail, usually in the form of a drawing or some other form of illustration to show exactly how a facility or detail is to be built.

A full understanding of the current situation will only be possible if different types of information and/or information from different sources are combined.

In recent years, there has been a tendency to focus on the social and institutional aspects of sanitation provision and to assume that physical aspects will take care of themselves. However, physical aspects of sanitation provision remain important and often require spatial and definitive information – the first to indicate the location of existing facilities and the second to define the technology options that are available to improve sanitation conditions. So, the need for spatial and definitive information should not be ignored.

Information requirements

Basic requirements

Whoever you are and whatever the level at which you are working, you are likely to need to know something of:

○ the existing situation – what facilities and services exist, how they perform and who has access to them

○ people's attitudes – particularly their views on sanitation and their willingness to pay for improved facilities

○ the options for change – including available technologies and their costs

○ available resources – including physical, financial, institutional and human resources.

The key to informed decision making is to have access to sufficient information to allow the main issues and options to be identified. Too little information will mean that decisions are ill-informed. Too much information, collected in an unfocused way, may hinder decision making because its sheer volume makes it impossible to see what is and is not relevant to the decisions to be made. Collection of excess information may divert the limited resources that are available away from more urgent tasks.

The form that information takes is also important. Dudley (1993, p. 71) notes that a new idea is only likely to be adopted if 'it fits into a person's existing structure of knowledge'.[1] This principle is equally true of information – if people do not recognize what it is and what it is for, they will not use it. Community members and those working with them will already use information in an informal way, weighing up options on the basis of what they already know and what they can see. They are likely to have little experience of complex quantitative forms of information and may not recognize its value even when they see it. Conversely, city planners and policy makers often do not recognize the value of qualitative information obtained through participatory appraisal processes. They may not accept, and indeed may be unable to use, information unless it is expressed in more or less quantitative form. So, information intended for use by planners and policy makers should be collected in a form that allows it to be quantified.

The point here is not that community members should never use quantitative information while policy makers should always rely on it. Rather, the need is to work with stakeholders to develop information systems that mean something to them. As with other aspects of sanitation planning, this means starting from an awareness of the existing situation and, where necessary, taking action to inform stakeholder perceptions.

Information requirements of different groups

A person's information requirements will depend on who they are and the level at which they are working.

Those working at the local level will require information on the local situation, any external factors that influence that situation and the options for intervention in it. Much of this information may be qualitative but, where necessary, it should be supplemented by simple maps, graphs and tables. Information on possible technical options should be kept as simple as possible.

Those working at the municipal level will need sufficient information to be able to compare what is happening in different areas and link the actions proposed for those areas into a coordinated whole in order to take strategic decisions relating to the city as a whole. Qualitative information will provide them with a feel for problems and people's perceptions of them. Spatial information will tell them where services are in relation to the people who need them. Quantitative analysis of subjects such as sanitation coverage in different areas, income levels and willingness to pay for services will help them to identify priority action areas and decide on the most appropriate interventions to improve services. Information on sanitation technologies will guide sanitation choices and ensure that people are aware of their management requirements.

Those who are concerned with policy and/or national sanitation programmes need information that allows them to understand what is happening in the country, state or province to which the policy or programme is to apply, together with any variations between regions and/or cities and towns. The information must be in a form that allows them to compare different situations, identify priority concerns, frame policies to address those concerns and monitor their implementation.

Information needs at different stages in the planning process

Planners should recognize that information needs will change and develop in the course of the planning process and plan their information collection activities accordingly.

At the understanding problems stage, the focus should be on obtaining sufficient information to develop a general understanding of problems and opportunities. Experiences from Andhra Pradesh in India described in Box 7.1 illustrate the importance of field observation as a means of understanding problems.

> **Box 7.1 The value of field observation – an example from India**
>
> The Andhra Pradesh Urban Services for the Poor (APUSP) project is an integrated urban project, supported by DFID, which aims to bring about improved access to 'appropriate and sustainable services' for poor people living in the 32 'Class 1' towns (those with over 100 000 population) in the Indian state of Andhra Pradesh. State government officials initially suggested that the project did not need to cover sanitation as this was already catered for by the Indian government's Integrated Low Cost Sanitation Programme (ILCS). This involves the provision of latrines with two pits, which are intended to be used alternately, giving time for their contents to decompose and become harmless to health before they are removed.
>
> Early site visits revealed many problems with the ILCS programme. Some latrines had never been finished. Many were not being used. Even where latrines were being used, initial conversations with members of the households that owned them revealed that they had no idea of the sequence in which the pits were to be used. In some cases, pits were being used in series, with the effluent discharged to an open drain, rather than in parallel as intended.
>
> These initial investigations, taking only a few hours in total, clearly revealed that the sanitation needs of low-income people were not being catered for by the ILCS as it stood and should not be excluded from the APUSP.

Where possible, existing (often referred to as secondary) sources of information should be used. However, it is important to recognize that:

○ secondary information may be out of date or otherwise inaccurate

○ official statistics and system plans will not normally provide information on the condition of facilities and how they are operated and maintained.

Secondary information should be checked by observation in the field and by talking to key stakeholders. The latter should include users of existing and proposed sanitation facilities.

When developing solutions or preparing local plans, the main need will be for more detailed information on the areas in which action is focused. It may also be appropriate to start to collect more general information about the town or city as a whole. Indeed improving the information base will often be a key activity at this stage of the process.

Mapping may be required in order to establish an understanding of overall drainage patterns and develop a basis for future drainage proposals. Later, the information gained from pilot projects may provide useful qualitative information on issues such as community attitudes and capacity for operation and maintenance.

City-wide plans should, as far as is possible, be developed on the basis of accurate information rather than conjecture. The focus at this stage of the process should be similar to that during the developing solutions stage but with a greater emphasis on institutionalizing information systems, making sure that information is regularly collected, easily accessible and provided in a usable form for the whole of the town or city.

The same general principles will apply when developing policy. The initial need will be to develop an overall understanding of the existing situation and the problems and possibilities that it presents. Follow-up investigations can then home in on specific problems and issues.

The systems used for information collection, storage and analysis of information should be compatible with those that already exist in the organizations charged with maintaining and using it. There is no point, for instance, in producing a detailed computerized management information system to a municipality that has few computers and no history of routinely using information for planning purposes. Where there is a need to introduce more sophisticated information management systems, this should be done systematically, making adequate provision for staff orientation and training.[2]

The importance of triangulation

Wherever possible, information should be cross-checked or 'triangulated'. Chambers (1994) uses the term triangulation to mean 'cross-checking and progressive learning and approximation'. It involves assessing and comparing findings obtained using different methods and disciplines, at different places and times and by different investigators. For example:

- o 'Rapid assessment' involving transect walks and discussions with residents in representative areas will provide a check on the information provided by official records, perhaps revealing the existence of schemes that have been initiated and managed by people themselves.

- o Discussions with different informants may reveal different perceptions about the causes of sanitation problems. For instance municipal officials may blame community members for lifting manhole covers and allowing storm water to drain to the sewer. Local people may see this as a better option than letting their houses flood. Talking to different people and checking their statements against your own observation will give you to a better understanding of the situation and how problems might be resolved. It will be particularly important to listen to poor, excluded and marginalized groups such as tenants, low-caste people and female-headed households.

- o Showing a summary of official statistics and records to community members may enable them to provide a critique of the official view and help everyone to obtain a better understanding of 'where we are now'.

If initial checks reveal that there is a problem with existing information, it will be necessary to consider how more accurate and relevant information can be obtained. It may be that this has to be built into the developing solutions stage of the planning process.

Sources of information

Maps that provide information on physical features such as hills and rivers, main roads and railways and political boundaries should be available with the municipal authorities, although the quality of these maps will not always be good.

Information on the nature and form of existing development may be available with the municipal planning authorities. (In the case of smaller towns, responsibility for physical planning may rest with a state/provincial level planning agency.)

Specialist agencies and departments that have been set up to deal with the specific needs of low-income areas may have information on 'slums' and 'squatter settlements'. If they are available, aerial photographs can reveal settlement patterns and help you to distinguish between planned and unplanned areas.

Unregulated settlements in peri-urban areas are likely to be poorly recorded and the best way of defining their locations and limits may be through 'windscreen' surveys – driving around and recording what you find on the ground.

Specialist agencies should have good records of the routes of existing collector sewers and drains but it may be that information on existing tertiary systems will have to be obtained in the field.

Information on ongoing and proposed sanitation programmes should be available from the organizations that are responsible for funding, implementing and monitoring them. General information on centrally funded projects and programmes should be available with the government departments that are responsible for them. Municipalities and other local stakeholders may hold more detailed information on the implementation of programmes in their own town or city. NGOs may hold information on programmes which they have either initiated or supported.

Information on technologies and standards should be available with specialist agencies and government departments. Research institutions and consultants may hold information on innovative technologies and may also have conducted assessments of existing projects and programmes.

Recording, analysing and presenting information

In order to be useful, information must be recorded in a way that the intended users can understand. Some examples of what this might mean in practice are given below.

Photographs and videos can be used to provide a qualitative record of conditions and problems. These may be particularly useful in the initial understanding problems stage of the planning process. They can be used as part of presentations designed to provide an overall picture of sanitation problems and introduce possible solutions.

Information on the location of public sanitation facilities should normally be presented on maps and plans. When plotting information at the municipal level, use the best base map available. Maps and plans relating to specific local communities do not have to be exactly to scale, as long as they reflect the overall layout of streets and facilities and, where appropriate, record the lengths of sewers and drains.

Basic information on physical and social conditions, sanitation coverage, institutional arrangements and available resources might be presented in the form of a digest of the available information for each town or city. Municipal authorities would be responsible for preparing the digest of information, drawing upon any information held by those working more locally. Those working at the centre would be responsible for bringing the digests for various towns together to provide an overall picture for a state, province or country.

Once recorded on plans, spatial information can be analysed to produce quantitative information on services. For instance, the lengths of sewers shown on a plan can be measured and compared with the total length of sewer necessary to serve all houses, thus allowing an estimate to be made of the percentage of a settlement that is sewered.

Information on available technologies and their costs might be presented in a simple manual. This should include detail drawings showing the various possible technologies and standard details, together with cost information in the form of bill-of-quantity type cost schedules. Each component or standard detail could then be represented on a left-hand page of the manual with the schedule of quantities required to construct the detail shown on the facing page.

Guidance on the application of the technology and constraints on its use should be provided. When intended for use by community members, this information should be provided in the local language. Some preliminary work to explore the ways in which community members collect and use information will normally be appropriate to ensure that the guidance materials mean something to them.

Techniques exist for quantifying qualitative information. For instance, it is possible to ask a number of people how they rate the quality of a service on a scale from very bad to very good, as shown below.

Very bad	Bad	Satisfactory	Good	Very good
1	2	3	4	5

This will often be the best way of assessing views on the quality of a service. Once the results have been obtained, they can be analysed and the average score can be determined. This will tell you what the overall view is about the question being asked.

Once available, quantitative information from different sources can be brought together to provide a better understanding of the current situation. For instance, population data can be compared with that on the number of solid waste workers in each ward to obtain an idea of staffing levels in different areas. This was done as part of a solid waste management study in Faisalabad, Pakistan. It revealed that, officially at least, in inner city wards, each worker served a population of around 500, regardless of whether these wards were predominantly high- or low-income. In wards on the city fringe, the number of people per worker sometimes exceeded 2500. Such information can be useful when deciding how to deploy the existing workforce and, perhaps, where to use additional private sector resources.

Information for local and municipal plans

We now turn to the ways in which the principles outlined in the first part of this chapter can be used to inform the development of plans at the local and municipal levels, bearing in mind the need to understand problems and develop solutions before moving into a full plan for a city, town or district, at all times matching information systems to available resources.

Information requirements for understanding problems

In Chapter 3, we suggested the following four basic questions as a framework for understanding problems:

o Who is responsible for providing existing services?

o What sanitation problems do we face?

o What are the causes of problems?

o What resources do we have?

We now suggest an approach to gathering the information needed to answer these questions.

Initial contacts

Initial information on official responsibility for sanitation provision can be obtained through interviews with government officials. These initial contacts may lead you to other sources of information. However, it will usually be the case that individuals and organizations other than government provide many sanitation services. Individual householders are usually the largest providers and managers of on-site facilities.[3] People may cooperate to provide shared services at the local level. NGOs may provide support to these people and the community organizations that represent them. These 'self-help' efforts are most likely to occur in 'informal' low-income areas. So, concurrently with initial contacts with 'formal' sanitation providers, efforts must be made to identify and talk to those who can provide information on informal approaches to sanitation provision. These might include local politicians, recognized community leaders and NGOs with close links with the community.

When interviewing government officials and other secondary stakeholders, you should explore their views on the other three questions. What are the main sanitation problems, what are their causes and what resources might be available to tackle them? Ask particularly about:

o charging policies and arrangements for recovering costs from users

o any schemes that might provide funding for the sanitation-related activities of municipalities and other stakeholders.

Secondary information

At the understanding problems stage, the aim should be to collect secondary information that throws light on sanitation problems and available resources. This might include:

o copies of the laws and ordinances that set out the duties and responsibilities of local government

o information on the location and socio-economic status of low-income areas

o statistics on existing sanitation coverage

o plans showing the extent of existing service provision

o budgets and other documents that throw light on the current financial status of the municipality, particularly the extent of its dependence on transfers from higher levels of government and the percentage of current expenditure that is devoted to capital works.

Field investigations

Initial interviews with secondary stakeholders and secondary information will provide a partial understanding of sanitation problems.

However, they will not give any indication of what people think about sanitation and may not accurately reflect the situation on the ground. For instance, there may be no official house-to-house solid waste collection service, but it may be that households are paying municipal sweepers and/or micro-entrepreneurs to collect waste from their houses.

Rapid appraisal in the field can help to provide a more complete understanding of sanitation problems and possibilities. This might include:

o Transect walks in representative areas, particularly those that are thought to suffer from inadequate sanitation, poor drainage and poor solid waste collection services. During these walks look for evidence of initiatives to improve sanitation facilities and services, even if these are unsatisfactory in some respects. For instance, it may be that the wastewater discharges from several houses are connected to a local sewer.

o Inspection of existing facilities and services, including existing drains and sewers, pumping stations, solid waste transfer points and waste disposal facilities. For instance, to reduce costs, operators often maintain the water level in pumping station wet wells above the crown of the incoming sewer, thus reducing flow velocities in upstream sewers to well below those assumed by designers. Look particularly for evidence that facilities are not being used as intended by their designers, and where possible investigate the reasons for this. Specialist support should be sought for this task.

o Informal meetings with community members and government employees. While carrying out transect walks and inspections, talk to community members and government employees. Explore their sanitation-related concerns and ask them to provide further information on any interesting points that you have observed. In the case of the houses connected to a local sewer as described above, discussion with community members will quickly establish who built the sewer and what, if any, support they received. These initial discussions may well lead on to informal interviews with key stakeholders in the initiatives that you have identified, which will add to your understanding of available resources.

When meeting community members, it will be important to explore a range of viewpoints. Make sure that some of the people visiting the community are women as they should be able to talk to women in the community and obtain their view of problems. It is also possible that women will see issues and problems that would be missed by men.

Further information on a number of participatory methodologies for developing a shared understanding of local problems is given in Appendix 3.

The best results will be obtained if the results from field investigations in different areas are brought together to provide an overall understanding of the existing situation (see Box 7.2).

Investigating demand for improved sanitation

During field investigations, look for evidence that there is a demand for improved

Box 7.2 Field investigations in Quthbullapur, Andhra Pradesh

Quthbullapur, with a population of around 200 000, is located close to Hyderabad, the state capital of Andhra Pradesh. A workshop was held to explore the sanitation problems of the town and simultaneously to introduce the concept of strategic planning to local stakeholders. In order to develop an understanding of problems, the workshop participants were divided into groups and each group was asked to visit a selected location in order to investigate the sanitation problems in that area.

The areas used for the field visits were selected to illustrate a range of situations and problems. They included:

o low-income areas in which varying degrees of effort had already been made to improve sanitation services
o a middle-income area in which sewerage had been provided under a Government of Andhra Pradesh programme of assistance to community initiatives
o an area traversed by a main drain and trunk sewer with potential to serve much of the town.

Each group presented its findings to the workshop and this exercise proved to be very useful in identifying problems and possibilities. The workshop organizers then located the various field-visit areas on a map of the municipality and encouraged participants to discuss the wider implications of their findings in relation to the other areas. This exercise revealed that the effluent from the sewers in the middle-income area flowed into drains which then passed through one of the low-income areas into a marshy area that was causing problems for surrounding settlements. This highlighted the need to look at drainage problems in terms of drainage basins rather than individual areas. The group visiting the trunk sewer found that there were few connections to it, reinforcing the perception that there was a need for a municipality-wide approach to wastewater disposal.

sanitation. This evidence may reveal itself in a number of ways.

1. Through what people do. Is there evidence that people have built, are building or are trying to build new or improved sanitation facilities? Are there septic tanks in streets or connections to drains that look as if they may be from WCs?

2. Through what people say. Conversations with community members and interviews with key informants (for instance local masons and suppliers of sanitary fittings and, not least, typical householders) may provide information on activities and initiatives that might not be obvious through casual observation from the street. Since different people are likely to have different views on sanitation, it will be necessary to talk to representatives of different groups within society.

3. Through requests for action to improve sanitation. Local councillors and other people and organizations with access to funds will know if people are coming to them with requests for help with improved sanitation, drainage or both.

Where some people show an interest in improved sanitation, they can provide a starting point for the development of more general demand within the community. For instance, it is not uncommon for visual surveys to reveal groups of houses with improved sanitation, suggesting that one householder has built a latrine and in doing so has influenced his or her neighbours to follow suit. So, look for patterns of sanitation improvement, which will help you to understand the dynamics of the improvement process.

Initial assessment of problems and resources

Once problems have been identified and resources have been identified, the next step will be to carry out an initial assessment in order to:

○ identify priority problems and their causes

○ explore possible responses to those problems

○ establish what further information will be required to develop a comprehensive strategic plan.

Encourage stakeholders to carry out this assessment together. This will help to develop a shared understanding of problems and inform discussion on the development of information systems during the developing solutions stage of the strategic planning process. As already indicated, it will normally be best to do this during the initial planning workshop.

Priority problems and their causes

The causes of some problems may be unclear. For instance, frequent sewer blockages might be due to the lack of fall on the sewer, poor construction and/or misuse of the system, particularly the dumping of solid waste into the sewer at manholes. In such situations, the causes of problems should be explored in a systematic way.

This may be done by recording problems on cards. These are then placed on a board or sticky cloth (see Chapter 9 for further details) and moved so that relationships of cause and effect can be seen, effects being placed above causes so that the reasons for problems are at the bottom and the problem to be solved is at the top. This is known as a problem tree analysis. Figure 7.1 illustrates how this might work out in practice in relation to solid waste accumulation in residential areas.

Problem trees are sometimes used as the first stage in developing a logical framework – a comprehensive approach to tackling a problem or achieving a goal (see Chapter 10 for further details). When used in this way, the aim is to bring all problems into one complete tree, which identifies an overall goal to which the plan or programme should be directed.

It will often be more appropriate to carry out more limited analyses, designed to lead to immediate actions that will solve immediate problems and throw light on the approach to be taken to solve more deep-seated problems.

The example in Figure 7.1 illustrates how this might work in practice. It identifies one cause of problems that is internal to the community – the lack of awareness of the danger to health posed by uncollected solid waste. This might be overcome by a health education campaign. However, it also identifies the fact that the problem is caused in part by waste being brought in to the area from the outside, suggesting that the causes of the problem lie partly outside the community. So, action to solve the problem will be required at the municipal level. Note that some of the root causes of problems may emerge after discussion among workshop participants.

Problem trees can appear rather complicated, because causes and effects can be difficult to determine precisely. A simplified approach was used during the first planning workshop in Bharatpur. Participants were asked to write down sanitation and drainage-related problems on cards. The cards were then collected and grouped under appropriate headings. Repeated cards were then removed and similar ones were edited so that each subject was covered by a

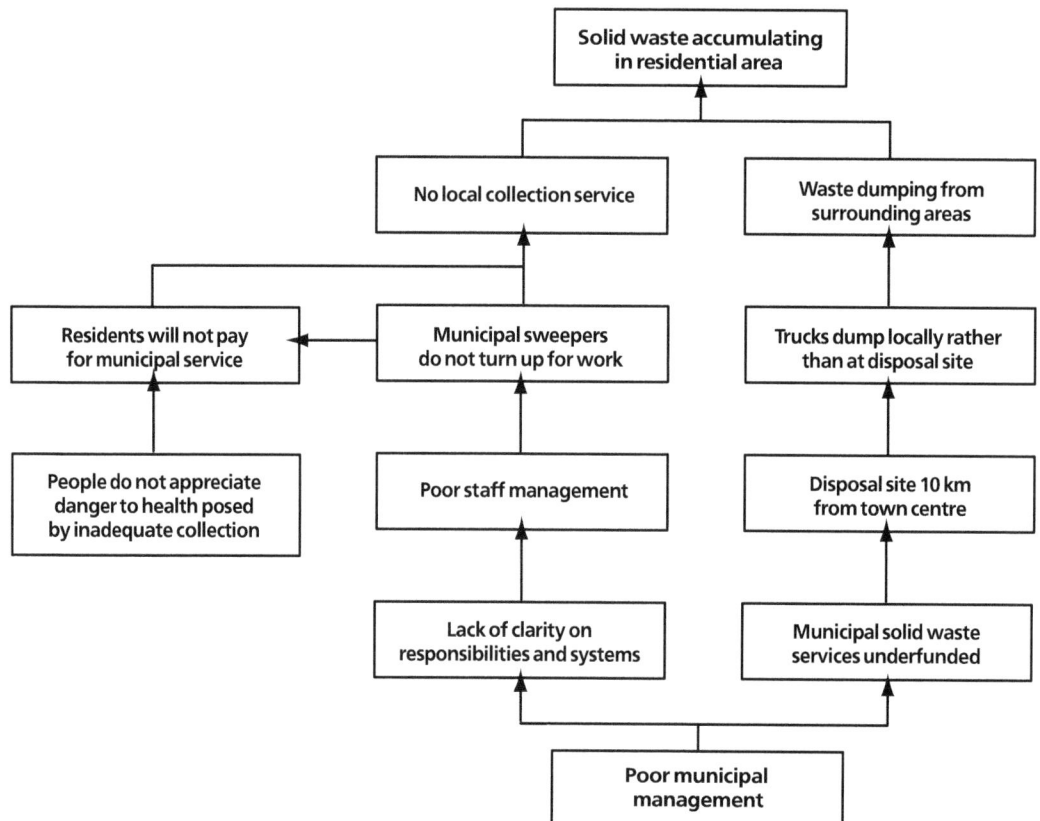

Figure 7.1 Example of problem tree analysis

single card. The cards were next arranged into three groups, relating to:

○ factors that could not be changed
○ the primary causes of sanitation problems
○ resulting problems with water and sanitation facilities. This rather less detailed analysis is probably more appropriate than a full problem tree analysis for use in understanding problems.

Available resources
Assessment of existing provision will give an idea of the extent and nature of existing sanitation problems and current activities and responsibilities. However, they will tell you little about the opportunities for change. In order to assess the latter, information is required on available resources. In particular, the aim should be to establish answers to the following questions:

○ Which organizations, groups and individuals might take an increased role in sanitation provision?
○ Are there any gaps in the availability of knowledge and skills, for those relating sanitation and hygiene promotion?
○ How might improved sanitation services be financed?

Organizational resources
A good way to start to assess organizational resources and identify gaps will be to develop a matrix of tasks to be carried out in relation to different sectors and at different levels. This might be developed in the course of the first planning workshop, drawing on the results of information collected during the understanding problems stage. Workshop participants would be asked to identify tasks and to write them on a card, using different coloured cards for different organizations. These cards can then be displayed within an overall framework of the type shown in Table 7.1.

This will give workshop participants a clear picture of who is responsible for what and remind them that government is not the only provider of sanitation services.

The next task will be to make an initial assessment of the resources that are available within each organization. When undertaking this task, the aim should be to identify:

○ available knowledge and skills
○ the extent to which current institutional structures and systems allow those resources to be used
○ any areas in which resources are lacking.

This can also be done in a shared session, placing cards in the appropriate places on a table displayed where all workshop participants can see it (see Table 7.2). A particular task for the facilitator will be to encourage participants to identify locally available resources, both current and potential. In Bharatpur, the participants broke into two groups, one to deal with community involve-

Table 7.1 Framework for identification of existing tasks and responsibilities

	Solid waste management	Drainage	Excreta and wastewater disposal	Hygiene education
City level				
Zonal				
Neighbourhood				
Household				

Table 7.2 Bharatpur resource analysis

	Drainage	Water supply	Solid waste management	Sanitation	Hygiene education
Lead/ nodal agency	Bharatpur Municipal Council (BMC)	Public Health Engineering Dept hygiene education (PHED)	BMC	BMC	Med/integrated Child Development Scheme
	Proposed nodal agency	*Should come under proposed agency*			*CARE*
Support agency	BMC, Urban Improvement Trust, Housing Board	PHED	ACORD (local NGO), other NGOs *Small scale enterprises*	Sulabh (national NGO), UNICEF	Anganwadis, schools, Adult Educational Programmes, CBOs
Available personnel	Yes	Yes	Yes	Yes	Yes
Technical expertise	Yes, but needs improvement	Yes, but needs improvement	ACORD, IIRD (NGOs), CPCB, small enterprises	Sulabh, UNICEF	UNICEF, CARE, Information, Education and communication cell (Health Dept)
Extension skills	Yes, but needs improvement	*NGOs, other social organizations*	NGOs and CBOs	NGOs and CBOs *Government agencies*	NGO, Angan, ANM, health workers *Youth clubs, children's groups, media*
Capital Funds	*Needed from bilateral and multilateral agencies*	Bi- and multi-laterals, state	[WB-UNDP, CPCB, HUDCO]	BMC-inadequate Sehbhagi Vida Yojan UNICEF, WB, HUDCO	UNICEF, Health Dept, CARE
Operation and maintenance funds	*Bi- and multi-laterals; MCB, state, user*	Users/state	*User charges (sharing basis)*	User charges	ICDS, WHO, UNICEF *Donations, clubs, social Institutions*

Note:
- shaded boxes indicate that resources are currently lacking in that area
- items in italics are suggestions or potential new resources

ment, drainage and water supply and the second to consider solid waste management, low-cost sanitation and hygiene education. For each aspect of sanitation, participants were asked to identify a possible lead agency and support organizations and the resources available. In subsequent discussion, the group suggested potential new or additional resources to fill gaps in current provision.

At this stage, it may be useful to encourage people to think about existing systems and incentives. Do these encourage individuals to use their knowledge and skills creatively? If the initial investigations reveal problems and issues with existing incentives, options for introducing improved systems should be investigated during later stages of the planning process.

At a more local level the aim should be to identify any individuals already working on aspects of sanitation provision who might be able to contribute to an expanded and improved programme.

Financial resources

Initial assessment of financial resources can be built around answers to the following questions.

○ Is there clear information on the current financial capacity of the municipality?

○ What are the possible sources of external finance and how might they be tapped?

○ How much are users already paying for sanitation services, both officially and unofficially?

○ Would it be possible to raise funds locally to supplement official programmes and, if so, how? For instance, is there a possibility that private sector organizations might be willing to provide funds for sanitation improvements?

It may be useful to carry out some rough calculations to determine the number of sanitation units that the various sources of finance might provide and how far this provision might go in meeting overall sanitation needs.

Methods for estimating unit costs and people's willingness to pay for improved sanitation are introduced in Chapter 8.

Developing solutions: Improving the information base

As indicated in Chapter 3, the developing solutions stage will normally include action to improve the information base. Possibilities in this respect are now briefly discussed.

Improvements in the map base

These will be a priority if existing maps are old and/or poorly detailed. Aim to develop a single base map (or set of maps) for the whole town. This should be at a scale in the range 1:5000 to 1:20 000 and should show information on topography, roads, railways, canals and other physical features and the limits of built up areas. Larger scales, typically in the range 1:250 to 1:1000 will be required for detailed planning at the local level.

Supplementary maps and plans, using the same base map, can then be produced. These might provide information on political boundaries, the areas covered by different types of development (formal and informal, recognized and unrecognized, etc.) and information on infrastructure networks and facilities.

Before commissioning new maps, check on those that are already available. It may be, for instance, that good quality maps exist but are held by state/provincial government departments so that they are not available to those working at the municipal level. In other cases, specialist organizations such as water supply agencies may have good map information. It is quite likely that one of the tasks to be undertaken during the developing solutions stage will be to ensure that such information is made available to municipal stakeholders.

It must be possible to reproduce base maps. This means that they must be available in either digital form or as negatives. If existing negatives have to remain with a central department, explore the possibility of making copies of the negatives. While this can be an expensive process, it will be money well spent. International development agencies should consider making funds available for this purpose.

Records of existing sewerage and drainage networks

Informed decisions on improvements in sewerage and drainage provision, operation and maintenance cannot be made in the absence of information on existing sewerage and drainage networks. Where existing records are inadequate, a high priority should be given to recording networks.

In order to match actions to available resources, consider the possibility of taking a step-wise approach to mapping the network. This might involve:

○ an initial assessment of the whole system, focusing on drainage boundaries and problem areas, with the results plotted on a city-wide base map

○ more detailed assessment of drainage basins in which there are frequent flooding problems. This should cover the location of existing drains and drainage boundaries, and ground and drain invert and top water levels.

The information should then be plotted on a suitable base map. In order to understand problems and possibilities relating to collector drains, longitudinal drain sections will be required. These should *always* be linked to a plan with chainages (distances from the start of the drain) clearly marked on both the section and the plan. The section should also show easily identifiable features such as changes in direction and road crossing points.

Detailed surveys of existing sanitation services and programmes

These will be required to obtain more detailed information on problems and issues identified during the understanding problems stage of the planning process. They might include:

○ structured observation

○ interviews with key informants

○ focus group discussions around key problems and issues

○ participatory mapping

○ conventional questionnaire surveys.

(See Appendix 3 for further details of these survey methods.) A combination of survey methods should be used in order to obtain an overall understanding of the current situation, covering not only physical provision but also people's attitudes to improved sanitation and the way in which services are operated and maintained (see Box 7.3). At the developing solutions stage, it will normally be appropriate to focus survey efforts on some of the wards and/or areas in which the greatest problems occur.

Similar methods can be used to assess the performance of existing sanitation programmes. The key questions to be answered are:

○ Is the programme meeting its objectives in terms of the facilities provided?

○ Are those facilities being used as intended?

Box 7.3 Investigating local solid waste collection services – Faisalabad, Pakistan

In Faisalabad, as in all Pakistani towns and cities, there is no official house-to-house solid waste collection service. In practice, house-to-house collection services are common in high and middle-income areas and are not unknown in low-income areas. These services are provided by both municipal sweepers, operating beyond their official remit, and private sweepers. The term 'sweeper' is used throughout south Asia to denote people who sweep the streets and collect waste from communal dustbins. In both cases, householders pay the sweeper directly for providing the service.

As part of the Faisalabad solid waste management study, a detailed investigation of house-to-house collection services was carried out for one housing block in a lower middle-income area containing about 500 households. A team was trained to observe the number of collection workers entering the area and follow-up interviews were held with these workers to obtain information on their working practices. The survey revealed that many householders were paying for solid waste to be collected from their houses and that about 20 sweepers were engaged in this activity, some but not all of whom worked for the municipality. Contacts between individual sweepers and their customers had developed in a rather ad hoc manner, as would be expected with such informal activity, so that most sweepers had customers scattered throughout the area rather than being concentrated in 'blocks'. This meant that collection routes were unnecessarily long. There appeared to be some scope for swapping of customers between sweepers in order to reduce the length of collection routes and thus to reduce the level of effort required to earn the same income.

Municipal finances

Investigations of municipal finances should build on the initial investigations carried out in the understanding problems stage with the aim of developing a better understanding of current income and expenditure patterns and thus identifying the possibilities for change and improvement. The focus at the developing solutions stage should be on expenditure on the provision, operation and maintenance of sanitation facilities, including analysis of the costs of any services that have been contracted out to either the private sector or community organizations.

It may be that information is not available in a readily usable form. Where this is the case, there will be a need to investigate how existing information systems can be improved. If possible, those with responsibility for financial systems should be involved in these investigations. This will ensure that outside investigators develop a good understanding of existing systems and at the same time helps to make local stakeholders aware of the need for change and the possibility of achieving change. Where there are clear deficiencies that cannot be rectified immediately, the development of improved systems may have to be included as an element in the sanitation plan itself.

Documenting pilot projects

It will be important to ensure that pilot projects are well documented so that none of the lessons are lost. In particular, make sure that the information is available on:

o the situation before and after implementation of the pilot

- any special features of the area chosen for the pilot
- the costs of implementation and subsequent operation and maintenance
- particular problems that arise during the implementation and subsequent operation and maintenance of facilities.

As with other types of information, the information collected from pilot projects should be triangulated. In particular, efforts should be made to obtain the views of the people who use the facilities and services provided through the pilot. This might involve a combination of interviews with individual residents, focus group discussions and small questionnaire surveys. When planning for interviews and focus group discussions, bear in mind the need to obtain the views of all users and not just dominant groups. In particular, women may have different views than men on the convenience and suitability of sanitation facilities.

The conventional way to document the findings of a pilot project is to produce a short report, detailing what was done and the key findings. In some cases, it may be appropriate to document the findings of a pilot in a short video. This has the advantage that it is not dependent on the written word and should be accessible to all people in the community.

Developing an integrated information base

In institutions that lack a strong information culture, there is a real danger that the results of investigations will be lost over time. This suggests a need to go beyond individual information collection exercises to think about the development of an information system which not only stores information but also allows information from different sources to be brought together as and when required. One way of doing this is to superimpose information from different sources on a base map so as to develop a better understanding of its meaning. For instance, superimposing information on service coverage on a map showing areas with different types of tenure might show that people with formal tenure are more likely than those with insecure tenure to be provided with basic environmental sanitation services.

In Bharatpur, this idea of superimposing information from different sources to provide a better understanding of sanitation conditions and their causes was formalized in the concept of social and technical mapping, as described in Box 7.4. The aim was to bring together the spatial information traditionally used by engineers and physical planners and the social information collected by social specialists to form an integrated whole. This process might be started in selected areas during the developing solutions stage. However, social and technical mapping for the town as a whole should normally be incorporated into the strategic plan proper.

The uses and limitations of Geographic Information Systems

The system of overlays described in the previous paragraphs is, in fact, a simple form of Geographic Information System (GIS). While a geographic information system does not have to be computerized, the term GIS is normally used for a computer-based information system that allows data from different sources to be brought together on a geographical base, in effect overlaid, as in the simple system described above. GIS can also be used to link different types of information so that, for instance, qualitative and quantitative information on a particular low-income housing area can be stored in a database and related to the location of that

Box 7.4 Social and technical mapping – the approach proposed in Bharatpur

In Bharatpur, social and technical mapping was proposed as a way of collecting and presenting information on sanitation conditions in the city as a whole, with a particular focus on the areas that were worst affected by sanitation deficiencies. The aim was to provide information on maps in a form that facilitated decision making on the priorities for action. This would ensure that funds and other resources were directed to the areas that were the most deprived and contained high numbers of poor people.

The information was to be presented in two parts.

City maps
A base map and a series of overlays, all to the same scale, which could be laid over one another as described on the previous page. They should include:
- A social map showing colonies, *mohallas* (neighbourhoods), and 'informal' areas. Information on incomes and other socio-economic indicators would be related to the areas shown on this map.
- A technical map showing solid waste facilities and problem areas (particularly areas not covered by municipal facilities), unofficial dumping sites and areas that vehicles could not reach.
- A technical map showing the location of public toilets, areas with low levels of latrine coverage, areas with high incidence of service (primitive dry) latrines, etc.
- A technical map showing the principal drain lines, areas experiencing severe blockages and low-lying areas prone to flooding.

Neighbourhood profiles
A profile for each neighbourhood comprising:
- A summary sheet (one page) with essential data and a weighting/points score to show whether problems are high, medium or low priority compared with the rest of the city.
- Community drawn maps showing facilities and problem areas. (The basic community-drawn maps might be developed into something more 'polished' with the help of professional draughtsmen.)
- Basic social and demographic data.
- Details of sanitation problems.
- Information on community preferences for improvement.

The aim was to keep the profiles brief so that they would be accessible to those who might be interested in using them.

A range of participatory survey methods, including several of those covered in Appendix 3, was proposed to collect this information.

---

housing area on the overall city map. For further information of GIS systems, see Masser and Sliuzas (1999), but for the moment, note the following important points.

- A GIS system requires a map base, which must be digitized if it is to be held on the computer.
- Given the large effort needed to digitize

the map base, there is little point in digitizing an inaccurate map.

Where an accurate map base is not available for the whole of a town or a city, it will generally be better to develop a less sophisticated information system. For instance, it should be possible to produce a database containing information on different communities, giving each community a number and relating this to a numbered map or plan showing the approximate locations of communities *without digitizing the map base*.

This might be the first stage in developing a GIS system for the town. The next stage might be to develop an accurately referenced base for the town, showing key features such as main roads, railways and canals but without infill details in the first instance. It should be possible to fill in the detail for specific areas as and when accurate information on those areas becomes available.

An example of the pro-forma for a neighbourhood profile is given in Box 7.5. Use this as a starting point for developing your own pro-forma but do not hesitate to modify it to reflect local conditions and experience.

Information for policy makers and programme planners

Like strategic plans for specific areas, towns and cities, sanitation policies should be developed on the basis of information rather than conjecture. The aim should be to develop information systems that:

o assist decision makers to make sensible policy choices

o provide a baseline against which change can be measured

o allow progress with policies and programmes to be monitored.

Information requirements for policy development

Information requirements for policy development are likely to include the following.[4]

Background information on area and population. In particular the number of people living in urban areas, the urban growth rate and perhaps the spread of population between different sizes of settlement and between different areas of the country. This will help to put other types of information into context. It should generally be available from official reports and statistics.

Existing sanitation services. Information on the coverage of existing services will provide some indication of the scale of the problems to be faced. Basic information on service coverage may be available in official reports and statistics. However, these are unlikely to give much information on the other ways in which services might be deficient (see list of possible deficiencies in Chapter 1.) This information is important if the policy is to address real rather than perceived needs. In particular, information on access to existing services will help to decide whether the policy needs to make provision for the particular needs of marginalized groups.

Where this information is not available from 'official' sources, investigate other sources, for instance NGOs working in low-income areas. If initial investigations reveal gaps in the information base, surveys of representative areas should be commissioned in order to develop a more detailed understanding of existing services, where they are, how they perform and who they reach.

The existing policy environment. Study of existing policy documents and legislation will reveal the extent to which the current policy environment is potentially supportive of a more strategic approach to sanitation planning. In addition to existing sanitation

Box 7.5 Example of pro-forma for neighbourhood profile

Mohalla Summary Sheet	Date of assessment:
Name of *mohalla* (neighbourhood)	Ward no.
Name of elected representative	

	Details	Comments
Population		
Main income group		
Main ethnic/social group		
Type of development (approved, unplanned, notified slum, unrecognized slum)		
Tenure status		
Range of plot sizes		
Latrines		
Estimated percentage of households with a latrine (excluding *katcha* and service latrines)		
Is area served by a public toilet?		
Estimated number of users of toilet		
Condition of toilet		
Estimated percentage of households using open defecation		
Solid waste management (garbage)		
Estimated percentage of households served by municipal collection service		
No. of bins/collection points		
Frequency of collection		
Can vehicles gain access to streets and lanes?		
Cleanliness of drains and open areas		
Drainage		
Adequacy of natural drainage (does water drain away easily due to slope or good soil permeability?)		
Highest level of water table		
Details of any flood problems (do they affect public space, access routes or private plots)		
Water supply		
Estimated percentage of homes with house connection		
Water pressure (above plinth, at plinth, below plinth)		
Hours supplied per day		
Details of other sources of water		
Community Willingness to participate in sanitation programme		

Priority weighting	high/medium/low
Latrines	
Solid waste management	
Drainage	

policy (which will often form part of a joint water and sanitation policy), investigations should cover policies on land tenure and regularization of informal development, since these influence the approach taken to sanitation provision in what will often be the poorest areas. Particular attention should be paid to current incentive systems and their impact on approaches to sanitation provision.

Existing roles, responsibilities, activities and programmes. Information on official roles, responsibilities and programmes should be available from official sources. However, as at the municipal level, it will also be important to take account of other less official activities, particularly those of householders, NGOs and 'formal' and 'informal' sector private operators. This will help to ensure that policies are based on realistic assumptions about who is likely to provide services. The investigation should look for any overlapping of responsibilities and for differences between what is meant to happen and what actually happens in practice.

Information on current operation and maintenance practices, or indeed the lack of them, should help policy makers to explore the ways in which policies might address the need for improved operation and maintenance.

Information on the environmental impact of existing approaches to sanitation provision might lead to the conclusion that policies and programmes should promote the use of environmentally friendly technologies.

Information on the impact of existing programmes will provide guidance on any changes that might be needed in those programmes to make them more effective. When assessing programmes, it will be important to consider whether they are properly focused. For instance, a programme might be very successful in providing new sewers but will only have value if householders are connecting to those sewers.

Information on available technologies and their costs will be required in order to assess the overall cost of different policy options. Once this information is available, it can be used in conjunction with any available information on willingness and ability to pay to determine the viability of those options. For instance, there will be no point in developing a policy that is based on widespread sewerage provision if the available information suggests that sewerage is unaffordable to the majority of the population.

Resources. These include the financial, institutional and human resources that might be available for sanitation provision. Information on the financial resources available for sanitation service improvements should include but not be limited to the resources available with government. You should aim to assess:

○ expenditure on sanitation-related services by municipalities and other government departments, distinguishing between locally and centrally raised funds

○ possible sources of private sector finance

○ resources available with sanitation users and the organizations that represent them.

Consideration of institutional and human resources should include but not be confined to government agencies. Investigations should also cover:

○ private sector organizations – contractors, consultants and financial institutions

○ civil society organizations – NGOs and CBOs.

It may be useful to commission studies to assess the capacity of typical organizations in the various sectors. What are the current resource needs of these organizations in terms of both finances and human capital and what is constraining their ability to contribute to the provision of better sanitation services?

Support systems. Higher levels of government may provide support to sanitation providers in the form of specific programmes (e.g. the Integrated Low Cost Sanitation programme in India). They may also provide support in the form of training and/or through special national, state or provincial government units charged with providing technical back-up to those working at the municipal level. What support systems exist and how do they operate?

Information needs at different stages of the policy development process

An incremental approach to information, similar to that proposed for planning at the municipal level, will often be appropriate for the development of policies and programmes. Within this overall process, the first task should be to ensure that an information culture exists. Where this does not already exist, development of the policy itself should not start until it has been possible to convince senior decision makers of the importance of information and to show them examples of the part that it can play in developing effective policies and programmes. National NGOs and international agencies can play a part here in stressing the importance of information and, even better, in providing examples of successful information-based sanitation initiatives.

The next stage in the process should be to collect sufficient information to obtain an overall picture of the situation. As far as is possible, the focus at this stage should be on existing information. Possible sources of such information include official government records, sector profiles prepared by international agencies and studies carried out by national and international consultants and NGOs. It may be worthwhile to engage a consultant to bring together information from different sources and to assess the reliability of that information. Before doing this, be clear about what you want to achieve and make sure that this understanding is reflected in clear terms of reference.

Do not go into too much detail at this stage. The aim should be to ensure that you are approximately right. Avoid placing reliance on seemingly accurate information that later proves to be precisely wrong. For instance, officials may base their assessment of the success of a particular low-cost sanitation programme on the number of low-cost sanitation units built through the programme. However, this information will mean relatively little if most of the intended users are not using the units, as is too often the case. The principle of triangulation is important here. Relatively unstructured qualitative assessments of existing programmes, based on looking at what actually happens and talking to people, can provide more useful information than large formal surveys that do not ask the right questions.

Where initial investigations reveal gaps in existing information, the policy development process should allow time and space for those gaps to be filled through a process analogous to the developing solutions stage of the planning process at the municipal and local levels. The WASPOLA process described in Box 4.4 provides a good example of this step-wise approach to the assembly of information with early review of existing information leading into the commissioning of case studies designed to explore specific areas of concern. These case studies will normally focus on specific towns and may involve investigation of representative areas within those towns. While existing information may provide a starting point for the investigations, there will often be a need for additional surveys. A study of existing training provision and its relevance to the needs of municipalities and other service providers may also be required.

Key points in this chapter

1. To be strategic, planning must be information-based.

2. Information can be qualitative, quantitative, spatial or definitive. In most situations, it will be useful to combine information of different types and from different sources.

3. A person's information requirements will depend on their role in sanitation provision. The information collected should be relevant to the needs of its intended users and available in a form that is accessible to them.

4. Information needs will also vary with the stage reached in the planning process. At the understanding problems stage, the need is for mainly qualitative information on the current problems and the options for dealing with them. As the planning process proceeds, more detailed information will be required.

5. A good map base is important, particularly for drainage and sewerage planning. Maps should be available at the municipal level in a form that can be copied.

6. Studies in specific areas, perhaps linked to proposals to develop improved services, can be useful first step in developing an improved information base.

7. In the medium to long term, the aim should be to bring the results of such studies into an integrated information system. If an accurate map base, computers and computer skills are available, this might take the form of a GIS.

8. Like municipal and local plans, policies should be information-based. A staged process, which allows proposals to be developed as information becomes available, will often be appropriate for policy development.

Chapter 7 endnotes

1 The concept of 'recognizability' is just one of a number of interesting concepts discussed by Dudley (1993).

2 The drive to provide improved information systems often comes from external stakeholders. All too often, municipal managers see these initiatives as being self-contained entities that have little to do with the other aspects of the municipality's other management systems.

3 For instance, information provided by the municipal authorities in Bharatpur showed that most households disposed of their wastewater to individual septic tanks. Most or all of these septic tanks had been provided and financed by householders themselves.

4 This list is loosely based on the list of requirements identified by the USAID Environmental Health Project (EHP) and its partners in the course of its work on the development of materials to assist the development of national sanitation policies. Details of this work and other activities undertaken by EHP are available on the EHP website www.ehproject.org/.

CHAPTER 8
Choosing an appropriate sanitation technology

IN CHAPTER 2 we suggested that the choice of an appropriate technology helps to ensure that sanitation services are affordable to their users and thus operationally sustainable over time. However, there are many approaches and technologies and the choices between them may appear anything but clear at first sight. The first part of this chapter suggests a logical approach to ordering choices while keeping in mind the need to consider and, where necessary, inform the demands of sanitation users.

Sanitation technologies can only be considered appropriate if they are affordable and users are willing to pay for them and so the latter part of the chapter focuses on affordability and willingness to pay. Both require an understanding of the cost of the proposed sanitation option and so an introduction to methods of assessing sanitation costs is provided. This leads into discussion of methods for assessing willingness to pay for sanitation services and, where necessary, reducing costs to a level that is affordable to intended users. Brief details of specific technologies are given in Appendix 2.

Approaches to sanitation selection

In the past, the accepted approach to sanitation selection was based on the assumption that the professional knows best. This approach, which is closely linked to the planning model introduced in Chapter 1, makes use of specialist knowledge but pays little attention to the knowledge and concerns of the intended users. It therefore risks providing people with services that they do not want. In theory, it has been displaced by more demand-based approaches to sanitation selection although in practice it is still followed by many government officials.

As we have already seen, the current 'received wisdom' is that sanitation choice should be demand-led. Sanitation is seen as a commodity, to be sold like any other commodity, for instance a car. People should be offered a menu of sanitation choices, including sewerage, pour-flush latrines and pit latrines from which they can choose. This approach is flawed in that it assumes that all, or at least most, sanitation technologies are equally possible and appropriate in any given situation. As we will see shortly, this will rarely be the case. We have already noted in Chapter 1 that this 'market driven' approach to sanitation provision ignores the fact that people's sanitation choices may impact on their neighbours and that different stakeholders may have different objectives. Also, there is a real danger that the choices of community members will relate to their immediate needs and ignore the wider environmental implications of their sanitation choices.

Others would argue that users should be allowed a completely free sanitation choice. This approach is demand-based but pays little attention to the need to inform demand, and underestimates the value of 'professional' knowledge. It assumes that all stakeholders have the same priorities and will act as a coherent group at the local level. The focus on local demand means that the approach encourages local ad hoc activity at the expense of overall planning.

In practice, the best approach to sanitation choice will be one that:

○ recognizes that existing conditions, particularly the availability of water, are likely to favour some sanitation technologies and preclude the use of others

○ takes account of the knowledge, concerns and priorities of both sanitation users and professionals.

When considering sanitation choices, ask yourself 'how might the technology fail?'.[1] This question will provide a framework for considering all the factors that might affect the performance of a particular technology in any given situation and in particular whether the financial and institutional resources needed to ensure its success are available.

People will only adopt ideas and hence technologies that they consider to be compatible with their own image of themselves. So, it is important to explore what the intended users think about the various sanitation options that might be offered to them. Bear in mind the fact that different groups are likely to have different assumptions about the advantages and disadvantages of different approaches. For instance, women may attach more importance than men to having facilities available at the household level. Do not assume that the views of potential users will be fixed. Indeed, throughout this book we emphasize the need to inform demand so as to ensure that the right choices are made.

Categories of sanitation technology

Sanitation technologies can be categorized in terms of whether they are:

○ 'Wet' or 'dry' – in other words whether they are or are not dependent on water to transport excreta.

○ On-site, hybrid or off-site. On-site systems retain both liquid and solids on or near the point at which they are produced. (Most on-site options deal only with excreta and separate arrangements may have to be made for the removal of sullage water.) We use the term 'hybrid' for systems that retain solids on or near the plot but remove wastewater. They can be used either for WC wastes alone or for all waste flows. Off-site systems remove both excreta and sullage water from the vicinity of the plot for disposal elsewhere.

Table 8.1 shows how various sanitation technologies fit into these categories.

A step-wise procedure for sanitation choice

Bearing in mind the categorization of sanitation technologies given in Table 8.1, we now suggest a simple logical process for choosing the most appropriate technology for any given situation. This process is built round a number of key questions, as indicated in Figure 8.1. The first question is about the level of service to be provided while the others concern the technology to be used to deliver that level of service. Each is now considered in more detail.

At what level should sanitation facilities be provided?

Whenever possible, sanitation facilities should be provided at the household level. This option provides the best results in terms of convenience and impact upon health. It is often assumed that, despite these advantages, household-level sanitation facilities cannot be provided because of lack of space, lack of funds or both.

CHOOSING AN APPROPRIATE SANITATION TECHNOLOGY

Table 8.1 Categorization of sanitation technologies

	Dry systems	Wet systems
On-site	Various forms of pit latrine, composting latrines, dry box and dehydrating latrines	WCs/pour-flush toilets connected to leach pits and via septic tanks to soakaways
Partially on-site (hybrid systems)		WCs/pour-flush toilets connected via interceptor tanks to drains and sewers
Off-site	Bucket latrines and their variations (generally considered unacceptable on health grounds) Vaults and cartage systems (used in Japan but not currently feasible in developing countries)	WCs/pour-flush toilets connected to sewers Cess pits and tanks (from which liquid and solid wastes are removed regularly)

But latrines can be provided on very small plots. For instance, World Bank-funded sites and services schemes in Mumbai, India provided individual pour-flush toilets on plots with areas as small as 22 m². In other Indian cities, household-level sanitation has been reported on plots of just 14 m² (Cotton and Saywell, 1998) (see Figure 8.2).

Where it seems that people cannot afford household-level facilities, consider ways of reducing the cost of sanitation facilities. Look first at the latrine superstructure. Why should this be constructed in brick if every other building on the plot uses cheaper materials? The use of simple pre-cast pit latrine slabs in Mozambique (Box 4.3) shows how creative thinking can reduce costs to an affordable level.

Regardless of this, the increased convenience and health benefits associated with household facilities justify some

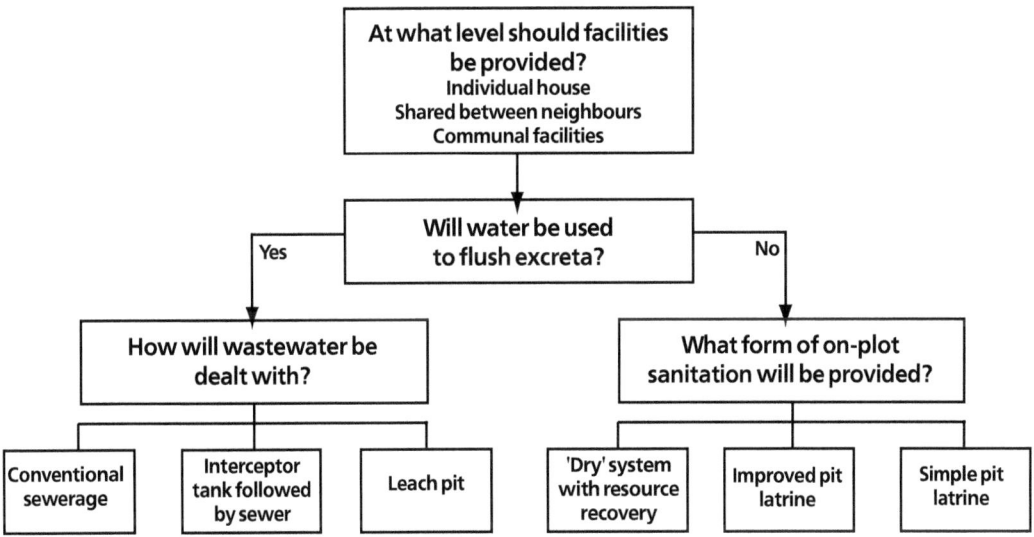

Figure 8.1 Key questions to inform sanitation choice

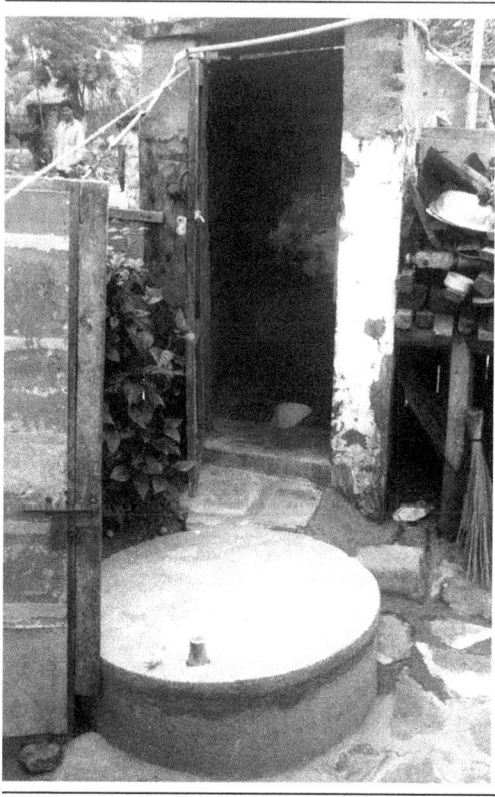

Figure 8.2 On-plot provision does not need much space

This latrine has been constructed on a small plot. The latrine itself occupies less than 1 m². In this case, the leachpit is located within the plot but it would also be possible to locate the pit or pits in a street or lane immediately outside the plot.

[Photo: Darren Saywell]

degree of capital subsidy where users would otherwise not be able to afford them. Where this is not possible, it may be worth introducing a scheme that encourages users to save towards the cost of improved facilities.

There could be situations in which infrastructure improvements, including the provision of household level sanitation, lead landlords to increase rents and/or attract higher income people to an area so that existing occupiers are squeezed out in a process of 'gentrification'. In areas in which most residents are tenants, it may be that shared or even communal facilities offer a safer option for existing residents.

Shared facilities can be used where there is insufficient space on-site for individual household latrines but where it is possible to identify places close to plots where groups of toilets can be built. Access to these toilets can be controlled by either:

o locating toilets in 'semi-private' space, which is only accessible to the intended users[2] (see Figure 8.3), or

o providing intended users with keys.

Some sanitation programmes still start from the assumption that communal facilities offer the only affordable option for low-income people. In practice, communal facilities may not be that much cheaper than household level or shared facilities, a point that is illustrated by the construction details of the three examples shown in Figures 8.2 – 8.4. Communal facilities are often poorly maintained and at worst can become so unpleasant that people stop using them. This can make them very expensive in relation to their useful life. Where a user charge is made, this may be set at a level that discourages people from using the facilities on a regular basis. Indeed, the cost to users over time may be greater

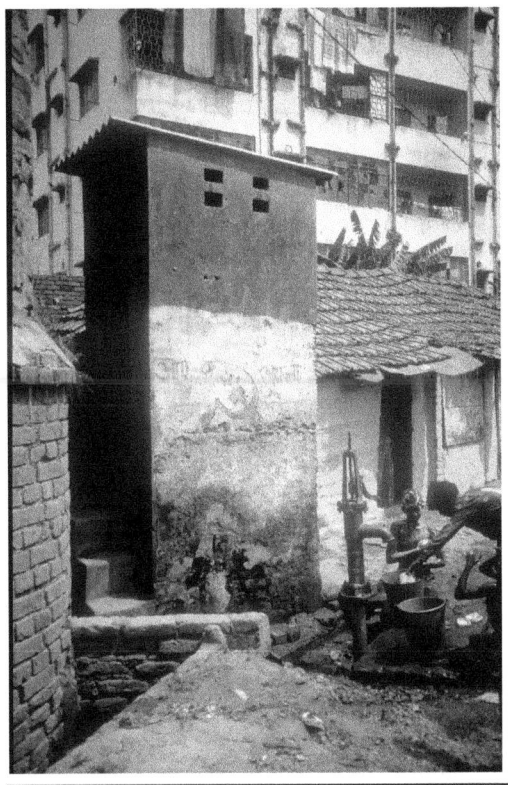

Figure 8.3 Shared toilets may be appropriate

This toilet block is typical of many found in 'slum' areas in Kolkata, India. The thika tenancy holdings house 10–20 families in one-room huts clustered around a central open space. The entrance is narrow so that the central space and toilet are not accessible to outsiders.

Figure 8.4 Communal facilities in public places

A public toilet in Pune, Maharashtra, operated by the NGO Sulabh International. Comparison of this toilet with that shown in Figure 8.2 suggests that communal latrines are not necessarily cheaper than on-plot facilities.

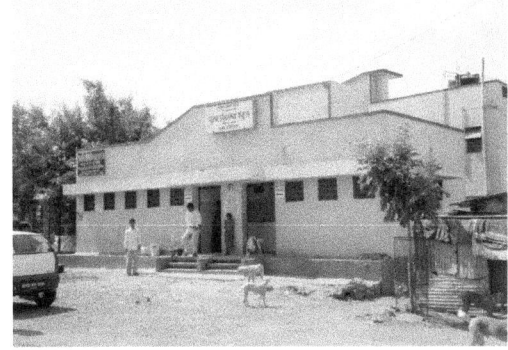

than that of household or shared facilities.

Where they are used in public places such as markets, communal latrines should be viewed as a supplement to good sanitation in or close to the home and careful consideration should be given to the way in which they are to be managed.

Where there is no alternative to the use of communal facilities, perhaps because people's tenure is not secure or a settlement has grown so dense that there is no room for any other options, explore options for involving users in the management of latrines. This approach has been successfully adopted by the NGO SPARC in Mumbai and Pune (see Box 10.3).

Will water be used to flush excreta?

Sanitation facilities can be broadly divided into wet systems, those that use water to flush faeces, and dry systems, those that do not require water. Do not assume that a wet system will automatically provide a higher level of service than a dry system. Unless water is available on or close to the plot, a dry system will usually provide a better level of service because a wet system will not work.

As a first step to choosing between wet and dry systems, ask the following questions:

○ Is water available on or close to sanitation facilities?

○ Do people use water for anal cleansing?

If the answer to both questions is yes, a wet system will normally be the best system, although there will be a need to consider how to deal with the wastewater produced.

Where people use water for anal cleansing but water is not available close to sanitation facilities, the preferred option may be to improve the water supply to the level at which pour-flush toilets can be used. Even where people do not use water for anal cleansing, people will often choose a wet system with a pour-flush toilet, which they see as a higher level of service. If water is available close to the plot, the wet system should be possible. Nevertheless, you should at least explore with them the possibility of using a dry system with separate arrangements for the disposal of sullage (wastewater from kitchens and bathrooms). This has the advantage that the polluting effect of sullage water on receiving waters will be less than that of the combined discharge of WC and sullage water.

If the answer to both questions is no, the best option will normally be a dry system and the key issue becomes whether this should be a simple pit latrine system or something more complex and ambitious.

How will wastewater be dealt with?

This question is important for wet systems, which produce faecally contaminated water that:

○ is potentially harmful to the health of anyone who comes into contact with it

○ will cause pollution and environmental degradation unless arrangements are made for its safe disposal.

Even where a dry on-plot system is used for excreta disposal, there may still be a need to deal with sullage water although the problem of disposal will be greatly reduced.

As indicated in Table 8.1, the options for disposal of contaminated water fall into three broad categories.

○ On-site systems which allow wastewater to percolate into the ground from some form of leach pit, perhaps preceded by a septic tank. Faecal solids digest in the pit or tank but eventually have to be removed and disposed of in way that is hygienic and does not harm the environment.

○ Hybrid systems, which remove faecal solids in an interceptor tank located on or close to the plot. The effluent from the tank is then transported in a sewer or open drain to the disposal/treatment point. (The latter system is unsatisfactory in many respects but is common in informal areas in some parts of the world.)

○ Conventional sewerage, which transports both liquid and solid wastes away from individual plots. Note that sewerage transports wastewater rather than treating it and suitable treatment will normally be required if the wastewater is discharged to the environment or used for irrigation.

Factors influencing the choice between these options include:

○ The availability of water. Sewerage requires more water than the other systems, typically at least 60 litres per person per day as against the 25–30 litres per person per day required to transport wastes to a local leach pit or interceptor tank.

○ Population density. In general, the higher the population density, the more difficult will it be to dispose of wastewater on-site.

○ The likelihood of pollution of either ground or surface water. In general:

• sewage treatment will be required to ensure that the effluent from off-site and hybrid systems does not harm the environment and/or crops irrigated with waste water

• pathogens from leach-pits and drain fields will present a risk to health if they enter groundwater that is used for drinking purposes. This will only be a problem where either the ground is fissured or the groundwater source used for drinking is close to the surface. Even then, the health risk may be less that that caused by allowing untreated black water to flow through housing areas.

○ The capital and recurrent costs of the various options and the way in which these are divided between users and institutional providers. We will return to this later in this chapter.

○ The skills needed to construct, operate and maintain systems. In general:

• on-site systems can be constructed by individual households or local artisans and have simple management requirements
• off-site systems require greater construction and management skills, and it is particularly important that sewers are laid to constant gradients, that pipes are properly jointed and that unwanted solid materials are excluded from the system
• interceptor tank systems are less susceptible to blockages caused by irregular falls and poor workmanship than conventional sewers and thus fall somewhere between the other two options in terms of their skill requirements.

○ The degree of cooperation needed between the different stakeholders. On-site systems require less cooperation between users than other systems.

Bearing in mind the information given above, Figure 8.5 provides a simple algorithm for determining the most appropriate wastewater disposal option. It is meant for guidance and the figures are recommendations and should not be taken as absolute. Use it with discretion rather than as a rigid tool.

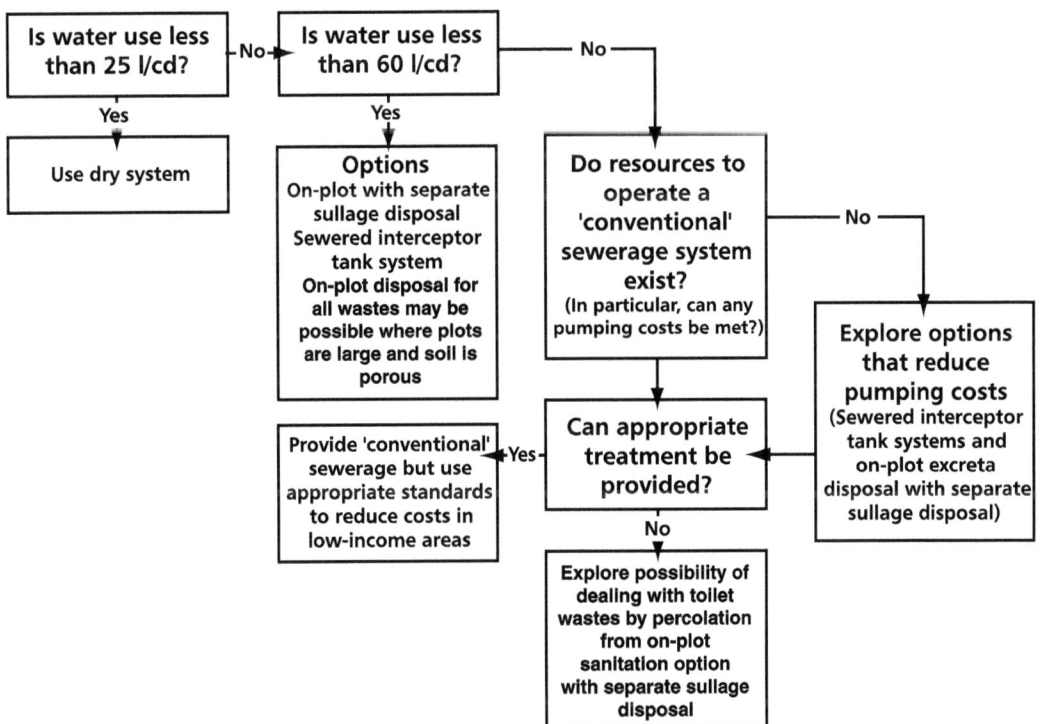

Figure 8.5 Algorithm for wastewater disposal from 'wet' sanitation systems

What form of dry on-site sanitation will be provided?

If initial assessment suggests that a dry system offers the best option, the basic choice is between different on-site options. Off-site options do exist but these are either insanitary (bucket latrine systems and their variations) or unsuitable for use in developing countries (vault and cartage systems such as those found in Japan).

The choice is then between a basic pit latrine, some form of ventilated improved latrine (VIP) and some form of 'ecological' sanitation offering resource recovery. Further information on these options is given in Appendix 2. The choice will be influenced by cost, acceptability to users and the possibility of utilizing wastes as a resource for agriculture.

Explore the advantages and disadvantages of the different options with local people. Make sure that they understand how each option is meant to work and what operation and maintenance commitments they will be required to make. Where there is no local experience of an approach, it should always be piloted and demonstrated on a small scale before attempts are made to introduce it more widely. This is particularly important for ecological approaches, which perhaps require a greater level of user commitment than simpler methods.

If considering an ecological approach, ask whether people will use the toilet as intended, diverting urine and spreading ash on the chamber contents? Will they be willing and able to use the pit contents as a fertilizer or soil conditioner? The answers to these questions are more likely to be positive if there is a tradition of dry sanitation and excreta reuse, as in Vietnam and China. In the case of VIPs, a key question is whether or not people will be willing to use a latrine with a dark interior.

Costing viable sanitation options

Following the procedure described in the previous pages will help to eliminate unsuitable sanitation choices, leaving a choice between the limited range of technologies that might be feasible in the local situation. The next stage in the planning process will be to consider the costs of possible technologies. Only when these costs have been calculated will it be possible to go on to assess whether they are affordable to their intended users.

When considering the cost of providing a sanitation service it is necessary to take account of:

○ its capital cost, what it costs to build it

○ its recurrent cost, that of operating and maintaining it.

If recurrent costs are ignored, there is a real danger that the sanitation service will not be sustainable.

When comparing the costs of different options, bear in mind that existing facilities represent 'sunk' costs, in other words those that have already been incurred, and so do not need to be taken into account when calculating the capital costs. It may be, for instance, that every house has a septic tank from which wastewater is discharged into an existing drain. It would be possible to fill in these septic tanks and replace the whole system with conventional sewers. Alternatively, the septic tanks could be connected to small-bore sewers to create a sewered interceptor tank system. When comparing the options, the cost of providing the septic tanks does not need to be taken into account because they are already there. The cost of periodically emptying the tanks, on the other hand, must be included in the financial comparison.[3]

There are two broad approaches to the estimation of both capital and recurrent costs.

- Calculate the cost of a single unit and multiply this by the number of units required, to calculate the cost of the whole scheme.
- Calculate the cost of the whole scheme and then divide by the number of households served to arrive at an average cost per household.

The first should be used for on-site technologies and the on-plot components of networked schemes.

For networked systems, such as sewerage, drainage and solid waste disposal, the normal procedure is to calculate the capital and recurrent costs of the whole scheme and then divide these by the number of households to be served to arrive at the average costs per household of the public or shared components of the scheme. To obtain the total capital cost per household, the cost of any on-site facilities required to complement off-plot improvements will have to be calculated and added to the cost of public components in order to arrive at the total capital cost per household.

Unit costs for on-site technologies and components

The simplest option for estimating the cost of a standard unit (for instance a pit latrine to be produced to a standard design) is to ask several contractors to give you an estimate of their all-in price for building it. Unfortunately, this gives you no information on the costs of the different components of the unit and this makes it difficult to decide how much to adjust the price to allow for any modifications required on site.

A better approach will be to break the cost down to in relation to the various activities to be undertaken. (In the pit latrine example given above, components would include the pit, any pit lining, the slab and the superstructure walls, etc.). The quantities and costs for each individual item can be recorded on a simple schedule, in the form of a standard bill of quantities, as indicated in Box 8.1.

The costs for individual activities may be estimated from either:

- market rates for complete items, including the cost of labour and any contractors' profit (taken from the prices quoted by contractors for previous schemes), or by
- building up an estimate of the cost of a particular item from the quantities of materials and labour inputs required to complete it. Standard rates can then be obtained for each unit of material or labour and the cost obtained by multiplying each quantity by the appropriate standard rate. In some countries, this information may be available in the form of a standard schedule of rates. The total amount for that activity is then obtained by multiplying the quantity by the rate.

If you are not familiar with cost estimation methods yourself, you should seek advice from an engineer who is familiar with local costs and costing methods.

If the work is being carried out or managed by the community, it will be useful to monitor the implementation of some typical units at the pilot stage. The purchase costs of materials and the labour inputs required to complete the work should be recorded. Ideally, this information can be developed to give unit costs for future estimation purposes.

Estimating the cost of a networked system

The first step in estimating the cost for a networked system is to establish a hierarchy of components. The costs of the different

Box 8.1 Standard bill of quantities type schedule for a ventilated improved pit (VIP) latrine

Item no.	Description	Quantity	Unit	Rate	Amount Qty × rate
1	Excavate in laterite soil to depth of 5 m and for pit diameter of 1.25 m.	6.94	cubic metres		
2	Provide and lay brickwork in collar below slab	0.8	cubic metres		
3	Provide and place concrete in 75mm deep cover slab, including allowance for forming opening in slab and footrests as shown on the drawing	2.4	square metres		
4	Provide and lay 112mm thick brickwork in superstructure	10	square metres		
5	Provide and fix door and frame, dimensions 1.9 m by 0.75 m	Item	–		
6	Provide and fix roof, galvanized steel sheeting	2.25	square metres		
7	Form ventilation opening in superstructure, 0.5 m by 0.3 m	Item	–		
8	Provide and fix 150mm diameter plastic vent pipe, in accordance with specification	Item	–		
9	Provide and securely fix plastic-coated wire mesh at top of vent pipe	Item	–		

components can then be estimated as follows.

The cost of primary and secondary facilities, such as main drains and collector sewers, should be calculated on a case-by-case basis. Prepare unit costs for drains and sewers of different sizes and calculate the length of each size required. Costs can be summarized in a table giving the length of each sewer or drain leg, its size, its cost per unit length, any additional costs required, for instance for road reinstatement. The total cost can then be derived from these data. Make separate allowance for items such as pumping stations. It will often be advisable to seek professional assistance for the design and costing of any primary and secondary facilities required.

Estimate the cost of tertiary level facilities (local sewers and drains) using the following procedure.

1. Choose a number of locations that are typical of different types and densities of development and determine their areas.

2. Determine the number of households

contained within each area (or the number that can reasonably be expected to be contained in the area if all vacant plots are developed).

3. Design a tertiary sewerage and/or drainage system to serve that area, assuming that the system will connect to a secondary facility at the edge of the area.

4. Prepare and cost a schedule of quantities or estimate the materials and labour that would be required for this tertiary system. The cost estimate should exclude house connections, which should be included in household-level estimates.

5. Divide the total calculated cost by the area covered to provide the average cost per hectare and by the number of households within the area to give the average cost per household.

The results for areas having the same or similar character should be averaged. These results can then be used to estimate the average cost of tertiary facilities for all areas having similar characteristics.

The cost of household-level components (WCs and house drains) can be calculated on the basis of typical house layouts, using the same approach as that used for self-contained on-site technologies. The cost of these components will normally be borne directly by the householders, as will the cost of connections to sewers. They do not, therefore, have to be considered when estimating public costs but do have to be taken into account when estimating affordability to users and willingness to pay for improvements.

Recurrent costs

Recurrent costs are those that are incurred for the operation and maintenance of facilities, including overall management costs. Recurrent costs will vary from place to place, depending on local conditions. For instance, the cost of operating and maintaining a sewer is likely to be much higher in flat areas with poor solid waste collection than in an area with good gradients and adequate solid waste collection services.

Where limited information on recurrent costs is available, as will often be the case, it may be necessary to introduce model operation and maintenance procedures in a range of representative areas and to record the costs. The stages in doing this would be as follows.

1. Select suitable areas or facilities – the areas should be large enough to enable meaningful comparisons to be drawn, perhaps a whole ward or housing development.

2. Agree on the operation and maintenance procedures to be followed.

3. Implement those procedures over a period of weeks, monitoring the costs, the quality of service provided and any problems that are encountered.

4. If necessary, make adjustments to operation and maintenance procedures and repeat the exercise to obtain a better idea of the relationship between inputs and the outputs achieved.

5. Extrapolate the results of the exercise to the town as a whole.

Table 8.2 provides an introduction to the types of operation and maintenance cost that are likely to be incurred for a range of typical sanitation technologies.

Table 8.2 does not include tasks such as keeping pit latrine slabs clean and routine building maintenance. For household facilities, these will normally be carried out

Table 8.2 Operation and maintenance costs for different technologies

On-site technologies[4]	Sewers	Sewered interceptor tank systems
Pit latrines (and other dry systems), leach pits, septic tanks, etc.		
Pit emptying (frequency can be calculated on the basis that each person using the facility produces 40 litres of sludge per year)	Pumping costs (including pump maintenance where required)	Interceptor tank emptying and treatment of contents
	Operation and maintenance of treatment facilities (including power costs for technologies such as activated sludge)	Perhaps some pumping costs but should be possible to avoid pumping in most cases
Repair of access covers		Rehabilitation and repair. (Probably less than for conventional sewers because of fewer access points.)
Replacement of vent-pipe screen (VIPs)	Rehabilitation and repair, for instance replacement of manhole covers and (occasionally) replacement of broken sewer pipes	Operation and maintenance of treatment facilities. Possibly some reduction in cost incurred when compared with 'conventional' sewers because interceptor tanks remove some of the biochemical oxygen demand (BOD) load.
	Cleaning and desilting. For conventional sewers laid to self-cleansing falls, these costs should, in theory, be low. In practice, many sewers in low-income areas receive high silt loads and are laid to low gradients. In such circumstances, cleaning and desilting costs may be high	

by family members and will not incur financial costs. For communal latrines, cleaning the latrine will normally be part of the caretaker/attendant's job and the cost to be considered will be his or her salary. However, there may be a need to allow for the purchase of cleaning materials.

Those who are concerned with either policy development or sanitation planning at the municipal level will need to estimate all of these costs.

Those working at the local level may not need to estimate all the costs from first principles. For instance, if you are considering the cost of local sewers, connected to a municipal system, your concern will be with the tariff that you will be charged rather than the cost of treatment and operating and maintaining the municipal sewer system.

Willingness to pay for improved sanitation services

Up to this point, we have been concerned with the selection of an appropriate sanitation technology and estimating the cost of that technology. We now turn to the important issue of willingness to pay for improved facilities.

It will normally be necessary to estimate willingness to pay for sanitation services when either:

○ users are currently paying much less than the full cost of sanitation services or

○ there are plans to improve the level of

service and/or protect the environment by providing improved facilities, thus incurring increased costs.

User willingness to pay for improved services will mean little if service providers are unwilling to charge for those services.[5] So, it will be equally important to assess willingness to charge for services. Willingness to pay studies may play a part in changing the mindsets of service providers and bringing about increased willingness to charge but only if:

o resistance to raising charges stems from an unproved belief that the poor cannot pay higher charges

o those who make decisions on charges are willing to accept the evidence offered by a willingness to pay study that people are prepared to pay more for sanitation services.

The second condition is important. Government decision makers may keep services charges unrealistically low for a number of reasons, not just a belief that the poor cannot pay. In many situations, these reasons are 'political' in that politicians believe that low prices help to maintain their popularity. In such circumstances, the initial focus should be on convincing key decision makers that the only way to ensure sustainable services is to raise charges to realistic levels and maintain them at those levels. A willingness to pay exercise might form part of the strategy for raising awareness but will rarely be enough, in itself, to change deeply entrenched ways of thinking. Rather, the initial focus should be on advocacy, perhaps involving demonstration of the improvements in service provision that can be achieved if greater efforts are made to recover costs and use the additional finances generated effectively.

Approaches to estimating willingness to pay

Four broad approaches to estimating willingness to pay are introduced and briefly discussed below.[6]

The simplest is the affordability rule of thumb approach. This is based on the assumption that people can afford to pay a set percentage of their income (typically set at 3–5%) for water and sanitation services. It is not accurate because income is only one of the factors that determine willingness to pay for water and sanitation services. On the other hand, where income data is available, the approach needs very few resources. Use it as a first check to determine whether the current tariff for water and sanitation services is unrealistically low. Where this is the case, rule of thumb figures may help to convince decision makers that there is scope to raise prices.

Revealed preference (RP) methods measure demand indirectly by examining current expenditure on services, for instance the amount paid to use a communal sanitation facility or to a private sweeper to remove solid waste. They may involve the use of a variety of methods, including participant observation, small questionnaire surveys, focus group discussions and key informant interviews.

Clearly, RP methods will not reveal the maximum amount that people are willing to pay for services if the price they are current paying is subsidized and/or they are only paying part of the true economic price of a service. Box 8.2 illustrates the point that not all subsidies are explicit. RP methods will, however, provide an indication of the minimum that people will be prepared to pay for a service and this in itself will be useful, particularly where the amount that poor people pay for services is considerably more than that assumed by officials and policy makers.

> **Box 8.2 Implicit and explicit subsidies – examples from sewerage schemes in Pakistan**
>
> As already indicated in Chapter 5, community-constructed lane (tertiary) sewers are common in many Pakistani cities. In most cases, the participating households pay the full construction cost of the sewer and their household connections and also pay for essential maintenance as and when it is required. Where a good fall is available, as for instance in Orangi, Karachi, sewage is discharged to the nearest natural drainage channel. In flatter areas, it is more likely to be discharged to a collector drain or sewer provided by the municipal authorities.
>
> The fact that community members are paying the cost of providing, operating and maintaining local facilities does not mean that there is no subsidy. Where sewage is discharged to the nearest natural watercourse, someone else is likely to have to bear the costs of the resultant pollution. Even where sewage is discharged to a municipal drain or sewer, it is still unlikely that it will be treated. In such cases, the sewerage tariff may cover the financial cost of operating the system but will rarely if ever cover any environmental costs resulting from the discharge of untreated sewage to natural watercourses.
>
> In flat cities, sewage almost always has to be pumped and someone has to pay the cost of that pumping (see Box 5.3). Where connections from community-built systems are unauthorized, as is frequently the case, community members make no contribution to the costs of the municipal system.

RP methods should normally be based on information from the area within which action is planned. It might seem a simple step to use similar methods to estimate willingness to pay in one area and then to transfer the findings to another similar location. For instance, if people in one low-income settlement have installed and paid for local sewers or leach pits, it would seem reasonable to assume that people in other similar areas should also be willing and able to pay for such facilities. Care is required when using this 'information transfer' approach since apparently similar areas may have very different characteristics. These may be social in character, for instance people in one area may have security of tenure and those in another may not. Physical factors may also be important. For instance, many people in informal areas around Cairo, Egypt, discharge wastewater to cess pits, which have to be regularly emptied.

Seepage from pits can allow an increase in the intervals at which the pit has to be emptied. People in areas with poor ground permeability, requiring more frequent pit emptying, are more likely to be willing to connect to a sewer than those living in areas with good ground permeability.

Despite these drawbacks, the information transfer method is simple and, provided that it is used with due care, would appear to be a valid approach to the estimation of minimum willingness to pay at the municipal and local levels. Only use it where you are sure that the areas being compared have similar physical and socio-economic characteristics and, if possible, back up your findings using other methods. Where possible, local stakeholders should be involved in the investigation. This will help to ensure that factors affecting willingness to pay are not overlooked. It will also provide opportunities for the transfer of ideas and information between communities.

Contingent valuation (CV) methods involve asking people what they are willing to pay for different sanitation services in carefully designed and realistic hypothetical scenarios (Whittington 1998). The assumed advantage of CV methods is that they provide a way of estimating willingness to pay for different service levels.[7] The aim is to develop a 'demand curve' which provides information on the quantity of a commodity (such as water) that people are likely to demand at different price levels. With this information, it should be possible to assess the degree to which facilities have to be upgraded and extended to cover demand. This scenario does not work too well for sanitation. A pit latrine is not necessarily a lower standard of service than a WC connected to a sewer. If there is no water on or near the plot, it may actually represent a higher standard of service.

A more appropriate use of CV, which is closer to the use for which it was originally developed, is to assess willingness to pay for different levels of environmental protection. The key question then becomes how much people are prepared to pay to ensure that their liquid and solid wastes are treated or otherwise dealt with in a way that prevents harm to the environment. Do not be surprised if this amount is small. There is likely to be a need to inform users of the problems caused by untreated wastes and perhaps enforce environmental legislation that prevents people from discharging untreated wastes to the natural environment.

This brings us to an important point relating to informing demand. The amount that people are willing to pay is unlikely to remain static over time. In most cases, people's willingness to pay for a service will be influenced by the information that is available to them. Involving local people in investigations of what people are doing in other similar areas may well lead to an increase in their awareness and a consequent increase (or indeed decrease) in their willingness to pay for a service.

This very brief review suggests that CV methods can give misleading results unless a CV expert is involved in their design, implementation and analysis. Until now, most CV exercises have been carried out by a fairly small group of such experts, many of whom have been expatriates. Countries such as India are developing in-country expertise but the relatively high cost of CV means that it should be used sparingly.

Because of their relatively high cost, CV methods are likely to be useful mainly for the development of policy. If you are planning to commission a CV survey, think carefully about the information that you want from it. Sanitation specialists should be involved in the design of the survey alongside economists in order to make sure that the options offered are realistic.

Boxes 8.3 and 8.4 give examples of the use of different approaches to estimating willingness to pay, illustrating the point that there is no single right method and that even the simplest methods can yield useful results if used judiciously.

Options for reducing costs

A common response when the cost of a service exceeds its intended users' ability or willingness to pay is to reduce the level of service by opting for shared or communal facilities. This approach should be used with care, since the real cost of such facilities may be higher than expected if the facilities are poorly maintained and quickly fall into disuse. Also, user charges may deter poor people from using communal latrines.

> **Box 8.3 Triangulating the results of 'rule of thumb' and revealed preference methods**
>
> In Faisalabad, Pakistan, the standard monthly tariff for water and sanitation services in 2000 was Rs 65 per month. The average household income obtained from household surveys in the areas covered by the Faisalabad Area Upgrading Project (FAUP) was around Rs 3000 per month. The rule of thumb assumption that people will be willing to pay 4% of their household income for water and sanitation services, suggests that they should be willing to pay around Rs 120 per month for these services, around twice what they are paying at present. This simple calculation suggests that people could and should be paying more for water and sanitation services. This conclusion is supported by the fact that small surveys in one FAUP area revealed that some households were paying up to Rs 150 per month to purchase 'sweet' water from vendors. In this area, as in other areas in Faisalabad, the groundwater is saline and people do not like to drink it.
>
> This example also illustrates the main disadvantage of the information transfer method. Willingness to pay for vended water varies between different parts of Faisalabad, partly because the groundwater is some areas is more saline than that in others. In such circumstances, the results of the survey in one settlement cannot automatically be applied to other sociologically similar settlements. Despite this caveat, the investigations do suggest that there is considerable scope to increase water and sewerage tariffs in Faisalabad. Given the political reluctance to increase charges, more sophisticated investigations using CV methods would not appear to be justified at present.

A better option for reducing costs is to explore ways of reducing the cost of the preferred technology. An example of what this means in practice is provided by the example of 'condominial' sewerage in Brazil.[8] This reduces costs by:

○ locating tertiary (condominial) sewers at the back of plots, within the front boundary of plots or in the sidewalk as appropriate, so reducing the length of connections and eliminating or reducing traffic loads so that sewers can be laid at shallow depths

○ adopting appropriate standards, for instance allowing a minimum sewer diameter of 100 mm rather than the 150 mm or 225 mm minimum standard that is common in other countries

○ developing innovative details, for instance using prefabricated chambers and replacing some chambers with prefabricated plastic 'rodding eyes'.

Options for reducing the cost of on-site technologies include:

○ using lower-cost materials for the latrine superstructure – the latrine does not have to be built of brick or stone

○ using some form of 'san-plat', a light concrete slab that can be laid on top of a cheaper pit latrine cover, so reducing the cost of the cover while retaining a hard cleanable surface around the defecation hole.

These examples show that careful design, using standards that are developed to suit local conditions, can result in considerable cost reductions. However, as with reductions

Box 8.4 Contingent valuation and solid waste disposal in Chennai, India

Anand (1999) provides a good example of the use of contingent valuation. His work focused on solid waste collection in Chennai, India, and in particular on the Civic Exnora model for primary (local) solid waste collection. Civic Exnora units are found in all but the highest and lowest income areas in the city. Each unit covers one or more streets and is responsible for the management of local waste collection from households and its removal to a suitable disposal point, preferably a municipal transfer station.

CV was used to explore the interest of households in improved collection services, encompassing the introduction of a Civic Exnora service (in areas where these did not already operate), transfer of the waste to a suitable disposal point and final disposal in an environmentally acceptable way. They were also asked whether they would be interested in participating in a 'zero-waste' scheme, which involved composting the waste at the local level.

Analysis of the results showed that concern for waste management was not limited to middle- and upper-income groups and that:

○ most respondents were willing to pay for primary collection
○ a significant percentage was also willing to pay for transport and disposal of the waste to the edges of the city
○ respondents were least concerned with environmentally acceptable final disposal.

The last point links with another finding of the study, that 84% of respondents were unaware of how and where solid waste disposal took place. This suggests a need to inform citizens of the importance of environmentally friendly solid waste disposal. Willingness to pay studies should not be seen as an end in themselves but part of an ongoing process to develop and inform demand.

Respondents showed little interest in local waste disposal using vermi-composting (composting pits at the household level). Indeed, no-one who was already a member of a Civic Exnora group opted for vermi-composting. This might be because their waste was being collected so that they faced no problems. It could also be that their membership of a Civic Exnora group had made them more aware of the difficulties that could arise in pursuing local self-managed solutions to waste disposal. If this is true, it confirms that knowledge affects willingness to pay.

---

in levels of service, reductions in standards should be used with care. There is no point in reducing the capital cost of a sanitation facility to the extent that subsequent operation and maintenance become problematic and therefore expensive.

If you are in doubt about the advantages and disadvantages of changes in standards, it will be best to test the changed standards on a pilot scale before introducing them more generally.

Key points in this chapter

1. The key to successful sanitation service provision is to ensure that the technology

chosen is acceptable and affordable to users, and appropriate to the situation.

2. Sanitation choices will be affected by the existing situation, not least people's assumptions and attitudes.

3. It is best to take a shared approach to sanitation choice, drawing on the information and views of both professionals and community members – the intended users.

4. When selecting a sanitation option, the first question to be answered is where the sanitation facilities should be located and the second whether water will be used for flushing excreta. Answering these questions narrows the number of options to be considered and simplifies subsequent choices.

5. Choosing the most appropriate sanitation technology for any given situation will help minimize costs. However, it will also be necessary to estimate the cost of the technology, and establish whether the intended users are able and willing to pay for it. In some cases, it may be necessary to examine ways of reducing the cost of a technology to a level that is attractive to potential users.

6. It will not be possible to calculate the cost of every on-site facility and local network. So, the costs of such facilities should be calculated for representative situations and extrapolated over the area of a scheme as a whole. The costs of higher-order facilities such as collector sewers are location-specific and will normally have to be calculated on a case-by-case basis.

7. There are various methods for assessing affordability and willingness to pay. Some of these, such as contingent valuation (CV), are relatively expensive and may provide inaccurate results if not carried out by trained personnel. In many cases, simpler methods will be appropriate, even though they are theoretically less accurate.

8. In many cases, lack of willingness to charge is a greater problem than lack of willingness to pay. Where this is the case, the focus should be on convincing decision makers of the benefits of charging a realistic price for environmental sanitation services. The approach taken to this task will depend on the reasons for the unwillingness to charge.

9. Where the most appropriate sanitation technologies still appear to be unaffordable, it will often be possible to reduce costs by adopting standards that are appropriate to the local situation. These will often provide cheaper services than conventional standards.

Chapter 8 endnotes

1 For a more detailed exploration of this, together with the concepts of 'recognizability' and respectability, see Dudley (1993).
2 This is possible where several housing units are clustered around a central open space, as with courtyard houses in Ghana (Mitchell and Bevan 1992) and *thika* tenancy holdings in Kolkata (Thomas 1999)
3 The maintenance costs of the conventional sewer option will not necessarily be negligible. Experience in low-income areas with poor solid waste management services suggests that conventional sewers are subject to frequent blockages. In such circumstances, the provision of interceptor tanks may actually reduce maintenance costs by concentrating maintenance requirements in one place.
4 For further information on aspects of the operation and maintenance of on-site sanitation technologies see Watt (1984), and Cotton and Saywell (1998).

5 WSP/DFID (1999) provides a discussion of this in the Indian context.
6 More detailed information on approaches to willingness to pay is provided in the DFID Guidance Manual on Water Supply and Sanitation Programmes, published by WEDC on behalf of DFID in 1998. This publication can be accessed on the internet at http://www.lboro.ac.uk/well/gm/contents.htm.
7 See Altaf and Hughes (1994), Whittington et al. (1992), and Marchand (1999) for details of studies in Burkina Faso, Ghana and the Philippines to measure the demand for improved sanitation services and solid waste management.
8 See Watson (1995) for a review of experience with condominial sewers.

CHAPTER 9
Guidelines for holding a participatory workshop

THE PROCESSES DESCRIBED in Chapters 3 to 5 used workshops to bring people together to share knowledge, make decisions and assign responsibilities for action. This chapter provides guidance on preparing for and holding participatory workshops. First, readers are reminded of the ways in which workshops can be used to facilitate the development of sanitation strategies and policies. Next, attention turns to the tasks to be undertaken to prepare for a workshop. This leads into consideration of workshop logistics and guidance on facilitating the workshop itself. Finally guidance is given on recording the results of the workshop.

How and when can workshops be used?

At the beginning of the planning or policy development process, a workshop can be used to bring the various stakeholders together in order to:

- introduce the concept of strategic planning
- explore priorities and concerns
- assign responsibilities for investigating the existing situation.

Later workshops can help to ensure that everyone remains committed to the process and that stakeholders remain aware of each other's activities and concerns. In particular, workshops provide opportunities to:

- agree on the contents of a sanitation plan
- obtain feedback on the contents of a plan or policy
- review progress in implementing a plan or policy.

Workshops require resources and skilled facilitation. So, you need to think carefully about what a workshop is likely to achieve before committing resources to it. Only hold a workshop if you are fairly sure that it will lead to action that will involve or impact upon the people who are asked to participate in it.

Preparing for the workshop

When preparing for a workshop, you need to answer a number of questions about your expectations of the workshop, who should attend it and how it should be organized. These questions are introduced and discussed below.

What outputs do we expect from the workshop?

The workshop will only be successful if you are clear about the outputs that you hope to achieve and how you intend to follow up on the workshop. In general, the outputs should include:

- clear decisions on follow-up activities, which should respond to the problems and issues identified in the course of the workshop
- clearly defined responsibilities for carrying out and coordinating these follow-up activities
- agreed arrangements for managing follow-up activities.

How many people should attend the workshop?

The number of people attending the workshop should not exceed about 50 at the very most. The best results will normally be achieved with 25–30 participants.

What organizations and groups should be represented at the workshop?

The answer to this question will obviously depend on the level at which the workshop is being held. Local workshops should include representatives of both:

o primary stakeholders, those who will be directly affected by the outcomes of a sanitation policy or plan, and in particular the low-income people who suffer from inadequate sanitation facilities

o secondary stakeholders, those who are or may be involved in the aspects of sanitation provision that are to be addressed by the workshop.

Most participants in workshops at the municipal and state/provincial levels will be representatives of secondary stakeholders. It may be difficult to ensure that people representing primary stakeholders have an input into higher level workshops but it is not impossible. At the workshop help in Quthbullapur in Andhra Pradesh, India, women from areas selected for field visits attended the session at which the findings of the field visits were analysed and gave their views on the problems in their areas. This proved to be an effective way of obtaining at least some idea of the concerns of primary stakeholders and thus triangulating the findings of workshop participants.

Who should represent the various stakeholders?

For all but the smallest workshops, it will not be practical to ask everyone who may be affected by its outcomes to attend. So, the various organizations and groups with an interest in the outcome of the workshop should be invited to select and send representatives to the workshop.

Recognized leaders and 'official' representatives are likely to see themselves as the representatives of primary stakeholders and should be invited to workshops to determine local planning priorities. However, they should not be the only community representatives. Efforts should be made to ensure that the concerns and needs of various groups, particularly the poor and disadvantaged, are not ignored. The following checklist will provide a starting point for determining whether those attending the workshop are likely to be truly representative.

o Do community representatives include both women and men?

o Do they come from all parts of the area to be covered by the plan?

o Do they represent a range of ages and occupations?

o In areas with a mix of owned and rented houses, do they represent both owners and renters?

Workshop organizers should work with community members to develop this checklist and decide on the groups to be represented at the workshop.

Representatives of secondary stakeholders should be drawn from groups that are likely to have a direct interest in the preparation and implementation of the plan. For example, local solid waste collection workers should be represented at a local workshop because they will be directly affected by any changes in solid waste collection practices agreed in the course of the workshop. On the other hand, it will be more appropriate to involve senior managers from large municipalities in a state level policy-planning workshop.

How much notice should be given?

All those individuals and groups who are to be invited should be contacted in good time – at least a week before the workshop for local stakeholders and preferably at least two weeks before for those working at the municipal level and above. Each invitee should be told where the workshop is to be held, its starting time and its length. The purpose of the workshop should also be explained together with any actions required to prepare for the workshop.

Who will chair and facilitate the workshop sessions?

The success or otherwise of workshops depends on the way in which they are chaired and facilitated. The role of the chairperson is to ensure that everyone has a chance to talk, that sessions do not overrun and that participants do not stray away from the subject of the session. The same person does not have to chair every session of the workshop. Those chosen to chair meetings will often be senior, well respected figures. However, the basic requirement of a good chairperson is that he or she is firm and fair.

The facilitator's role is to ensure that people know what they are meant to be doing in the workshop and then to help them to do it. It is important that the facilitator has:

o knowledge of participatory approaches and methods

o good communication skills.

When selecting a facilitator, first look for someone with the required knowledge and skills within one of the organizations that are involved in the strategic planning process. If no such person exists, is there someone who has good communication skills and who could be trained as a facilitator? If not, it may be necessary to use the services of a suitable outsider, perhaps a specialist consultant. Never choose a person as a facilitator just because he or she holds a senior position.

How long should the workshop last?

The workshop needs to be long enough to give people time to come together as a group to address problems and issues in a participatory way. On the other hand, for most participants, time spent attending a workshop is time that is not being used productively elsewhere. Two days is a good length for a planning workshop, since it allows a day for problem identification and analysis and a day for the identification of possible solutions. Later workshops may be shorter, lasting at most one day and perhaps only half a day.

What will be the structure and content of the workshop?

Time spent at the start of the planning process to answer this question should pay dividends later. The following points should be borne in mind when planning the workshop.

o Workshop sessions should be built around 'natural' breaks for lunch and refreshments. These give participants a chance to relax and talk informally among themselves. Between these breaks, individual sessions should, as far as is possible, be devoted to a single subject or activity.

o Ample time should be allowed for the later stages of the workshop, which will normally be devoted to the important question of what to do after the workshop. Beware of compressing these later activities into a short time period because earlier workshop sessions have overrun.

o If there are doubts about what is to be included in the workshop, it will normally be better to provide more time for a limited number of activities than to fit a large number of activities into the schedule.

- It is easy to underestimate the time required for group work. People have to be given time to develop their ideas and reach consensus on what they are going to say when they report back to the other workshop participants.
- Pay attention to the time required for field visits. How far away is the field location and how long will it take to get there? Are there likely to be problems with traffic at certain times of the day? These and similar questions will help to determine the time allowed for field visits and when they should take place.

Where should the workshop be held?

Policy workshops are often held in the national, state or provincial capital. Holding at least some workshops in other locations will help to ensure that people outside the capital have a chance to contribute to the development of policy.

Municipal level workshops may be held in a central location, perhaps a government facility or a hotel. If you are inviting people from local NGOs and CBOs, try to choose a location at which they will feel comfortable. Avoid five star hotels. When considering the option of using a government building, assess the risk that participants who work in the building will be frequently called away on other business.

Local workshops should be held as close to the area to be planned as possible, ideally within it. A school or a community hall might be an appropriate location.

Preparing information to present to the workshop

In order to ensure that the workshop participants are fully informed, it will often be necessary to present information that has been prepared in advance of the workshop. As a general rule, adopt this approach only for information to which the workshop participants would otherwise not have access and which it will not be possible to obtain in the course of the workshop.

This might include information relating to the following.

- The needs and aspirations of primary stakeholders. This will be required mainly at the municipal and policy levels. In Chapter 3, we described how two of the NGOs involved in the Bharatpur planning process carried out a consultation exercise with low- and middle-income communities and presented the results of that exercise to the workshop.
- The current and planned activities of key service providers, as they relate to the area under consideration. These key service providers might include the municipality, line agencies and NGOs that are active in sanitation. Each might be asked to make a short presentation of its activities early in the workshop.
- Government policies, with particular reference to any impact that these are likely to have on the proposed plan.

If the participants of the workshop are new to the strategic approach, it will normally be useful to prepare some information on the characteristics of the approach, drawing on the material presented earlier.

Bear the following points in mind when preparing information for presentation to the workshop.

- It will be best if the people who have collected and analysed the information are responsible for preparing it for presentation and then presenting it to the workshop.

- As far as is possible, the aim should be to present information rather than opinions. To check that the material to be presented is indeed factual, the workshop organizers should run through it with the presenters before the workshop.

- Do not present masses of data, which is only likely to confuse people. Rather, try to draw out the main facts about the existing situation.

- Prepare information in a way that is easily accessible. This may mean using videos and recordings of interviews rather than written information.

- Consider the possibility of making key pieces of information available to workshop participants in written form after it has been presented in open session.

Further guidance on the form in which the results of previous investigations might be presented to workshops is given in Box 9.1.

Workshop logistics

The workshop will only run smoothly if the organizers pay careful attention to the workshop logistics prior to the workshop itself. Some points on workshop logistics are given below and on the pages that follow.

Basic attributes of the selected workshop location

The selected location should provide the following.

- Sufficient space to allow people to 'break out' into small groups for discussions and group exercises. Ideally, this 'break-out' space should be in separate rooms. If the main workshop room is big enough, it may provide enough space for a number of groups to work separately.

- Wall space for displaying cards.

- A reliable power supply.

- Blinds or other arrangements for covering windows so that the room can be blacked out for PowerPoint and slide sessions.

Last but not least, it should be reasonably quiet. Excessive noise from traffic or a noisy air conditioner can ruin a workshop.

Seating arrangements

The seating arrangements for the workshop should provide:

- reasonable levels of comfort, bearing in mind the fact that participants will be at the workshop for up to two days

- the opportunity for all participants to see and hear what is happening at the front during shared or plenary sessions – take particular care to ensure that women are not marginalized by encouraging them to sit close to the front and ensuring that they are actively engaged in workshop sessions

- flexibility, so that people can break into small groups as and when required by the workshop timetable.

In order to provide flexibility, chairs should be light and movable so that they can face the front during plenary sessions and be moved into circles during small group sessions.

For local workshops, it may be possible for the participants to sit on mats or rugs on the floor. This helps to ensure that workshop participants treat each other as equals. On the other hand, the old and disabled may be inconvenienced by the lack of seating and their needs should be taken into account, perhaps by providing a limited number of chairs for those who want to use them.

Where chairs are provided, it will normally be useful to provide some tables, around which participants can sit for group sessions. Larger tables around the sides of the room may also be useful for writing,

Box 9.1 Options for presenting the results of previous investigations

A map or maps of the settlement, showing people's houses, the location of facilities and the location of problems such as flooding will provide an overall summary of the findings of previous investigations. Photographs and/or videos may be used to provide further detail. Basing plan information on a map base prepared in the course of community mapping exercises will increase local ownership of the presentation.

Simple graphs and tables may be used to present information on household-level facilities and conditions. The important word here is simple. Do not try to put too much information into one graph or table and concentrate on the overall picture rather than trying to show every last detail of what you know.

Information on possible technical options might be presented in the form of diagrams and drawings. However, be aware that not everyone at the workshop will be able to understand these diagrams and drawings. Photographs (in the form of slides) and models should be used wherever possible to illustrate points about technical options.

If examples of problems and possible solutions to those problems are locally available, it may be useful to take people to see them. Do not forget practical considerations. If transport is required, will it be available? Will it be possible for all participants to see what has to be seen?

preparing materials and perhaps displaying information that will be useful to the workshop participants.

Avoid formal layouts such as the horseshoe arrangements favoured by many organizers of formal conferences. Such arrangements tend to exclude those seated some distance from presenters and lack the flexibility required for small group sessions.

Equipment and materials for presenting, working with and displaying information

A workshop is a means of allowing participants to work with and present information. In order for them to do this effectively, arrangements have to be made for presenting, working with and displaying information.

Presenting information in plenary sessions

Options include flipcharts, whiteboards, overhead projectors, slide projectors and PowerPoint projectors. The advantages and disadvantages of the various options are listed in Table 9.1. Use this table to decide the most appropriate option or options for your situation. So, for instance, if the power source is unreliable, you should discard options that rely on power, or at least have alternative options available.

When preparing presentations, make sure that what you write is legible. For overhead slides, it is best to use a computer. Use a large font, typically at least size 20 for overhead slides and size 28 for PowerPoint slides. Make sure that separate points are clearly separated by using bullet points or numbers. Take care to ensure that diagrams are clearly legible and understandable.

When considering the best way of presenting information, be aware of the expectations of the workshop participants. Some senior officials are likely to be familiar with PowerPoint and may view other methods of presentation as rather old-fashioned and will therefore be less inclined to take their content seriously.

Table 9.1 Advantages and disadvantages of the various presentation options

Advantages	Disadvantages
Flipchart	
Relatively easy to use	Not very flexible
Cheap	Will tend to look 'unprofessional' unless considerable care and effort used in preparation
Not reliant on a power source	
Can be used by anyone with the basic ability to write and draw	Cannot show photographs and images
Allows the use of colour	
Quite easy to transport	
Whiteboard	
Useful for noting key points to aid group discussion	Need special pens
	Not easily portable
May already be available in a training room or meeting room	Limited surface area
	Time required to erase writing before additional writing
Overhead projector (OHP)	
Relatively easy to use	Need a power source
Flexible – you can easily add points in response to comments and return to a slide that has already been shown	Can break down
	Sometimes difficult to position projector so that it does not obscure the view of some participants
Points can easily be masked so that they are only shown when the presenter gets to them	Photographs cannot be reproduced easily
Prepared slides can easily be carried	Requires a screen or suitable wall
Produce a reasonably large image	Keeping slides in order can be difficult
	Care needed to produce good images
Slide projector	
Good option for showing visual images (to be used where PowerPoint is not available)	Needs a power source
	Cannot be used for text so usually has to be used in parallel with other equipment, which can create logistical difficulties
	Can jam
	May obscure the view of participants
PowerPoint presentation	
Looks professional	Need power source
Can incorporate both writing and images	Needs PowerPoint projector
Once set up, it is easy for the presenter to move backwards and forwards between slides	Some skills needed to use (but these can easily be learnt)
Can be animated so that points are displayed in order, at the time that you want them	Might be seen by some as rather impersonal
Equipment relatively easy to transport	
Unlike OHP slides, slides cannot be mixed up	

Bear in mind the possibility of using different options:

- alongside each other, for instance displaying key findings from a previous session on a flipchart as an aide-memoire to workshop participants
- at different times in the workshop, for instance scheduling a session of PowerPoint or slide projector images to illustrate particular points about existing conditions.

Using cards in participatory sessions

The disadvantage of all the options introduced above is that they cannot be used in a participatory way and so are of limited use when participants work together to identify and analyse information. Flipcharts provide perhaps the best option for allowing workshop participants to present information but even these allow only one person to present information at any given time.

The use of cards rather than flipchart paper allows contributions from different participants to be brought together and then analysed, edited and re-ordered by the workshop participants acting as a group. The workshop facilitator may still have to intervene where necessary to ensure that everyone's viewpoint is considered and that vocal individuals do not dominate the discussion. He or she may also be required to inform the discussion from time to time, introducing important facts and raising issues that would otherwise be missed by the participants. Examples of such issues include the need to consider improvements in hygiene and the extent to which problems can be solved within the boundaries of the project area.

The cards should be about 200 mm by 100 mm in size. Different colours of cards can be used for different purposes, for instance it might be appropriate to use one colour of card for problems and another colour for resources. Workshop participants will only be able to work with cards if they can see them and read them. This will only be possible if the information written on the cards is legible and workshop participants are sitting close enough to the cards to read them.

Rules for ensuring legibility are as follows:

- write one issue point per card
- use key words and not sentences
- write clearly
- use a maximum of three lines per card.

The options for displaying cards include specially prepared pin boards, to which cards can be attached with drawing pins, sheets of plain paper to which they can be stuck, and 'sticky cloths' (see Box 9.2). Once there, they can be moved around to reflect different relationships and priorities in response to suggestions from participants.

If the room is too large and formally arranged, it may be difficult to bring people close together and this makes working with cards difficult. Think about this potential problem and the options for overcoming it before the workshop. An example of what this might mean in practice is provided by a strategic planning workshop held in Quthbullapur in Andhra Pradesh, India. The workshop room was rather long and narrow. So, after the initial more formal presentations, sticky cloths and a flipchart were placed near the centre of one sidewall of the room and participants were asked to turn their chairs and face across rather than down the room. This helped to ensure that all the participants could see the information that was being presented.

Microphones and other electrical equipment

For small workshops, it may be possible to rely on people's unamplified voices. Indeed, this may be the best option since it may be

Box 9.2 Sticky cloths – how to prepare and use them

Sticky cloths are bed-sheet sized cloths that have been sprayed on one side with an adhesive of the type that is used for mounting photographs. Two coatings of adhesive are normally applied at an interval of a few hours. Once the cloth has been sprayed, it is and remains 'sticky'. It can be hung in a suitable place. Cards placed on the cloth will stay in place but it is easy to remove them and move them around. After the workshop, it can be wrapped up and then pulled out and made ready for use again so that it can be used for several workshops, although it may be necessary to spray it again after a few uses.

difficult to ensure that everyone has access to the microphone. However, there will be situations in which the use of microphones is advisable, for instance where the shape of the room means that those at the back are some distance from the speaker and/or there is some extraneous source of noise. In such situations, a cordless microphone should ideally be available so that all participants have access to microphone facilities. Where this is not possible, the seating should be laid out in a way that makes it reasonably easy for all participants to come forward to the fixed microphone when they wish to speak.

Other electrical equipment required for the workshop is likely to include an overhead projector, a slide projector and/or a PowerPoint projector for use with a computer. All electrical equipment should be set up and tested before the workshop starts. There is nothing worse, when making a presentation, than finding out that nothing happens when you switch the equipment on.

Other materials

Each participant in the workshop should be provided with a pen and a pad of paper on which he or she can record information and develop ideas in the course of the workshop. It will be best if these are given to workshop participants in a folder that contains details of the workshop schedule together with any other information that needs to be given to participants at the beginning of the workshop.

Plenty of marker pens should be available in a range of colours. It will generally be better if these produce a fairly thick line since this will ensure that the words written on cards and flip chart paper are clearly visible to all the participants. If whiteboards are to be used, make sure that markers suitable for use with them are available. (These produce marks that can be wiped off the whiteboard with a rag.)

It may be possible to buy suitably sized cards. If not, buy large sheets of light card and cut them up to the required size. If these have to be pinned, make sure that there is a good supply of drawing pins, and that there is a suitable surface to which they can be pinned.

Paper for use in group sessions and for subsequent presentations should be reasonably strong. It should typically be approximately A2 size (840 mm × 1176 mm).

Refreshment breaks

Regular refreshment breaks play an essential role in allowing workshop participants to relax, unwind and discuss issues among themselves. It will be best if refreshments are made available in a room other than the main workshop room so that participants are not distracted as the refreshments arrive. If this is not possible, try to set aside an area for refreshments at the back or side of the room.

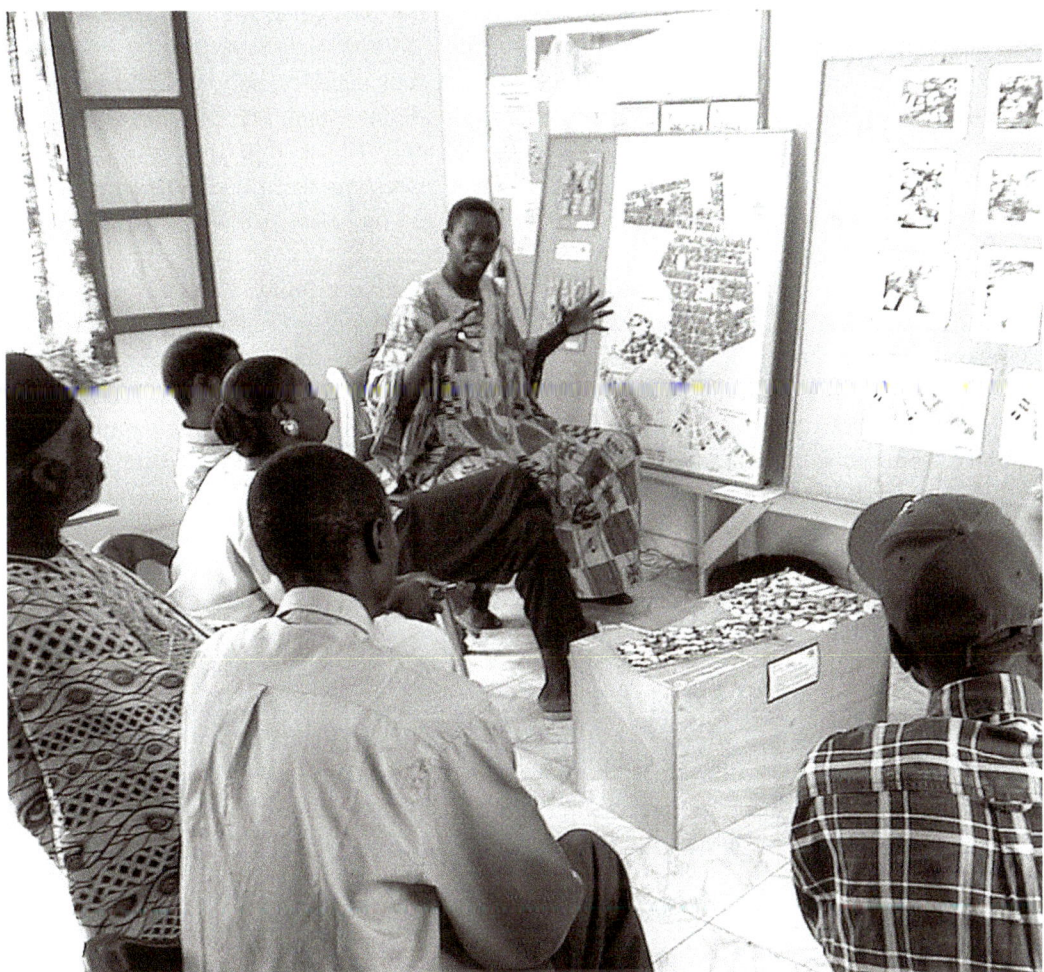

Figure 9.1 Participatory planning using plans and scale models
A participatory session in Yoff, Senegal. In the course of the project, community members used scale models to discuss the ways in which decentralized ecological sanitation systems might relate to housing sites, green space and pedestrian circulation. (Photo: Jerry Weisburd, Coterre, Philadelphia)

Ideally, the scheduling of breaks should be reasonably flexible to allow for overruns in the previous sessions (which certainly should not be encouraged but are sometimes unavoidable). There may be occasions, particularly during group sessions, when participants are asked to take their refreshments and return to their groups to continue discussions. This saves time and perhaps a cup of tea or coffee will lubricate the discussion.

The workshop itself

We have already suggested that the structure of most workshops will include an introduction, sessions devoted to the collection, presentation and analysis of information, assessment of available resources, agreement on action to be taken and allocation of responsibilities for taking that action. In previous chapters, we have given guidance on how some of these sessions might operate. In this section, we provide some additional information on specific points, focusing on the way in which the workshop is organized and run rather than the techniques used to identify and explore issues.

Introducing the workshop

The introduction provides an opportunity to set out the objectives of the workshop, at the same time ensuring that those attending are active participants rather than passive observers. Where it is felt necessary to have some form of formal opening of the workshop, it is best to keep this as separate as possible from the workshop proper.

Whether or not there is some form of introductory speech, the workshop organizers should introduce themselves and explain the purpose and proposed working methods of the workshop at the first possible opportunity.

Developing a sense of shared purpose

It will usually be a good idea to start the workshop proper with an icebreaker session, designed to introduce workshop participants to one another and to ease them into the active role that they will be expected to play in the workshop.

Where people do not know each other, a good way to encourage early participation is to ask participants to divide into pairs and find out about the other person and then introduce that person to the workshop. In order to do this, they must be prepared to listen, something that they will be required to do throughout the workshop.

Another icebreaker option is to ask workshop participants to divide into pairs. One person from each pair is then blindfolded and guided across the room by the other. This helps to build trust between participants and gives them an early experience of working together and trusting one another. However, not all participants will feel comfortable with such techniques.

Where participants already know each other, different icebreakers may be appropriate. For instance, people might be asked to divide into small groups and each person would then be asked to first draw something that represents them, their organization or their job and then explain it to the rest of the group.

Another possibility is to ask people to break into pairs or small groups and consider their concerns and expectations regarding the workshop. The main points emerging from this session can then be captured in a plenary session.

Bringing participants together in this way will help to ensure that they work well together throughout the course of the workshop.

Presentation of strategic principles

When a workshop takes place at or near the beginning of the planning process, it will normally be necessary to introduce the strategic principles set out in Chapter 2 and identify possibilities for applying them in the local situation. This can be done through a presentation on the need for a strategic approach. This will help to provide the context for problem analysis. It should be done in a way that is both understandable and relevant to the participants. With this in mind:

○ in workshops attended by a high proportion of non-technical people, efforts should be made to present the concepts relatively simply

○ for higher-level workshops, particularly those that are concerned with policy, a rather more technical approach can be taken, but the aim must still be to present concepts as simply and clearly as possible.

In both cases, it will be very important to explain the meaning of unfamiliar terms such as unbundling. It will also be helpful if examples can be given to illustrate concepts and ideas.

After presenting the principles, encourage discussion of their merits and their relevance to the existing situation. Some people may not accept all the principles at first, or believe that some cannot be applied in the short term. There may be good reasons for some of the doubts but the principles can nevertheless provide direction for the planning process and help participants to develop a vision of how improved sanitation services might look. Opportunities and constraints arising from this discussion should be taken forward and used to inform task identification.

Facilitating workshop sessions

Workshop facilitation is a skill that, to some extent at least, has to be learnt from experience. However, adherence to certain basic rules will help to ensure that the workshop proceeds smoothly and reaches useful conclusions. These include the following.

○ Explain what each session is about as clearly as possible at the beginning of the session. In particular, take time to explain the purpose of any field visits and what participants will be expected to do during and after the visit. Make sure that participants understand how the field visit contributes to the overall purpose of the workshop.

○ Where necessary, provide some information to get sessions rolling. For instance, for a session devoted to identifying resources, the facilitators might provide some guidance on the types of resource that might be available – agencies and organizations, personnel, technical and extension skills, funds for new works and those required to pay for operation and maintenance and so on.

○ Later intervene as necessary to move the discussion forward. In the first instance, encourage workshop participants to widen or shift the focus of their thinking rather than giving them ready-made answers. However, some more overt guidance and suggestions may be necessary when a session appears to get completely 'stuck'. When giving such guidance, stress that you are providing suggestions, which participants are free to accept or reject as they see fit.

○ Take time to periodically recap on workshop findings and summarize outputs. This may be done briefly at the end of each session but should always be done at the beginning of the second day of a two-day workshop. The session does not have to be long – not more than 15 minutes. After presenting your view of the outputs of the first day, ask participants if they agree with your presentation and whether they feel there are any other important points that they feel should be made at this stage.

○ Issues may arise once the workshop has begun and there may be calls to change the structure of the workshop to accommodate them. Do not rush into such changes. There is a real danger that the changes made to deal with particular problems and concerns may undermine the overall workshop structure. Lunch, tea and particularly overnight breaks provide opportunities for the workshop organizers to discuss the progress of the workshop and to decide whether any changes in structure and/or content are needed in order to reflect the way in which it is developing.

Agreeing on follow-up action

The workshop will only have been worthwhile if the actions agreed in the course of it are implemented. With this in mind, task identification and allocation should lead into discussion of the timetable for follow-up action. The time to be allocated to the various tasks identified in the previous session should be discussed in plenary session and deadlines for completion of the various tasks should be agreed. A time and date for a follow-up meeting at which the various stakeholders will report on progress with their tasks should also be agreed.

Closing the workshop

The workshop organizers should wrap up the workshop by thanking everyone who has attended and promising that the record of the workshop will be circulated to all participants. Set a time for completing this task and do not let it slip.

Recording the outputs of the workshop

The main outputs of the workshop should be recorded and then summarized in a short report, which should then be circulated to all workshop participants and to any other individuals and organizations with a possible interest in the workshop findings. For municipal and local workshops, these might include those working at higher levels of government who might be interested in the possible outcome of the workshop.

Two or three people should be assigned to type the information displayed on cards and display boards. It is best if this is done every evening after the completion of that day's sessions. The workshop organizers should check on the way in which information is being recorded. For instance, when recording the results of a problem tree analysis, it is not sufficient to type the information provided on cards. It is also necessary to record the order in which the cards were displayed and the links between them. It is possible to photograph the information displayed on display boards and sticky cloths. This will provide a record of the way in which information was arranged. However, you should not rely on photographs as the sole record of workshop outputs in case a photograph does not come out or cannot be read.

The report should include the outputs of the various sessions. For instance, if a problem tree or a matrix has been produced in the course of the workshop, it should be reproduced in the report. This will ensure that the basic findings of the workshop can be referred to in the future. However, the main purpose of the report should be to present the key decisions taken during the workshop in an easily accessible way. It may be that the best way to do this is to list the agreed action points in a brief main report and to include more detailed information on the outputs from the various sessions in an appendix.

A small team, not more than three people, should be assigned to produce the workshop report either before the workshop starts or at an early stage in the workshop itself. This will ensure that they are thinking about the need for the report throughout the workshop and so make sure that all necessary outputs are properly recorded.

When circulating the report, encourage those who receive copies to respond if they need clarification or think that one or more important points have been missed.

Other options for ensuring wide knowledge of the key workshop findings and recommendations should be considered, particularly when the workshop relates to local services that are of interest to community members. These might include:

○ holding a general meeting to communicate the main findings of the workshop
○ displaying the main findings in prominent places, such as local schools, health centres and community halls.

These options are not, of course, mutually exclusive.

Key points in this chapter

1. Workshops can be used in the course of planning and policy development processes to explore and identify possible responses to problems and issues, and agree responsibility for implementing those responses.

2. Workshops can also be used to elicit a response to specific plan and policy proposals.

3. The number of participants at a workshop should be restricted to a maximum of 50 and ideally to not more than 25–30 participants.

4. It will be hard to represent primary stakeholders, the end users of sanitation services, at workshops at the municipal level and higher. However, efforts should be made before the workshop to obtain an idea of their concerns and priorities and to present those concerns and priorities to the workshop. Do not forget the concerns of women, tenants and other less powerful groups.

5. The most successful workshops are those for which adequate preparations are made. Attention paid to getting the logistics right before the workshop starts will pay dividends during the workshop itself. Pay particular attention to the arrangements for any field visits by workshop participants.

6. As far as is possible, workshop discussions should be based on information rather than assumptions and prejudices.

7. Follow-up actions, together with responsibilities for carrying out those actions, should be agreed before the end of the workshop.

8. The outputs of the workshop should be recorded in writing and circulated to all participants as soon as possible after the completion of the workshop.

CHAPTER 10
Implementing the plan

THE PLAN WILL have no value unless it is implemented, at least in part. Even then, long-term gains will only be achieved if the lessons learnt in the course of implementation inform future plans and initiatives. Taken together, these points suggest a need to answer the questions:

○ How can we ensure that the plan is implemented?

○ How can we monitor its implementation?

○ How can we assess its impact and ensure that the lessons learnt are used to inform future plans and programmes?

This final chapter explores each of these questions in turn and then provides some ideas on how the experience of successful planning initiatives can be shared with other towns, cities and areas.

First steps

The first few months after the plan has been produced are perhaps the most crucial in the whole planning process. If implementation does not start during this period, there is a real danger that the plan will be sidelined as the various stakeholders respond to new challenges in the old ad hoc manner.

The group or committee that has taken overall responsibility for the plan should take steps to ensure that the concept of the plan is widely accepted and that stakeholder organizations are taking practical steps to implement it. Copies should be circulated as widely as possible and every opportunity should be taken to remind stakeholders of the existence of the plan and the need to implement it. Regular meetings, perhaps monthly in the first instance, should be held with representatives of the various organizations with responsibilities for individual plan components. Use these meetings to obtain feedback on progress and, where necessary, provide advice and guidance on taking work components forward.

Each stakeholder organization should ensure that it is in a position to implement the sections of the plan for which it is responsible, focusing particularly on first year activities and targets. Ideally, each organization should set up a small project team to oversee plan implementation. It may be appropriate for the team to report directly to the chief executive of the organization. Ideally, the team members should be relieved of other duties.

Setting targets

As already indicated in Chapter 3, setting intermediate targets will help you to monitor progress towards full implementation of the various plan components. Outline information on targets should already be available in the plan. Each organization should aim to develop a more detailed work plan for their particular components. These work plans should be available not more than two months after ratification of the plan. A meeting of the overall coordinating body should be scheduled for the end of this period to receive the proposals and, where necessary, provide advice and guidance on moving them forward.

Every effort should then be made to include plan components in the programmes and financial projections of the organizations that are concerned with those components. An even better outcome will be that these organizations apply the general principles underlying the planning process when establishing their own priorities and developing their internal budgets and work plans. This will help to mainstream the strategic approach so that it is seen as the normal way of doing business rather than an optional extra.

Developing detailed proposals

It will be necessary to develop detailed proposals for implementing the various components of the plan. These are likely to cover implementation of new works and improvements in operation and maintenance and financial systems, all of which are briefly considered below. They may also involve efforts to promote better sanitation and hygiene, as already described in Chapter 6.

Sufficient time must be allowed for proposals to be prepared and approved. In general, the larger and more complex the scheme, the longer the time needed to prepare a proposal and have it approved. Also, as a general rule, the larger the scheme, the higher the level at which it has to be approved.

Physical works

Proposals for physical improvements should include detailed drawings, estimates and contract documentation, which together provide sufficient detail to allow the proposed works to be implemented as intended. Drawings should be to scale, estimates should be as accurate as possible and contract documents should specify what has to be done in sufficient detail for the quality of work to be checked. The more accurate the documentation, the easier will it be to:

○ check that work is being executed as planned

○ agree and cost any changes required in the light of local circumstances.

Drawings
Although many local masons and petty contractors work without drawings, a drawing will help to make sure that the facility it depicts is built as intended and may also facilitate discussion on how designs might be improved. Standard drawings may be produced for on-site facilities such as double-pit pour-flush latrines. These can be linked to schedules, which provide information on quantities and space to enter standard costs (an example is given in Box 8.1). When working with local communities and masons, a series of simple illustrations showing the work to be carried out will be more useful than a formal drawing.

For more complex sewerage and drainage schemes, there will be a requirement for the following.

○ Drawings of standard system components, for example manholes, chambers and standard drain cross-sections. Typical scales should be 1:10, 1:20 or 1:50, depending on the size of the component and the amount of detail to be included in the drawing. These might be linked to standard schedules of quantities.

○ Plans and sections showing drain and sewer routes and levels. The plan and section should be shown on the same drawing so they can be related to one another. The horizontal scale should typically be in the range 1:250 to 1:1000 with a ten times exaggerated vertical scale for longitudinal sections. For local schemes, it should be possible to show all levels on a plan rather than producing sections for every sewer.[1] For small schemes, the plan does not have to be 100% spatially accurate, provided that distances and lengths are shown to scale.

o Information on the location and type of manholes and chambers and changes in cross-section or sewer diameter. This information should be included on plan drawings. Where a longitudinal section is provided, the locations of manholes and changes in cross-section and sewer diameter should also be shown on the section.

Drawings should be produced in a form that can be reproduced. Avoid the common practice of showing sewer and drain routes in coloured pencil on reproductions of original plans.

Specifications

The purpose of specifications is to regulate the quality of the work carried out on site. Larger schemes are likely to be implemented by formal organizations that either already have their own specifications or follow standard government specifications. It may be worthwhile to review these as there will often be scope for improvement.

For smaller schemes, these standard specifications are likely to be much too complex. For these schemes, the need is to provide guidance on good practice in a form that is accessible to the local stakeholders who are likely to be responsible for managing and/or implementing the work. This guidance might include information on:

o the minimum acceptable standard for purchased components such as pipes

o the type and quantity of materials to be used – for instance the type of sand, aggregate and cement to be used in a concrete mix and the quantities of each

o sources of components and materials of an acceptable standard

o good working practice – covering points like curing concrete, pipe laying etc.

This information should be produced in the first language of the people who are going to be responsible for the management and implementation of the work.

Packaging the work

Schemes involving a single facility, for example a new main drain or a municipal sewage treatment plant, will normally be best dealt with through the award of a single contract for all work associated with the implementation of the scheme.

Other plan components are likely to comprise a large number of essentially similar but unconnected works. This would be the case, for instance, in the case of a scheme to provide secondary and tertiary sewers to connect to an existing collector sewer. It is possible to divide such work into packages that can be managed by a number of smaller contractors rather than assigning it all to one large contractor. This will help to:

o provide an element of competition so that the few large contractors do not form a price fixing 'ring' and share the work out among themselves

o build local contracting capacity and hence enhance the resource base.

Improvements in operation and maintenance

The references to improved operation and maintenance in the plan itself are likely to be fairly general and there will often be a need to develop more detailed proposals in the period after ratification of the plan. These proposals should recognize the constraints inherent in the existing situation and address those constraints in a structured way.

The greatest constraint is often the fact that few stakeholders, least of all municipal decision makers, consider improved operation and maintenance to be a high priority. As with other aspects of the prevailing 'culture', this lack of concern with operation and maintenance is likely to be widely shared and deeply ingrained. Other important constraints are likely to include:

- inadequate information on where facilities are, what condition they are in and how they are meant to be operated and maintained
- inadequate finances
- poorly designed and constructed facilities (see Figure 10.1)
- lack of knowledge of what constitutes good maintenance.

Approach operation and maintenance in a logical manner that recognizes and deals with these constraints. It will be particularly important to convince senior decision makers of the benefits that can be achieved through improved operation and maintenance. You are more likely to be able to do this if your initial focus is on improvements that can be implemented fairly easily while demonstrating clear benefits.

A start on gathering the information required for improved operation and maintenance should have been made during the developing solutions stage of the planning process. It will normally be necessary to

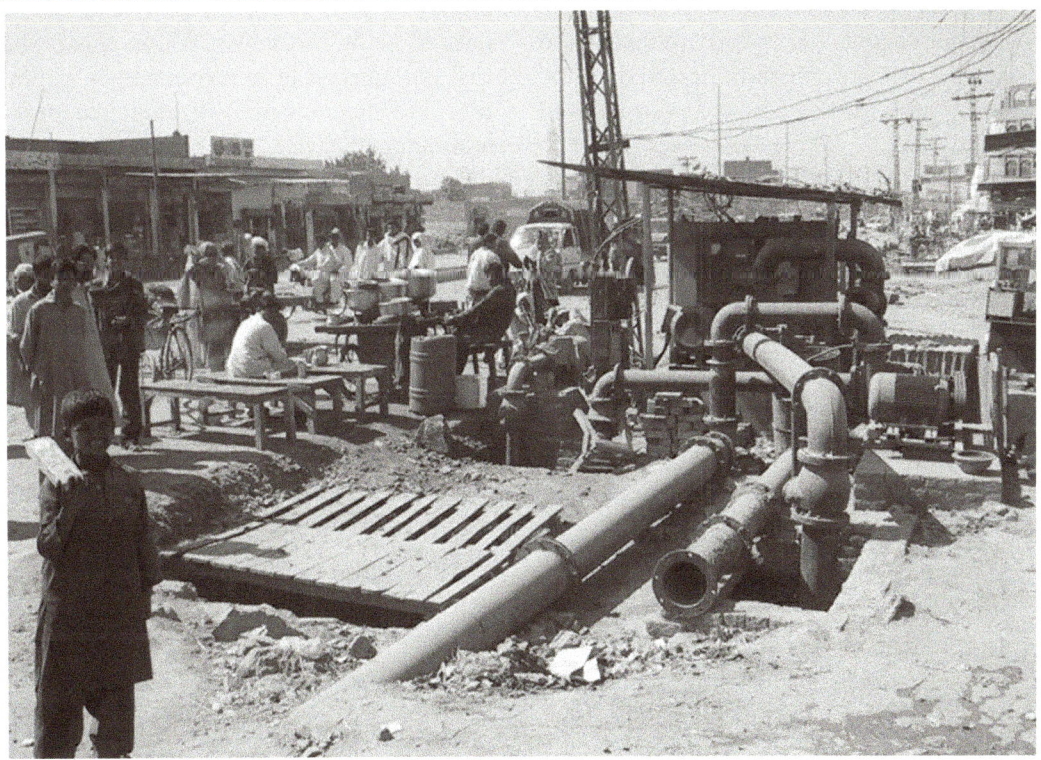

Figure 10.1 Poor design and construction inhibits good operation and maintenance
This pumping station in Faisalabad, Pakistan, is typical of many found in South Asia. Poor design and lack of proper fixing arrangements increase the possibility that pumps and motors will be misaligned, leading to excessive wear. The operators have no experience of operating a well designed pumping station with the result that good operation and maintenance is almost impossible.

further improve information on operation and maintenance as the plan is developed.

When developing detailed proposals for operation and maintenance improvements:

o Take account of existing incentives. Do they provide support for efforts to improve operation and maintenance or do they, as is often the case, encourage bad practice? If the latter, changes will be needed before operation and maintenance improvements can be sustained.

o Identify areas in which existing facilities are in operable condition. Avoid areas in which poor design or past neglect has resulted in conditions that make good operation and maintenance virtually impossible. For instance, it will be very difficult to demonstrate a good maintenance regime on poorly constructed sewers that have been neglected over the years and are now choked with silt and solid waste.

o Identify key operation and maintenance tasks. Look particularly for the 'big idea', the single concept or principle that defines the technology to be operated and maintained (Dudley 1993, p.19). If operation and maintenance deficiencies prevent the sustained achievement of the big idea, the facility will fail. The big idea of a leach pit receiving wastes from a WC is that liquid wastes are allowed to percolate through the walls of the pit while solids are retained for periodic removal. That of a sewer is that faecal solids are transported by water through a closed conduit, which excludes unwanted materials such as silt and solid waste.

o Consider the essential operation and maintenance practices required to ensure that the big idea of a technology can be achieved in practice over a period of time. For the leach pit, it will be essential to empty the pit contents when it is full, to do this in a hygienic way and to dispose of the contents in an environmentally acceptable way. The emphasis on the sewer being a closed conduit leads to the conclusion that replacing missing manhole and chamber covers before unwanted extraneous material has a chance to enter the sewer is a key maintenance task. The focus should then be on ensuring that these practices are carried out.

If assessment of essential practice reveals that the big idea of the technology cannot be achieved, it will be necessary to either change or modify the technology. In the case of the sewer, it may be that either water availability is too low or that the available ground slope is too flat to allow solids to be flushed along the sewer. Where this is the case, no amount of improvement in operation and maintenance will alleviate problems altogether. The only option in this case will be to remove the solids from the sewer, either by providing interceptor tanks on house connections or discharging WC wastes to leach pits. Where detailed investigations reveal the need for such action, it is likely that there will be a need to review the plan component to which they relate.

As far as is possible, detailed plans for improved operation and maintenance should be developed in consultation with those who will have to implement them (see Figure 10.2). Without this emphasis on consultation, there is a real danger that those who are currently responsible for operation and maintenance tasks will feel threatened by the proposals and will refuse to cooperate.[2]

As with new works, it may be advisable to break up operation and maintenance tasks into smaller packages. For instance, drain cleaning might be broken down into packages based on either drainage basins or political boundaries. Whether the work con-

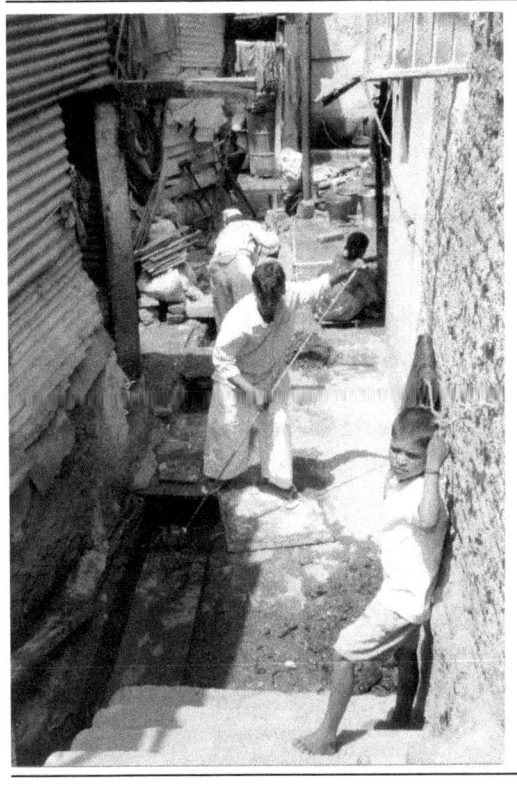

Figure 10.2 The need for improved practices

Drain cleaning in Pune, India. The equipment available for cleaning drains is often rudimentary. It may be appropriate to explore options for using improved equipment. However, the staff responsible for drain cleaning should be consulted about any proposed changes, both to reassure them that the changes will not adversely affect them and to obtain their insights into options for improving operational practices.

tinues to be carried out by the municipality, is contracted out to the private sector or is assigned to a community organization, division of the work into smaller packages will make it easier to compare the outputs achieved in particular areas with the inputs required to achieve them. This will provide a good basis for determining the cost-effectiveness of different approaches to operation and maintenance. Indeed, in the early stages of plan implementation it may be useful to manage operation and maintenance activities in different areas in different ways so as to assess the relative merits of different approaches.

Financial improvements

As for operation and maintenance improvements, it is likely that the plan will identify the general areas in which financial improvements are needed but will not spell out in detail how those improvements are going to be achieved. In the period following agreement on the plan, the various stakeholders should develop more detailed proposals for improvements.

The starting point will often be a more detailed assessment of existing financial systems. Do they provide information in a form that allows detailed assessment of where money is being spent and where savings might be made? In particular:

○ Do existing systems allow a clear distinction to be made between capital and recurrent expenditure?

○ To what extent do they provide a breakdown of both capital and recurrent expenditure in terms of both activities undertaken and/or tasks performed and levels of expenditure in different areas?

In the event that there is no clear distinction between capital and recurrent expenditure, the first priority should be to rectify this situation. If, as is more likely, this basic distinction is made but there is limited information on how and where money is spent, the aim should be to start to break down expenditure by area and/or tasks performed as appropriate. As with improvements in operation and maintenance, early proposals should focus on the options that are likely to have the greatest impact.

Training

The plan may include specific proposals for training. Where this is the case, post-plan activities will include contacting possible training providers and working out a detailed training programme. Regardless of this, there may be a need for training to inform stakeholders of the planning approach and improve their capacity to implement the plan.

Do not treat training activities as isolated events but rather look to integrate them with plan activities so that training reinforces practice and vice versa. Box 10.1 provides an example of a training programme developed by an NGO that illustrates this principle.

Training will yield few benefits if organizational structures and systems do not allow trainees to use what they have learnt after the training. So, training initiatives should be considered as part of wider efforts to improve human resources. These may involve changes in incentive systems, devolution of responsibilities to appropriate levels within government systems and changes in rules to ensure that, once trained, staff are not transferred to tasks that do not make use of their training. As a general rule, frequent staff transfers should be avoided.

Options for supervision and implementation

Overall responsibilities for managing the various components of the plan will already be set out in the plan itself. However, these organizations may wish to assign responsibility for implementing and supervising activities to other organizations. Table 10.1 summarizes the possibilities for supervising and implementing both new capital works and the operation and maintenance of completed facilities.

The exact boundaries between the responsibilities of individual householders, local organizations and government or some other central organization should be decided in the light of the local situation. When considering options, ask:

○ What is allowed/required by existing laws and regulations? In particular, do they provide scope for the involvement of civil society and private sector organizations in sanitation provision? If they do not, are they enforced and what scope is there for changing them?

○ Are there community organizations with the interest and capacity to undertake the tasks that could theoretically be assigned to them?

○ Are there private-sector organizations with the interest and capacity to undertake the tasks that could theoretically be assigned to them?

○ Will government officials and other formal sector stakeholders accept the involvement of community organizations and private sector operators (both formal and informal) in the supervision and implementation of activities?

Do not assume that a particular organization or individual will automatically elect to undertake a task just because they have the ability to do so. Experience suggests that it is more common for householders and civil society groups to hire small contractors and individual operators to carry out physical

Box 10.1 Training for managers and residents in Yoff, Senegal[3]

Yoff is situated on the outskirts of Dakar, the capital of Senegal. Originally a fishing village with a population of about 20 000, it is now part of Dakar. Its population reached 50 000 in 1994 and continues to grow at about 6.6% per annum (Weisburd, 2000). The village association Association pour la Promotion Economique, Culturelle et Sociale de Yoff (APECSY) is working in cooperation with the NGO CRESP Senegal to create a sustainable path to development, emphasizing sanitation, environment, community and capacity building. As part of its programme, it is developing a pilot *Cite Ecologique* to house about 1000 people. The sanitation system developed for this pilot area involves separate disposal of faecal wastes and sullage water. Faecal wastes are dealt with by either dry toilets with urine diversion or septic tanks. Sullage water is treated in reed beds. These facilities may be provided at the household level, but most will be provided as 'common stations' accessible to groups of residents. Training has been provided for:

○ a sanitation group, in effect the cadre for the project, which will be responsible for continuing the project, expanding the research and extending the approach to other parts of Yoff
○ residents, who will be responsible for operating and managing the common stations.

Training for the sanitation group was designed to create a core group of people with the skills to develop and maintain an integrated approach to sustainable sanitation provision. More specifically, it aimed to ensure that participants would be able to work with resident–user groups to plan, design, finance, construct, operate and maintain their common station. The course ran over about 70 hours, including evening sessions and several day-long weekend sessions focused on studio/design and field-based exercises. Participants were chosen on the basis of their prior interest or participation in the area and/or their possession of the specialist knowledge and skills required to carry the project forward. All were residents of Yoff, with almost 50:50 male/female participation. The course ended with a major demonstration project, field exams and written exams. Certificates were awarded based on overall performance. After the training, the trainees formed a formal association to conduct activities, with a small amount of funding from APECSY to cover its first year of operation.

The training for residents included hands-on instruction in maintenance and several meetings on management. Support materials were provided in the form of maintenance and inspection checklists, record-keeping tools, contact information for members of the sanitation group, copies of the maintenance manual and small posters on how the station works and what constitutes organic and non-organic waste. Some of this training was conducted by members of the new sanitation group.

---

improvements on their behalf. Even apparently unskilled tasks such as digging pit latrines and digging sewer trenches are often carried out by specialist labour, sometimes from a particular community. For instance, most pipe trenches in Pakistan are dug by Pushtoons from North-West Frontier Province.

Nevertheless, we have already seen in Chapter 5 that community groups, supported where necessary by NGOs, can take a leading role in managing the provision of local facilities. Box 10.2 illustrates how it is possible to contract out both the construction and subsequent operation and maintenance of facilities to NGOs and the

Table 10.1 Options for supervising and implementing new works and operation and maintenance tasks

	Type of activity	Responsibility for supervision	Responsibility for implementation
New works	Improvements to household level facilities	Householder	Householder or locally hired petty contractor
	Improvements to local facilities (tertiary drains and sewers, shared and communal sanitation blocks, etc.)	'Lane manager' operating on behalf of a group of households Community organization Municipal engineering department	Petty contractor Small formal contractor Community group Government through force account or departmental works procedures
	Improvements to higher-order facilities	Municipal engineering department or appropriate line department Consultant on behalf of above	Contractor Government through force account or departmental works procedures
Operation and maintenance	Household level facilities	Householder	Householder
	Local facilities	Community organization Ward councillor or equivalent Municipality or line agency, perhaps through local unit	Community organization Petty contractor Conventional contractor Municipality or line agency, perhaps through local unit
	Higher-order facilities	Municipality or appropriate line department Private-sector operator (normally through some form of public-private partnership agreement)	Municipality or appropriate line department Formal private-sector contractor

communities with which they work.

It may be appropriate for the municipality to register small contractors to carry out on-site tasks. For instance, Colombo Municipal Corporation in Sri Lanka licenses small contractors, mostly one-man operators, to lay the on-site pipework required to connect new consumers to the sewer network. This work is carried out on behalf of householders, who are responsible for paying the contractors. Many contractors are also registered to make the connection from the plot boundary to the public sewer on behalf of the municipality.

Contractual arrangements for work inside the plot boundary should generally be kept simple. In some cases, all that will be required is a simple verbal arrangement between the householder and the specialist labourer. It may be worthwhile to provide guidance as to how this relationship might be made slightly more formal.

Contracts for local shared facilities such as tertiary sewers and community sanitation blocks should also be simple. Box 10.3 suggests a number of possible contractual arrangements for such works.

Table 10.1 also indicates the possibility of using force account (sometimes referred to as direct labour or departmental works) methods to implement new works. In this approach, no contract is let. Rather, the government department itself takes responsibility for purchasing materials, providing or hiring labour and managing construction. International agencies do not favour force

Box 10.2 Community toilets in Pune

In Pune, most community toilet blocks had fallen into disrepair by the mid 1990s. In 1998, the newly appointed municipal commissioner proposed an investment programme to introduce significant improvements to the city's basic service infrastructure and waste management facilities. Under the new Demolition and Replacement Scheme, a massive Rs230 million (approximately US$5 million) expenditure programme for refurbishment of the city's sanitation services was initiated to construct 271 new community toilets (latrines) throughout the slum areas of the city. Each toilet unit is designed to serve 50 people and the programme as whole aims to serve 250 000 people.

A number of NGOs have been employed by Pune Municipal Corporation (PMC) to implement the programme on the assumption that the involvement of NGOs will reduce project costs and improve project effectiveness and sustainability. Different NGOs have taken different approaches to managing facilities. Although the NGOs are charged with managing the toilet blocks for 30 years, there are no formal contractual agreements. PMC provides a free water supply and makes no charge for sewerage (where the latrine is connected the city sewer system) or for septic tank cleaning (where discharge to a sewer is not possible).

Some of the NGOs have taken full responsibility for construction, operation and maintenance, operating their toilets on a 'pay-and-use' basis. Others charge a nominal flat rate per household per month. The revenue collected will cover operation and maintenance costs, but no attempt will be made to recover PMC's capital outlay for construction. The Mumbai-based SPARC/NSDF/Mahila Milan 'partnership' has encouraged local communities to take the lead in construction and then to appoint a community representative to manage the facilities. It reports considerable success with this approach.

(Burra 2001; Hobson 2000)

Box 10.3 Possible contractual arrangements for community-managed schemes

1. The contractor provides labour and tools only, with all materials being provided by or through the community. Often, the contractor will quote a lump sum for such labour-only contracts.
2. The contractor quotes a lump sum for the provision of labour, tools and materials. This approach reduces the amount that the community has to do for itself but at the same time introduces the need to check that the materials provided are satisfactory. There may be problems in agreeing on the price adjustment required if changes from the agreed scheme are made in the course of implementation.
3. The contractor quotes prices against a schedule of standard items such as trench excavation, laying sewers and constructing manholes and chambers. This type of contract needs more preparation but is better able to deal with variations than a lump-sum contract.

Investigations in Pakistan conducted in the course of the Faisalabad Area Upgrading Project revealed that communities usually use the first option. However, it may be worthwhile to explore the other options at the time that the first local facilities are being provided.

> **Box 10.4 Service provision by local entrepreneurs – a case from South Africa[4]**
>
> In South Africa, the Durban Metropolitan Council has subcontracted solid waste management services to small entrepreneurs in informal settlements. An example of this arrangement is provided by the case of Noma and Dombi Cleaning and Catering Services. This is a small company, owned by two women from Bester informal settlement. It has been contracted by the Durban Metropolitan Council to collect household waste from around Bester at a fee since 1998. The company employs 17 women who help in the distribution of refuse bags on a weekly basis and who also collect the waste dumped by households in selected locations around the settlement to skips. The Durban Solid Waste trucks collect the refuse from the skips on a weekly basis.
>
> Households are responsible for making sure that they pack their domestic waste in the plastic bags and deposit them at selected dumping points close to their homes. Waste collection is done on different days in the various areas of Bester.
>
> When the service began, many households did not stick to the waste collection timetable and there were problems because dogs and cats tore the bags, causing waste to be spread around in an unhygienic way. This problem was resolved by intensive civic education in the area and now people know that even when their plastic bags fill up prematurely, they have to keep them in their yards until their day of collection comes.
>
> Following the success of the Durban initiative, other local authorities are planning to start similar programmes.

account methods, seeing them as anti-competitive and easily manipulated by corrupt officials. However, competitive bidding processes for conventional contracts are not always as transparent as they seem and force account methods should not be dismissed out of hand.

One interesting variation on the force account approach is that developed by the Sindh Katchi Abadi Authority in Pakistan, which uses departmental works procedures for the provision of secondary sewers (Khaild and Aiddiqui 2000). Local people are hired to do the work and an NGO provides overall guidance and supervision.

In recent years, considerable attention has been paid to community contracting – awarding contracts for local works to organizations that represent the communities that are to benefit from the works (Cotton et al. 1998; Jinchang 1998). Community contracting should be used with care. Most small contracting firms are started by entrepreneurs and community organizations may lack the dynamism required to sustain a contracting business. Experience in the field suggests that, in the absence of a strong tradition of community cooperation, it is easy for community contracting initiatives to be 'captured' by one or two influential people. In such circumstances, a better option may be to encourage entrepreneurs from low-income areas to set up small businesses to provide services. Box 10.4 provides an example from South Africa of what this might mean in practice. Note the support to the process given by the civic authorities.

The need for formal agreements

Where locally-managed facilities are dependent on higher-order facilities provided by others, it is important that there is agreement as to who does what and who pays for what. This will normally require a formal agreement, setting out the rights and responsibilities of the partners. Take, for example, the case of a locally constructed and managed sewer connected to a collector sewer provided and managed by a central authority. The central authority has to bear the cost of operating the downstream system, including any sewage pumping and treatment that is required. It will be reluctant to approve the connection from a community-managed sewer unless it receives some revenue from community members to cover these downstream operating costs. At the same time, the community can argue that they should not pay the full tariff because they are managing the local part of the system and thus reducing the cost to the central authority. In such a situation, there should ideally be a standard agreement that the tariff will be reduced by an appropriate amount to allow for the fact that the community is managing its own local facilities.

The situation is often complicated by the fact that existing sewerage tariffs cover only a small fraction of operating costs. Where this is the case, it will still be desirable to reach some sort of agreement on a reduced tariff for those who manage their own local facilities. This will ensure that the principle of shared responsibilities has been established for future reference. Where this cannot be achieved, the community should be prepared to pay the full tariff since it is only by doing so that they can reasonably ask the authority to operate the downstream facilities regularly and efficiently.

Monitoring the progress of the plan

As implementation of the plan progresses, it will be important to monitor progress. This should be done at a number of levels. Those responsible for the overall plan must have overall information on the progress of each plan component. Those responsible for individual components need more detailed information on the progress of their component. More specifically, they need to know whether it is proceeding within an acceptable time-frame, producing the required result within the budgeted cost in a way that ensures that those intended to benefit actually do benefit (Hosain et al. 1999).

You will only be able to monitor effectively if you:

o identify objectives and estimate the time required to achieve them

o provide clear guidance on the quality of output required

o keep good records of what has been done, when it was done and how it measured up to expectations.

Using a logical framework to identify objectives and monitor progress towards them

Overall and intermediate objectives for specific plan components can be set out in a logical framework. In essence, this is a four by four matrix. The left-hand column of the matrix provides information on the following:

o The overall development objective to which the project is intended to contribute – its *goal*.

o The project's specific objective – its *purpose*. This should be one of the specific objectives defined in the plan. There may be more than one objective for any one component of the plan. Box 3.4 provided some examples – to introduce a primary collection service in specified wards, to establish a properly managed disposal site and to extend secondary collection services to all areas currently unserved. Each objective will require its own logical framework.

o The *outputs* or intermediate objectives that have to be reached in order to achieve the purpose.

o The *activities* required to achieve each of these outputs.

The basic difference between an activity and an output is that an activity takes place over time while an output represents a specific objective that has to be reached on the way to achieving the overall purpose.

The goal, purpose, outputs and activities are linked as shown in Figure 10.3.

The second column of the matrix provides information on *indicators* that can be used in assessing whether activities have been completed and outputs, purpose and goal have been achieved. Indicators for outputs should include an assessment of the time by which the output is to be achieved.

The third column provides information on the means to be used to *verify* that the indicators have been achieved. Progress with activities and the achievement of outputs will often be recorded in project files so it is important that information is stored in these files and that they are kept up to date.

The fourth column provides information on the *assumptions* that have been made in formulating the project and any *risks* that might threaten the successful completion of the project. If you have no means of justifying an assumption, it becomes a risk, threatening the successful achievement of the objective or completion of the activity to which it relates. Where a risk seriously threatens the success of a project or programme, an output designed to address that risk should be included in the first column of the logical framework.

Defining the quality of output required

Guidance on the quality required for new works can be provided through specifications. Written guidelines on quality requirements for operation and maintenance tasks will also be needed. Developing these guidelines for the various plan components will often be an early objective.

Local works, including maintenance tasks, may well be assigned to people who are not used to reading documents. For such people, even the simplest specifications are likely to be of limited use. An alternative, and perhaps more effective, way of defining the required quality for new works is to construct a facility to the required standard at the beginning of the project, agree with all concerned that this is the required quality and then use it as the standard against which all subsequent work is measured.

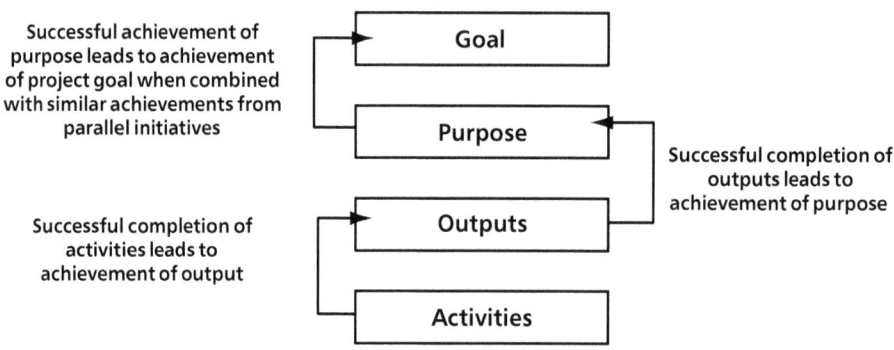

Figure 10.3 Links between activities, outputs, purpose and goal

A similar approach can be used for operation and maintenance tasks. A 'model' maintenance regime can be developed in one or more representative areas and staff from other areas can then be provided with training in this area. When doing so, it will be important to listen to any comments and suggestions made by the trainees. No matter how careful you are in choosing representative areas, there are bound to be areas with different characteristics. Operation and maintenance staff may well have useful insights about the impact of these differences on their work and the ways in which potential problems can be overcome.

Checking the progress and quality of work

Good records should be kept as a matter of course. An early objective for each plan component should be to develop simple pro formas to provide information on points such as the starting date, materials purchased, people assigned to various tasks, expenditure incurred and so on.

Problems that are not dealt with when they arise have an unfortunate tendency to turn into bigger problems. Good monitoring and supervision arrangements should facilitate the early identification of problems. However, identifying a problem does not guarantee that it will be dealt with promptly. Indeed, identifying problems early and dealing with them as they arise will often require fundamental changes in the ways in which public officials think. One of the objectives in the early stages of implementation should be to develop a more proactive approach to identifying and dealing with problems. This will often require training on the points to look for when checking works and procedures for dealing with faults and deficiencies. For example, it should be an absolute requirement that site engineers check the invert level of every manhole or chamber on a new sewer line and confirm that the sewer is free of construction debris before it is commissioned. This is an obvious point but one that is regularly neglected.

This training will have to be backed up by incentives to ensure that tasks are actually carried out. In the example of the sewer given above, good practice will be encouraged by a requirement that the engineer or technician responsible for site supervision must be able to produce a record of his or her checks on the invert levels manholes and chambers at any time. Such requirements must be supported by the sanction of disciplinary action for any engineer or technician who has not ensured that a contractor follows basic aspects of good practice.

People from the community can be very effective in monitoring the quality of work. After all, the facilities will serve them and it is often their money that is being spent. However, it is important that they are given guidance on the quality of work required. It is usually best if the community is asked to nominate a small group of people to monitor works on their behalf. These people can then be given appropriate training. It is not good if everyone oversees the contractor's work. Another option is to appoint people from the community to act as work supervisors. The danger with both of these approaches is that government engineers will ignore community concerns, but this danger can be reduced if both parties to the agreement are involved in the planning process from the outset.

Assessment

As one phase of the planning process, represented by a particular three or five-year action plan, draws to its close, it will be necessary to start thinking about reviewing overall objectives and developing a follow-up action plan to cover the next five years.

Assessment does not have to be a drawn-out process and should never be carried out for its own sake. Rather, the aim should be to gain knowledge that will help you and others to plan and develop better sanitation schemes in the future. Look for answers to the following questions.

○ How much did the initiative actually cost and was the cost any different from that originally estimated?

○ Is it operating as intended and what effort is required to manage its operation?

○ Has it brought about the expected benefits – in other words, what impact has it had?

○ Are people happy with what has been done or would they do some things differently if they were to be done again?

Answers to these questions can be obtained from various sources. Information on costs should be available from the records kept by the individual or organization responsible for managing implementation. You can find out whether a facility is operating as intended by observation and by talking to the people who use it and/or are responsible for its operation. It will be harder to assess the wider benefits, particularly those that relate to health. You may wish to take advice on this aspect of evaluation. It may well be that you learn some important lessons by asking people whether they are happy with what has been done and what they would do differently next time. Consult widely and do not restrict your contacts to community leaders.

The results of assessment should be made available to those who are working for further improvements in sanitation and related services.

Sharing experience

If you have successfully implemented a sanitation plan in a city, town or neighbourhood you have experience and information that should prove useful to those facing similar problems. Indeed, the growth of strategic planning will be largely dependent on the willingness of those with experience to share that experience.

What experience do you want to share?

The main focus should be on positive experiences with successful outcomes. No one will be particularly interested in hearing about your failures. This does not mean that you should present your experience as one long story of effortless achievement. It almost certainly will not have been that, and other people are likely to learn most from descriptions of the difficulties you faced and the actions you took to overcome them. It may be useful to use the following questions as a framework for identifying the messages that you want to communicate.

○ How did our approach aim to solve the problems that it set out to tackle?

○ What problems did we encounter?

○ How did we overcome those problems, or how would we seek to overcome them in the light of our experience?

When exploring these questions, you should look at the different aspects of sanitation provision as an integrated whole rather than dealing with them in isolation. For instance, if you have been involved in a scheme to provide new sanitation facilities using a particular technology, perhaps double-pit pour-flush latrines, you should describe not only the technology but also the arrangements made to implement and then operate and maintain it and how related issues like hygiene promotion and drainage were managed. Did any groups face problems with the approach adopted and the facilities provided?

It may be useful to consider your experience in terms of the project cycle – how did you:

o identify the need for sanitation improvements (establish demand)
o develop an understanding of the options (inform demand)
o implement the project or programme (respond to demand)
o operate and maintain services over time (sustain achievements)
o assess the effect of your work.

At each stage, think about what you were able to do yourself and where you found it necessary to seek help from other individuals and organizations. How were your relationships with these people and organizations defined? How did you overcome any communication difficulties and ensure that responsibilities were clearly defined and agreed?

With whom do you want to share your experience?

Those working at the local level will be interested in sharing experience with others working at the local level, for instance NGOs, CBOs and councillors. They may also wish to disseminate information to officials who have shown an interest in local action to improve sanitation. Municipal stakeholders should share their experiences with representatives of other municipalities.

Neither group should neglect to share its experience with representatives of central government and international agencies. Development is a practical discipline and those who make crucial decisions on development issues have much to learn from those working in the field. Conversely, the findings from policy-related studies and initiatives should be made available to municipal and local stakeholders.

The information to be shared may vary depending on the group with whom you want to share it. It may be worthwhile to develop a two-stage approach to information sharing. In the first stage, you might put out general information on what you have done. As groups come to you for further information, you can tailor information to their needs, as identified in discussions with members of the group.

How can information be shared?

Just as the content of the information to be shared should reflect the interests of the group for whom it is intended, so the methods used to share it will depend on the target audience. In general, written material will be more appropriate for municipal authorities, national NGOs, policy makers and planners, while the spoken word and visual material will be more appropriate for those working at the local level. Of course, you can use a variety of methods for any one target group.

Some specific routes for sharing information include:

o *Written material.* Articles and reports are a useful way of providing information on your experiences, including what you have achieved and the lessons that you have learnt. However, they will only be useful to others if they clearly identify the problems that you have faced and the ways in which they were overcome. They should also be very clear about any constraints that might limit the applicability of your approach. You should always write about what you did rather than what you intended to do, although a comparison between the two may be useful.

o *Videos* allow people to see what has been done but will only have an impact if they are edited so that key points are clearly brought out. It may be worthwhile to employ a professional video maker.

> **Box 10.5 'Face-to-face' community exchanges**
>
> The Asian Coalition of Housing Rights (ACHR) and Slum Dwellers International have been supporting community-to-community exchange programmes for the past decade. After a few years of experimentation, this methodology of sharing and learning generated such an impact that it was formalized into a training process for ACHR. Along with exchange pioneers in the SPARC alliance, India, and friends in People's Dialogue, South Africa, community-to-community exchanges have now extended beyond Asia to include direct international sharing among poor communities. The experiences from these exchanges are documents in the *Face to Face* newsletter, which is available from the ACHR and can be downloaded from their web site (www.achr.net).

- *Talks* give more opportunities to expand on points than reports and videos. They also allow for people to ask questions and make comments. Like other methods of communication, talks need to be well planned and structured. It may be worthwhile combining a talk with the viewing of a video and distribution of written material.

- A *workshop* requires more preparation than a simple talk but offers a longer period in which to get key points across. It offers good opportunities for interaction and sharing and may be a very good way of communicating important lessons. Again, it is important to ensure that the event is well planned and structured.

- *Exchange visits* give community members the chance to interact so that those who have been involved in sanitation improvements can tell others about their experience. People may be more convinced by what is said by 'people like themselves' than they are by more polished statements by outsiders. These may involve in-country exchange visits or might involve international visits (see Box 10.5).

Experience suggests that, while all of these methods can be useful, none of them is likely to change hearts and minds on its own. Rather, the need will usually be for a range of dissemination methods as part of a planned programme for developing interest in strategic planning processes.

Networks as a means of sharing experience

While you can do everything discussed above on your own, you will be more successful in sharing experience if you are part of a network of people and organizations with similar interests and objectives. These networks may operate at the local level, holding regular meetings and exchange visits as described in Box 10.6.

The problems described in Box 10.6 suggest a need for an organization that is seen as neutral to take responsibility for organizing networking activities. This might be an international organization such as UNICEF or the Water and Sanitation Program but a preferable option will be a government department that is committed and engaged. Where neither of these options are possible, it may be that a number of NGOs and CBOs can cooperate to set up some sort of resource centre that will be responsible for coordinating networking activities.

There are also a number of international networks that can be useful resources for those with access to the internet. An introduction to a number of these networks, including contact details, is given in Appendix 4.

Box 10.6 Water and Environmental Sanitation Network (WESNET), Pakistan

The WESNET NGO network was originally proposed by the Youth Commission for Human Rights (YCHR), an NGO based in Lahore, Pakistan. The initiative had some success in bringing together the various NGOs and officials from government agencies that were working on sanitation and solid waste management issues in Punjab Province and to some extent beyond. Some government officials attended its meetings. However, it proved difficult to sustain the initiative, partly because of limited funding and partly because the network was viewed as belonging primarily to the organization that initiated it.

Key points in this chapter

1. The strategic plan will only have value if it is implemented.

2. The first steps in implementation are crucial. If the process falters at this stage, the plan is likely to be shelved and will quickly be supplemented by ad hoc responses to immediate problems.

3. The initial emphasis should be on achieving the first year objectives set out in the plan document. Responsibilities for pursuing those objectives should be allocated at an early stage.

4. An assessment of all possible sources of funding should be carried out as soon as possible after ratification of the plan. These may include both internal and external sources but priority should be given to the former whenever possible.

5. It will often be necessary to develop the outline proposals for the various plan components contained in the plan itself into detailed proposals.

6. When developing proposals for improved operation and maintenance, it will be important to consider constraints, not the least of which is likely to be the low priority currently given to operation and maintenance.

7. In order to convince decision makers of the benefits of improved operation and maintenance, early initiatives should focus on areas in which it is relatively easy to achieve improvements and on those improvements that are likely to have the greatest immediate impact.

8. Responsibilities for supervising the implementation of the various plan components should be decided in the light of available resources and current legislation and procedures.

9. If local facilities managed by community or private sector organizations are connected to higher-order facilities managed by a central provider, a formal agreement will be required to set out the rights and responsibilities of the partners.

10. It will be important to monitor the progress of the plan and to assess its achievements. The results of this assessment should feed into follow-up plans.

11. When sharing experience relating to a strategic sanitation initiative, it is important to identify the problems encountered and describe the actions taken to overcome them.

Chapter 10 endnotes

1 This approach was used for the tertiary sewerage component of the World Bank-funded North-east Lahore Upgrading Project in Pakistan in the late 1980s. Every chamber was defined in terms of its type (Type A, Type B, Type C) which could be cross-referenced to a standard detail sheet. Information was given on the sewer invert level (or invert levels if branches came in at different levels) and the existing and proposed ground levels at the chamber. The distance between chambers was specified, as was the diameter and approximate gradient of the sewer running between them. The latter was intended for guidance only since the actual gradient was determined by the invert levels at the chambers and the distance between them. A similar approach was developed independently for the Bandung component of the KIP programme in Indonesia (T.P. O'Sullivan and Partners, undated).

2 This is precisely what happened with private sweepers operating in the area chosen for the introduction of a house-to-house collection service in Bharatpur.

3 This box is based on information supplied by Claudia Bockman Weisburd, a planner and community development specialist who has been involved with the Yoff project since 1998. For further information on the background to the project and its approach see Weisburd (2000).

4 Information provided by Martin Mulenga, a PhD research student at Southampton University, UK.

APPENDIX 1
Links between sanitation and health

Sanitation and health definitions

Faecal–oral infections are infections for which the transmission route is from the faeces of an infected person into the mouth of another person.

Pathogens are the infective organisms excreted by an infected person, which can then enter the body of another person and infect that person. They may be viruses, bacteria or small invertebrate animals, including amoeba and worms.

An infection is *latent* when there is a gap between the time a disease-causing organism leaves an infected person's body and the time it can pass the infection on to another person. Many latent infections require an intermediate host, sometimes a snail or a fish. Other infections are spread by pathogens that can live for long periods outside a person if they find a suitable environment, for instance a damp, shaded area such as an infrequently cleaned latrine floor.

A *vector* is the organism by which a disease is transmitted from one person to another. Mosquitoes are vectors of malaria and filariasis. Rats are vectors for leptospirosis and pneumonic plague.

Helminths are small parasitical worms that live in the body, usually in the gut, and make people feel tired and listless.

Excreta-related infections

Transmission routes and the barriers to transmission

Most excreta-related infections are faecal–oral in nature although at least one, schistosomiasis or bilharzia, can be spread in an infected person's urine. The 'f' diagram can be used to represent the routes by which they can be transmitted from one person to another. This is reproduced on the left-hand side of Figure A1.1, while the right-hand side of the figure illustrates the role of improved sanitation and hygiene in creating barriers to disease transmission.

Figure A1.1(a) illustrates the following points.

○ Pathogens may reach a new host because he or she drinks infected water (the term fluids in the diagram refers to water) but the route through foods shows that there is also a risk if contaminated water is used for food preparation.

○ Pathogens may reach a new host via fields if either people defecate in the fields or untreated water is used to irrigate crops. The first is likely to be particularly problematic if certain areas are generally accepted as open defecation areas.

○ Flies can transmit pathogens from uncovered faeces on to food.

○ Pathogens can be transmitted from faeces on to fingers and then directly to a person's mouth or on to food.

Figure A1.1(b) shows two barriers to disease transmission.

○ The *sanitation barrier* prevents faecal material getting into the wider environment and thus creating a hazard for other

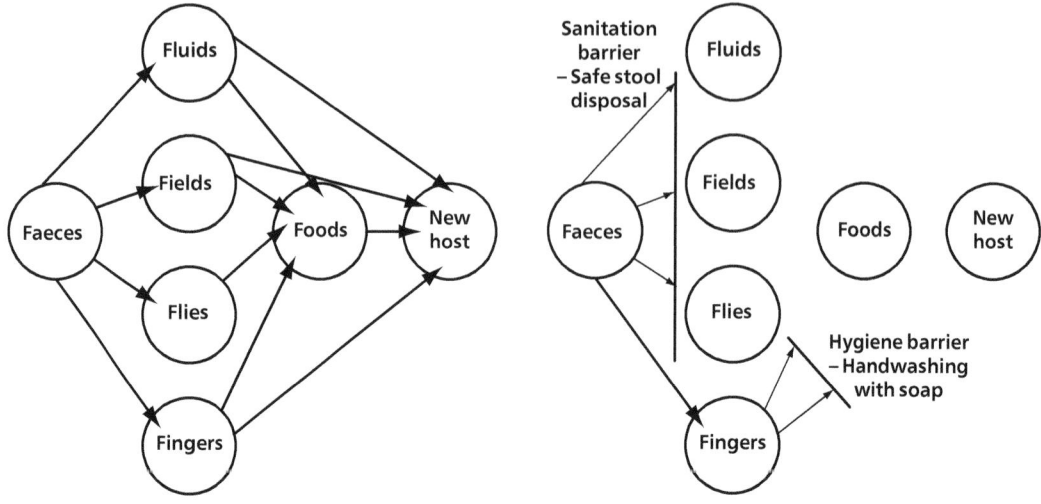

(a) Transmission routes   (b) Sanitation and hygiene barriers

Figure A1.1 Faecal–oral disease transmission routes and the role of improved sanitation and hygiene in breaking them

people. Sanitation systems must be designed to ensure safe stool disposal, which prevents pathogens from reaching water or fields and which keeps flies away from faeces.

o The *hygiene barrier* prevents pathogens finding their way from an infected person's hands via food or another person's hands, to the mouth of another person. The key to good hygiene is handwashing with soap after stool contact.

Blocking some transmission routes while leaving others open will not prevent the transmission of infections. So, planners must pay attention to the need for both improved sanitation and better hygiene.

Figure A1.1(b) also indicates that barriers to disease transmission should be placed as early as possible in the transmission route. Improvements at the household level, where people spend most of their time and are most likely to encounter pathogens, are likely to have the most significant impacts on health. Improvements in public facilities such as sewers will only have a significant health impact if they are linked with improvements within the household.

Categories of infection

Sanitation-related infections can be categorized in terms of their transmission mechanism as follows (Cairncross and Feacham, 1993):

1. Faecal–oral (non-bacterial)
2. Faecal–oral (bacterial)
3. Soil-transmitted helminths
4. Beef and pork tapeworms
5. Water-based helminths
6. Excreta-related insect vectors

Infections in the first five categories are associated with poor excreta disposal while excreta-related insect vectors can also flourish where there is poor drainage.

Infections in the first two categories are immediately infective. Those in categories three to five are latent. Many, but not all diseases in these categories require an intermediate host and all involve infection with some form of worm, with the degree of sickness depending on the number of adult worms infesting the patient. This means that the intensity of infection must be assessed in terms of average levels of infestation as well as the number of people infected.

Each of the six categories of infection is now briefly described, with particular attention paid to the ways in which the absence of good sanitation influences their transmission.

Faecal–oral infections are often referred to as water-borne diseases because they can be transmitted when someone drinks water that has been polluted by the faeces from an infected person (the fluids route in the 'f' diagram). These are not the only infections that can be transmitted via a faecal–oral route but they differ from the others in that they are immediately infective. Diseases in this category can be transmitted by all the routes shown in the 'f' diagram and so improvements in health will only be possible if planners pay attention to the need for both improved sanitation and better hygiene.

Faecal–oral infections can be further divided into two categories:

- *those spread by bacteria*, including cholera, typhoid, salmonellosis and shigallosis, a form of bacterial dysentery
- *those spread by other organisms*, including viruses and a range of small animals including amoeba and giardia. Non-bacterial infections include poliomyelitis, hepatitis A, rotavirus diarrhoea, amoebic dysentery and giardiasis.

The significance of this division lies in the fact that bacterial infections only lead to disease if a person ingests a relatively large number of infectious bacteria. In technical terms, they have a high infective dose. These infections can be transmitted both by direct contact routes, via fingers and food and through contaminated drinking water. So, prevention of these diseases requires both good hygiene and the provision of clean drinking water. Sanitation improvements can have a secondary impact in reducing the amount of pollution reaching drinking water sources and fields but will only be effective in breaking transmission routes if everyone has a form of sanitation that prevents pathogens from reaching drinking water sources.

Most non-bacterial infections will lead to disease if a person ingests much smaller numbers of infectious organisms. In other words, they have a low infective dose. Diseases with a low infective dose are likely to be transmitted by a direct contact route, via fingers and food. Sanitation improvements are unlikely to have a significant impact upon the transmission of these infections unless they are accompanied by action to improve hygiene behaviour. Sanitation plans should emphasize the need to provide water for hand washing close to each latrine. In the case of some infections, for instance poliomyelitis, the best barrier against disease transmission is vaccination.

Properly designed and maintained sanitation facilities will prevent *fly breeding in excreta* and thus reduce transmission via flies. Poorly designed and maintained sanitation facilities may actually become a focus for insect breeding and thus increase the danger of infection.

Water-based helminth infections require an intermediate water-based host for part of their life cycle. In most cases, this is some form of snail although some diseases rely on plants or fish to provide a link in their transmission route. Sickness is caused by parasitic worms that live in the infected person, usually in the intestines. These do not kill people directly but weaken them and reduce their ability to work.

The most important infection in this

group is schistosomiasis, also known as bilharzia, which is caused by worms living in an infected person's veins. Eggs from the worms may be excreted or passed in the urine. They hatch in water and the larvae penetrate any suitable snail that they encounter. Once inside a snail, the larvae develop further and aquatic larvae known as *cercariae* emerge into the water after a period of 1–3 months. These live for a period of up to 48 hours in water and will penetrate any human skin that they encounter, subsequently developing into adult worms and starting the cycle again. Schistosomiasis can be a particular problem in irrigated areas and around water bodies that are used for fishing, since both require people to enter contaminated water.

The transmission route for schistosomiasis can be broken by:

○ on-site sanitation systems, which retain excreta and prevent it from reaching water bodies and irrigation channels

○ sewage treatment systems with a long retention time, for instance waste stabilization ponds.

However, infection will continue unless all faeces are prevented from reaching the watercourses. This means that sanitation improvements will rarely be sufficient on their own to deal with schistosomiasis. If it exists in your area, you should take advice on developing an integrated strategy, combining improved sanitation with measures to control snail populations and reduce people's exposure to contaminated water. The danger of exposure to contaminated water should be emphasised in hygiene education programmes and options for reducing exposure should be explored with community members, who will be best placed to know whether changes in behaviour to reduce exposure are possible in practice.

Beef and pork tapeworm infections are caused by parasitic worms that attach themselves to the small intestines of humans. Their eggs are excreted and eaten by cows or pigs. The larvae develop in the animal and can infect people who eat uncooked meat. They do not usually have severe effects in themselves but there is a danger that cysticercosis may occur in areas where the pork tapeworm is endemic. This is a severe disease that is contracted when a person ingests the eggs of the pork tapeworm.

Problems with beef and pork tapeworms are likely to arise when untreated or inadequately treated sewage is discharged onto land where cows or pigs are grazing or which is being used to produce fodder crops. Transmission can also occur when animals eat solid waste that includes human faeces removed from dry toilets. Improved on-site sanitation can break the transmission route, as can sewage treatment processes with a long retention time, such as waste stabilization ponds. The other important control measure is the complete cooking of food and this should be emphasized in public health programmes where tapeworm infection is endemic.

Soil transmitted helminth infections are caused by parasitic worms living in the intestines. The most serious infections are ascaris (roundworm) and hookworm. Infection results in general sickness and weakness rather than specific acute symptoms and for this reason may be widespread in the community without people being aware of it. In fact, surveys have revealed infection rates of over 50% in poor communities in countries as diverse as Venezuela, Bangladesh and Malaysia. Those in occupational groups such as refuse collectors and sanitary workers are particularly exposed to infection and are often unaware that they are infected.

The first stage in transmission occurs when an infected person excretes eggs produced by the infecting worms. The eggs hatch if they encounter a suitable environment, typically a moist shaded soil. The larvae can survive for long periods outside the body in suitable conditions and this increases the chance of infection. For ascaris, the infective cycle is completed when larvae are ingested from hands, food and utensils. One form of hookworm (*ascaris duodenale*) can be transmitted in the same way via unwashed vegetables, but all hookworm infections are spread by larvae penetrating the skin, usually round the feet and ankles.

The danger of transmission is greatest where some or all of the following occur:

○ people defecate on the ground, particularly where certain areas are commonly used for defecation

○ latrine floors become soiled and are not cleaned properly, particularly where the floor is earth

○ raw sewage is used to irrigate crops

○ small children are allowed to defecate in yards and compounds, particularly where there is no hard surface.

Immediate reductions in helminth infection can be achieved through chemotherapy – the use of de-worming medicines. However, for lasting effect, chemotherapy must be combined with longer-term measures. Good sanitation is important since it can prevent eggs from reaching the ground. It will only do this if *all*, including young children, use the facilities and this must be emphasized during sanitation and hygiene promotion. The effect of improved hygiene will be less than for more directly transmitted infections although it must have some effect where larvae are ingested from hands and food.

Sewage treatment facilities that retain sewage for several days, in particular waste stabilization ponds, can be effective in breaking the transmission route via irrigated crops. Undigested sewage sludge should not be used as a fertilizer since the pathogens will settle during the treatment process and be concentrated in the sludge.

Infections associated with poor drainage

Excreta-related insect vectors are generally associated with poor drainage, which allows pools of dirty water to form. These provide breeding sites for the mosquitoes that are responsible for the spread of a number of diseases (Kolsky, 1999). These include *bancroftian filariasis*, which is spread by mosquitoes of the type *culex quinquefasciatus*, which is the main nocturnal mosquito found in urban areas throughout the world (Lines, 2002).

Chemical spraying can be used as a short-term measure against mosquitoes but the best long-term approach to control is to drastically reduce the number of mosquitoes by eliminating breeding sites. Drainage improvements, designed to remove standing water, can play an important role in this. However physical improvements in themselves are not enough. Unless drainage facilities are maintained, there is a danger that no long-term improvement will be achieved.

Flooding can occur because of inadequate drainage. The risk of disease transmission will increase if floodwater becomes mixed with water from sewers, septic tanks and leach pits. When designing facilities, everything possible should be done to prevent this mixing from occurring. Pit latrines and leach-pits should be raised above the natural ground level to prevent the entry of storm water. Drainage systems should be designed to allow storm water to run on the surface rather than entering drains and sewers and causing them to overflow. Attention must also be paid to operation and maintenance. Flooding is more likely to occur if drains are not cleaned regularly and/or solid waste is allowed to accumulate in them.

Open drains carrying sewage and sullage water are potential sources of infection. Pathogen concentrations in sullage are likely to be a lot less than those in sewage but many drains that are nominally intended to carry sullage water receive sewage flows from WCs and septic tanks.

Health impacts of improvements in solid waste management

Uncollected solid waste in streets or at dump sites can provide a habitat for rats and flies and thus contribute to the spread of a number of diseases. Rats are the major vectors of plague and leptospirosis while flies provide a possible transmission route for faecal–oral disease. Discarded tin cans and tyres can collect relatively clean water and thus provide a breeding ground for *Aedes mosquitoes*, which transmit dengue and yellow fever.

Solid waste is also linked to faecal–oral transmission routes in other ways. The mixing of faecal wastes from primitive dry sanitation systems with other solid wastes can pose a health threat to sanitary workers. If the waste is used as a fertilizer or eaten by animals, there may be a risk of disease transmission via food. Uncollected solid waste often finds its way into surface drains and sewers, causing blockages, contributing to flooding and helping to create insect breeding sites.

All these impacts can be reduced by improvements in solid waste management. However, localized improvements will not eliminate problems. Where waste is collected in some streets but not in the surrounding areas, there is nothing to stop insects and rats crossing from one area to another and carrying diseases with them.

APPENDIX 2
Summary information on sanitation technologies

Short summaries of the various sanitation technologies are given in the pages that follow. They are grouped in accordance with the following categories.

Dry on-site systems: simple pit latrine, ventilated improved pit latrine (VIP), twin-pit VIP, and 'ecological' approaches, including 'dry box' systems with separate urine separation and dehydrating latrines.

Wet (water-flushed) on-site systems: single leach pit disposal, twin leach pit disposal, septic tank discharging to a soakaway or drainfield.

Hybrid systems: household septic tanks and leach pits used in association with open drains and sewered interceptor tank systems.

Wet off-plot systems: sewerage.

Researchers have also developed water-flushed systems including urine separation but these have not been widely used to date, certainly not in southern countries, and are not discussed here.

Dry on-site systems – simple pit latrine

The simple pit latrine is the simplest form of dry on-site sanitation (Figure A2.1). Its main components are:

The superstructure. All that is strictly required is an enclosure to ensure privacy. Most pit latrines include a roof and a door but these are not essential. Discuss the superstructure design with the intended users, taking particular account of the need to comply with local social norms and to minimize costs.

A pit cover slab with a hole for defecation. This will normally be a concrete slab covering the pit or a smaller slab (Sanplat) that is supported by a cover made from locally obtainable materials (mud and wood). It must be possible to clean the slab. The cover slab should be raised 150–300 mm above the surrounding ground level to ensure that floodwater does not enter the pit. A removable cover should be provided and placed over the defecation hole whenever the latrine is not in use in order to prevent flies and other insects from entering and leaving the pit.

The pit. The larger the horizontal dimensions, the greater the cost of covering the pit. Greater volume can be achieved without unduly increasing covering costs by making the pit longer than it is wide. A high water table or hard rock may limit the depth of the pit but the greater the depth achieved the longer the pit will last. In poor ground, the whole depth of the pit may have to be lined. The lining should be porous so that water can escape. In good ground, no lining will be required other than a collar round the top of the pit.

When to use a simple pit latrine. When the amount of water available on-site is less than about 25 litres per person per day and there are financial or cultural reasons why a ventilated improved pit latrine cannot be used.

Advantages. The main advantage of the simple pit latrine is its low cost.

Disadvantages. Insects, particularly flies will create problems and represent a possible health hazard unless the removable cover over the hole is replaced after each use of

184 URBAN SANITATION

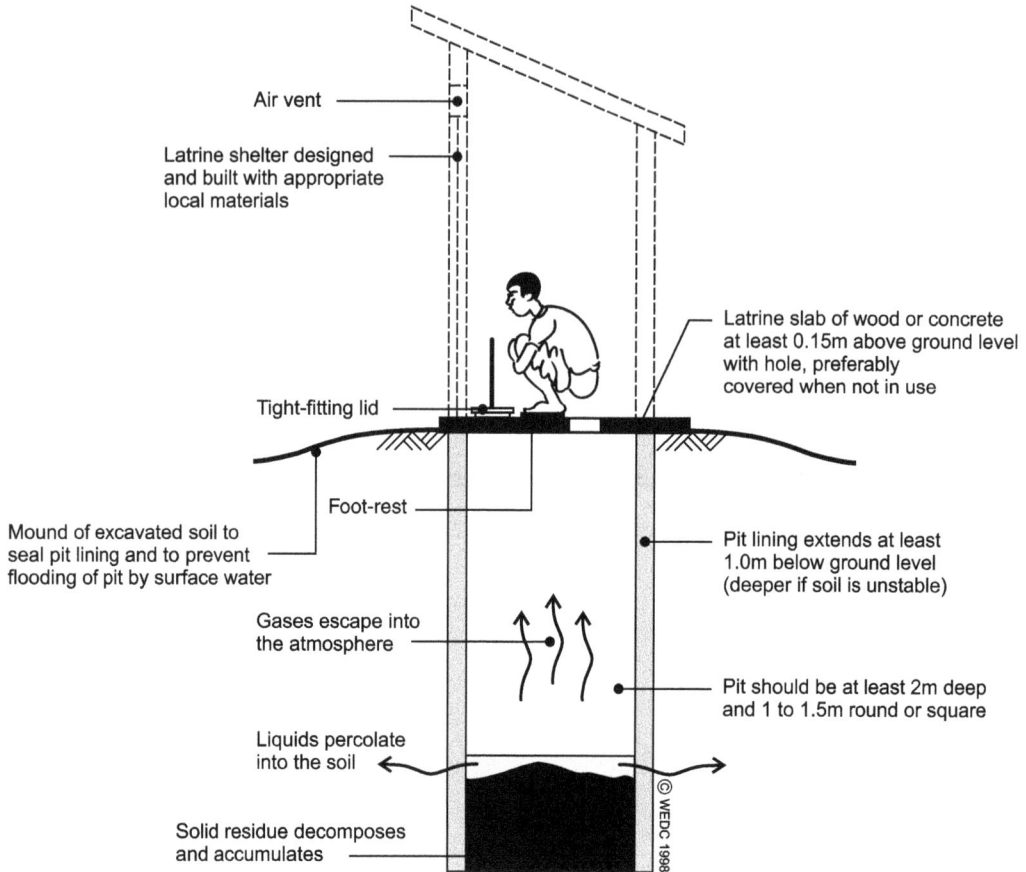

Figure A2.1 Simple pit latrine

the latrine. There may also be problems with smells.

Examples of good practice. A simple design of concrete cover slab has been developed and extensively used in Mozambique. The slab is very slightly domed to avoid the need for reinforcement and incorporates a tightly fitting cover for the hole. Slabs are produced at local casting yards and sold to sanitation users at a subsidized price.

Dry on-site systems – ventilated improved pit (VIP) latrine

The ventilated improved pit (VIP) latrine is a development of the simple pit latrine, designed to eliminate fly problems and reduce bad smells (Figure A2.2). It does this by drawing flies and smells from the pit into a vent pipe, at the top of which the flies are trapped by a screen and eventually die.

The points made about the design of the slab and the pit for simple pit latrines also apply to VIPs. Other key points are as follows.

The vent pipe should extend well above the roof of the latrine superstructure, as this will ensure a good draft of air up the pipe. Ideally, it should be at least 150 mm in diameter, painted black and located on the sunny side of the superstructure to increase con-

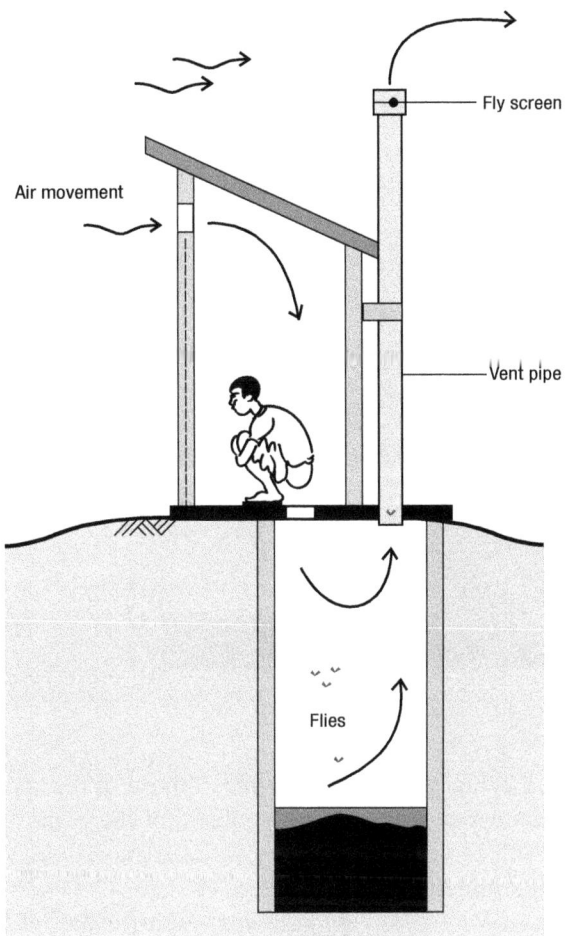

Figure A2.2 Ventilated improved pit (VIP) latrine

vection. The screen must be made of a material that is resistant to corrosion.

The interior of the superstructure must be dark so that flies are attracted to the light at the top of the vent pipe.

Access to the pit to remove the contents may be gained via removal of slabs located outside the superstructure. Alternatively, a hole can be provided in the superstructure wall through which a tanker suction pipe can be introduced (see Figure 6.2). This arrangement is more likely to be effective if the pit contents are wet.

When to use a VIP? When the amount of water available is less than about 25 litres per person per day, it is possible to dig a fairly deep pit – preferably at least 5 m deep, people are prepared to use a latrine with a dark interior, and non-corrosive material is available to make the fly screen at the top of the vent.

Advantages. Relatively low cost (but higher than simple pit latrine) and reduction in fly and smell problems when compared with most simple pit latrines.

Disadvantages. Users may not appreciate the need for a dark interior and may modify the superstructure to provide more light,

186 URBAN SANITATION

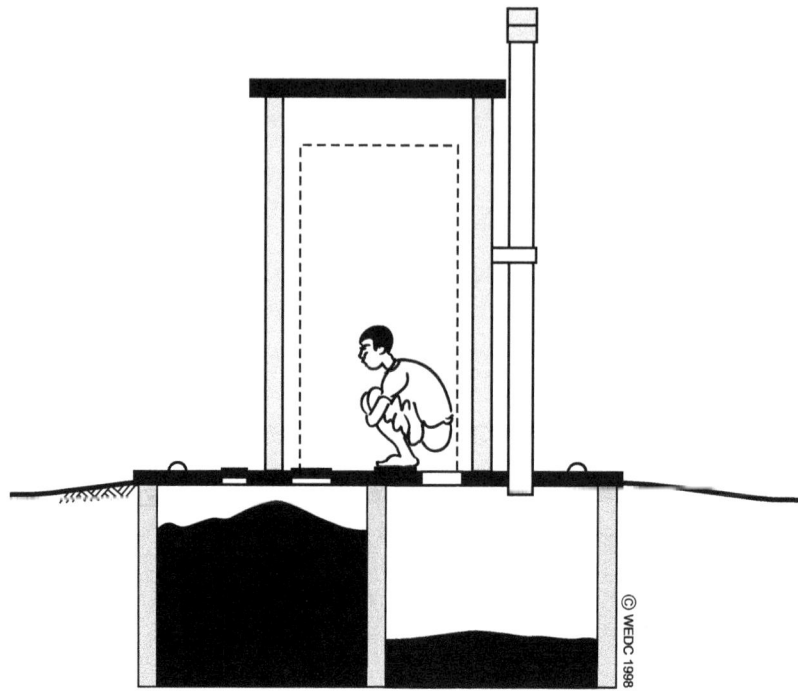

Figure A2.3 Twin-pit VIP latrine

thus undermining the basic rationale behind the design. The design is very dependent on a durable fly screen and health and convenience benefits will be undermined if the screen fails for any reason.

Examples of good practice. The Blair Research Laboratory in Zimbabwe has developed a range of VIP designs suitable for different conditions (Morgan, 1990).

Dry on-site systems – twin-pit VIP latrines

The design provides two pits or chambers with the intention that only one pit is used at any time. Once a pit is full, the contents are left in the pit while the other pit is being used. By the time the second pit is full, the contents of the first pit should have decomposed so that they are odourless and free of harmful organisms. They can then be removed without any danger to health.

The basic features of the twin-pit VIP are similar to those of the standard VIP, except of course that there are two pits, each with its own defecation hole, vent pipe and flyscreen. (Figure A2.3 shows the opening for the vent pipe for the pit that is not in use blocked off on the assumption that the vent pipe can be moved from one side to the other when required.)

The superstructure is shared between the two pits. The hole leading to the pit that is not currently in use should be covered by a slab or stopper.

It is not uncommon for the pits to be replaced by chambers located partly or wholly above ground level. Pits are normally designed to contain the excreta collected over a period of around two years.

The internal dimensions of each pit should be about 0.9 m square by 0.9 m deep.

Advantages. The design reduces the need to handle fresh faecal material and this has potential health benefits. It requires little water, which can be an important consideration where water resources are limited. Little depth is required so that the design is more suitable than conventional VIPs for areas with a high water table or very hard sub-surface rock.

Disadvantages. The twin pit VIP is rather more expensive than the conventional single-pit design. However, the biggest practical problems usually stem from difficulties in ensuring that the latrine is used as designed and in emptying the pits once they are full. When considering twin-pit VIPs, make sure that potential users understand the technology, accept it and are prepared to use it as intended. Also, make sure that the arrangements for emptying pits are generally understood and agreed and, if possible, have been tested.

Examples of good practice. Twin pits were used in a World Bank-funded project in Botswana in the early 1980s. They appear to have been reasonable successful in the short term but the users wanted piped sewerage and it seems that many have now been replaced. This illustrates the point that users often perceive on-site dry systems as inferior to other forms of sanitation, whether or not this is objectively the case. When introducing such systems, be sure to thoroughly explore their advantages and disadvantages with potential users.

Dry on-site systems – 'dry box' and dehydrating systems

Dry box systems are designed to separate faeces and urine and dispose of them separately. Most of the nitrogen contained in excreta is in the urine which transmits few of the diseases associated with human waste. (Schistosomiasis is an exception but is only a problem in some areas.) So, once separated, urine can be diluted and used as a fertilizer without treatment. Dry box systems fall within the wider category of 'ecological' approaches to sanitation, which focus on resource recovery rather than 'disposal' of wastes. Rather than 'flush away' or 'drop and store' wastes, it stresses the desirability of using wastes as a resource so as to complete the ecological cycle. Some commentators advocate the addition of straw and vegetable waste to faecal wastes in order to optimize the carbon to nitrogen ratio in the waste and thus speed up decomposition.

Most dry box latrines used in developing countries use the same two-chamber approach as that adopted for double pit VIPs. A good example is the Vietnamese double vault system (Figure A2.4). Note the provision for urine separation.

It is not uncommon for the latrine to be built entirely above ground level. This makes the design suitable for places with a high groundwater table or hard sub-surface rock.

Another traditional latrine design involving urine separation is the 'long-drop' system used in multi-storey buildings in Sana'a and other Yemeni towns. (In Sana'a at least, most of these traditional latrines have now been replaced by more conventional sewered sanitation.)

Other designs include a panel to catch and transmit solar radiation and heat up the contents of the vault or chamber and hence encourage water to evapourate. Some, but not all of these dehydrating designs also feature urine separation.

Advantages. Advocates of dry box systems claim that they achieve rapid pathogen destruction and that there is no smell or fly breeding at moisture contents below 20%. In theory, at least, they also allow nutrients to be recycled and are thus more environmentally sustainable.

Disadvantages. The performance of dry box and dehydrating latrine designs will be adversely affected if users do not use them as intended. They would appear to be more sensitive to misuse and neglect

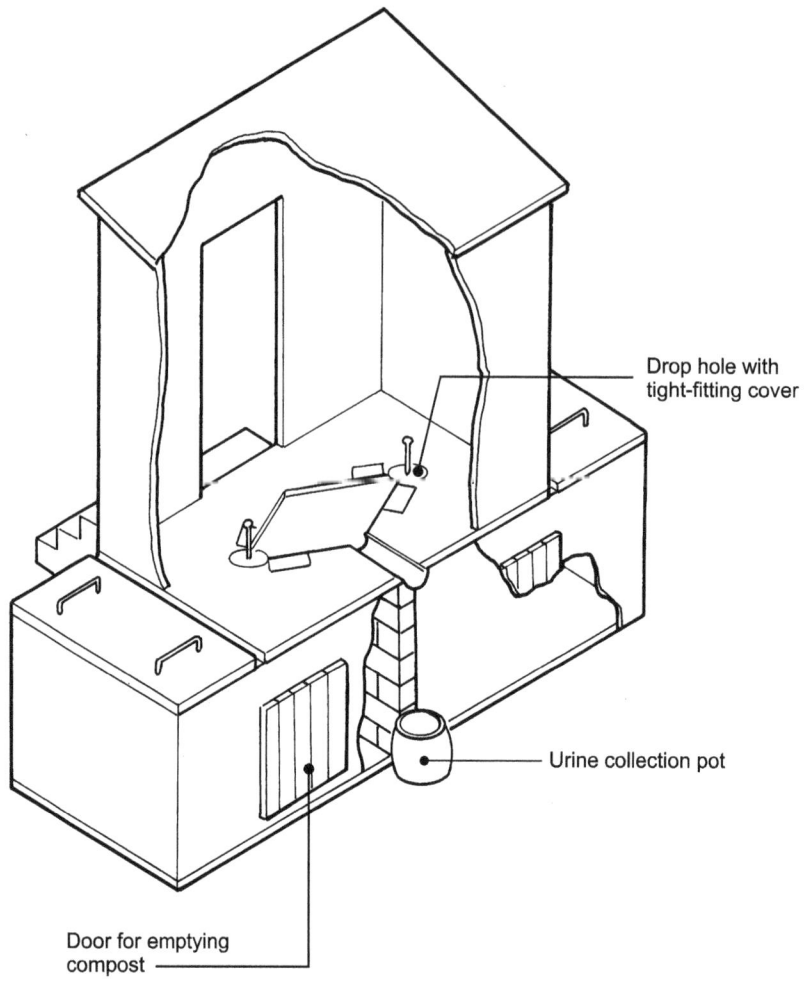

Figure A2.4 'Dry box' latrine

than conventional pit latrines. It is important that users are fully involved in the decision to adopt dry box latrines and understand how the latrines are to be used. This is, of course, something that should happen in any properly conducted strategic approach. More critically, there is a need for follow-up monitoring and support to ensure that the latrines are being used properly and this may be more difficult to guarantee.

In practice, there seem to be real barriers to the use of dry box latrines in urban areas in developing countries, not least the fact that many users are likely to be resistant to their use. Consider them only in areas where either there is already a strong tradition of the re-use of human excreta and/or there is an obvious potential to use wastes in agriculture. Always ask yourself what this system offers in addition to that which is offered by a simpler pit latrine system.

Examples of good practice. The greatest advances in dry box latrine technology have taken place in Sweden. This is a developed country and many of the reported technologies would appear to be too expensive for general adoption in low-income urban areas in developing countries. There are reports of

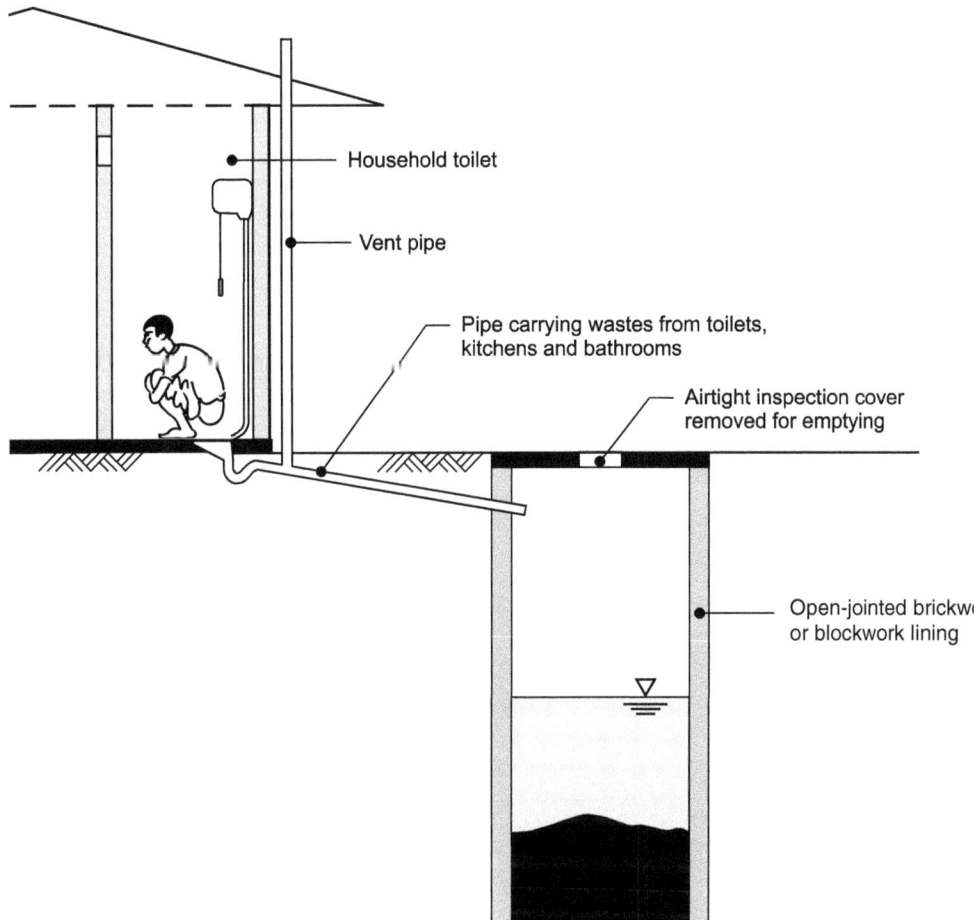

Figure A2.5 Single leach pit latrine

the successful use of dry box toilets in El Salvador, Ecuador and Mexico and larger scale experiments are currently continuing in China. A newsletter containing information on recent experience with ecological sanitation is available in English at www.gtz.de/ecosan/docs/nl6eng.pdf

Wet on-site systems – single leach pit latrines

Leach pits hold faecal material in the same way as the pit of a pit latrine (Figure A2.5). The pit lining should provide openings so that the flush water can percolate into the ground. The pit may be located under the latrine superstructure, as in a standard pit latrine design. However, it is easier to arrange for emptying the contents of the pit if it is off-set. Leach pits are not normally designed to cater for sullage water. If they are, the pit may not be able to cope with the amount of water discharged to it and flooding may be a problem as water use increases.

The key components of a single pit leach pit design are as follows:

○ The superstructure (see notes for pit latrines).

○ A WC pan incorporating a water seal. There are examples of pour-flush latrines

190 URBAN SANITATION

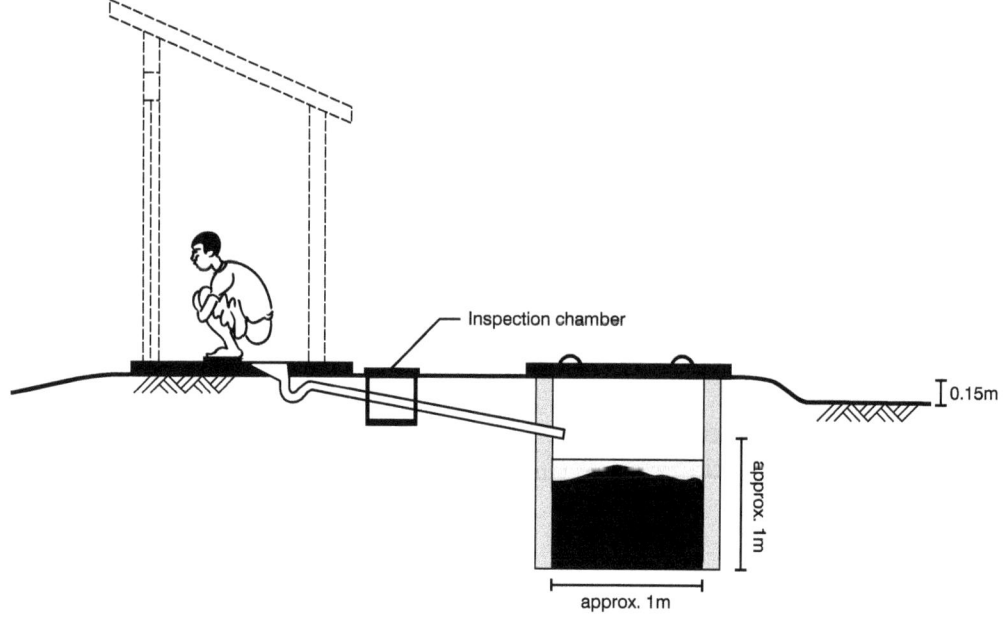

Section

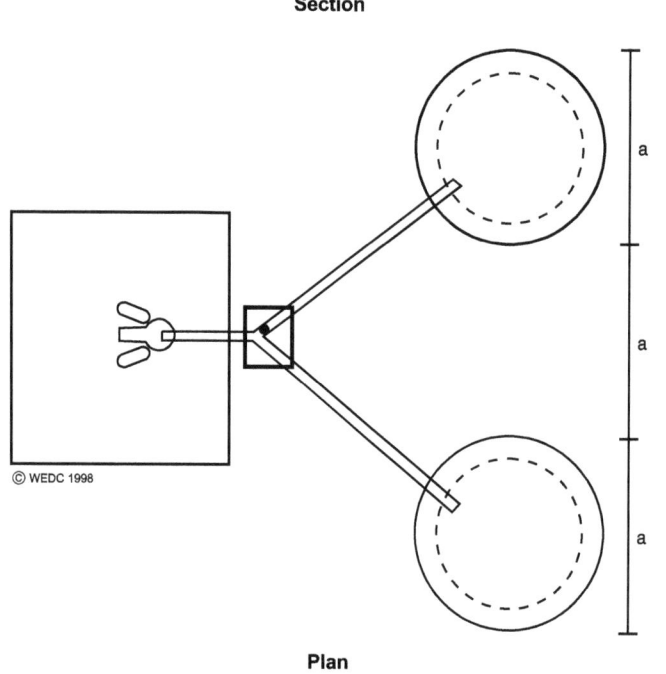

Plan
(Distance between pits (a) = width of one pit)

Figure A2.6 Double pit or twin leach pit latrine

that use a simple shute arrangement rather than a WC pan and water seal but the WC pan arrangement will always be worth the slight extra cost.

o The connecting pipe (for off-set designs). This should be 90 mm or 100 mm diameter and laid at a gradient of at least 1 in 20 (100 mm in 2 m).

o The pit. This should have as much capacity as possible but the plan dimensions should not generally be greater than about 1.25 m. A cylindrical pit will be the most economic arrangement and can be built with a single brick (112 mm) wall.

Small gaps should be left between bricks in the lower brick or blockwork courses to allow water to leach away from the pit. The cover slab should be removable. It may be advantageous to leave a small hole in the cover slab through which a rod can be inserted to check the level of sludge in the pit. Once the pit is full, it must be desludged. *When to use single leach pits?* When per capita water use is at least 25 litres per day and typically in the range 30–50 litres per day. At least 2 m should be available between the bottom of the pit and the water table. Equipment for emptying pits once they are full should be available, a point that is often overlooked.

Advantages. Single leach pits are simple and relatively cheap.

Disadvantages. There is a danger to health if the pit has to be desludged by manual methods. Another potential disadvantage is the need to make separate allowance for sullage drainage as water use rises.

Examples of successful use. The Baldia project in Karachi used single leach pits. The pits worked well initially but problems have been reported as water use increased and sewers have replaced at least some of them (Bakhteari and Wegelin-Schuringa, 1992).

Wet on-site systems – double-pit or twin leach pit latrines

The principle of twin leach pits is the same as that of twin pit VIPs (Figure A2.6). The two pits are used alternately with the contents of each being removed only after they have been left to decompose, typically over a period of perhaps two years.

Key design features include the following:

o WC pan and superstructure as for standard single leach pit design.

o Connecting pipe, incorporating small flow-division chamber with two outlet channels, one to each pit. The cover of the chamber should be removable so that the flow can be diverted into the 'working chamber. The other channel can be blocked off with a simple mud 'dam' or a more sophisticated stopper.

o The twin pits. The design of these should be as for a standard single pit design except that they will normally be smaller. Allow about two years sludge storage, which for a family of six will require a pit around 0.8 m in diameter by a little over 1 m deep below the inlet pipe.

o The pits may be located on the plot or in the road immediately outside it. Where possible, ensure that they can be easily be reached from the public right of way as this will reduce inconvenience to the household during emptying operations

When to use? Use the twin pit design when water use is at least 25 litres per person per day and the water table is at least 3 m below ground. It can be used where there is no official tanker desludging service since the contents are safe to remove by hand.

Advantages. Twin pit latrines are theoretically attractive because they eliminate the need to handle recently deposited faeces containing large numbers of pathogens.

Disadvantages and problems. Twin pits will only work well if the users know how they are meant to be used and are motivated to ensure that they are used as intended. In particular, people must be aware of the reasons why the pits should be used alternately and must be prepared to either empty pits themselves or pay to have them emptied.

Examples of good practice. The twin pit design is extensively used by a number of agencies and programmes. UNICEF sanitation programmes in urban and peri-urban areas are based on the use of the twin pit design and information should be sought from the nearest UNICEF office. Note, however, that some twin pit programmes have failed because users were not sufficiently informed on how they were meant to be operated.

Wet on-site systems – septic tank discharging to a soakaway or drainfield

Unlike leach pits, septic tanks are designed to be watertight. Solids settle in the tank and the liquid effluent from the tank is allowed to percolate into the ground from a soakaway or drainfield. The solids stored in the tank digest anaerobically over time, reducing in volume in the process. Conventional septic tank systems are designed to take both WC and sullage wastes.

The standard septic tank design is rectangular in shape with two compartments (see Figure A2.7). The division into two chambers reduces the possibility of solids being carried through the septic tank as most settle out in the first chamber. Providing tees at the inlet and outlet from the tank further reduces the possibility of carry-through of solids.

Septic tanks have to be sized to provide space for settlement of solids, for digesting solids and for storage of digested solids. Various formulae are available for calculating the size of septic tanks. In general, household septic tanks should be designed for 24 hours retention plus the volume required for sludge storage.

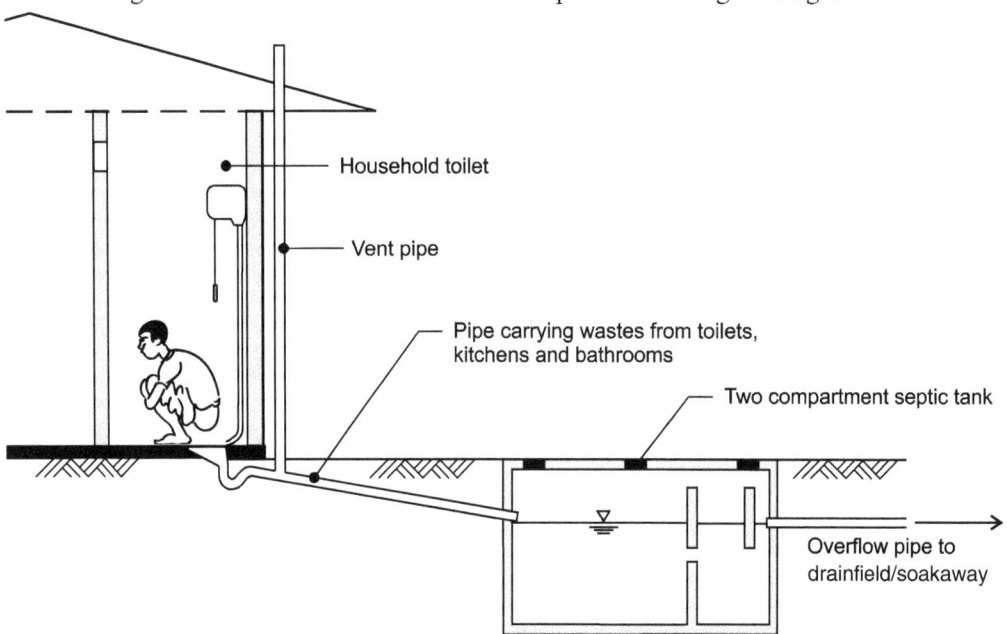

Figure A2.7 Septic tank discharging to a soakaway or drainfield

In theory, settled wastewater should be discharged to a soakaway or drainfield – a hole or trenches in the ground filled with stones or broken bricks. An open-jointed pipe should be provided in the bottom of each drainfield trench to ensure that wastewater is evenly distributed.

Advantages. Because solids are removed in a separate sealed compartment, septic tanks should be hydraulically more efficient than leach pits. In other words, there should be fewer problems with ensuring that wastewater leaches away into the ground.

Disadvantages. The biggest disadvantage of septic tank systems is their cost, which will normally be greater than that of an equivalent leach pit design. A fair amount of space is required if the soakaway or drainfield is to deal with all household wastewater.

Septic tank systems discharging to soakaways are widely used in some south-east Asian countries. However, many systems in other parts of the world involve disposal of the septic tank effluent to an open drain.

Hybrid systems – septic tanks discharging effluent to open drains

In many cities, people living in unsewered low and lower-middle income settlements solve their immediate sanitation and waste disposal problems by installing a WC and connecting it to a household septic tank. The effluent from the septic tank is discharged to an open drain running along the side of the street. The septic tank may be located just inside the plot or outside the plot in the public street. The normal practice is for the septic tank to deal only with WC wastes, with sullage wastes being discharged directly to the drain.

Most professionals condemn this system on the basis that it allows septic tank effluent containing a high concentration of dangerous pathogens to run in the street, where people may come into contact with it. While this system is better than the alternative of having no sanitation at all, there are better alternatives. These include:

○ replacing the open drains with shallow small-bore sewers

○ installing leach pits, designed to deal only with black water and leaving open drains to deal with sullage water.

The first option is considered below. A variation on the second approach has been used in some DFID upgrading schemes in Kolkata, India, where black water is discharged to leach pits and sullage and storm water is carried in shallow sewers.

Hybrid systems – sewered interceptor tank systems

The defining feature of sewered interceptor tank systems (SITS) is that solids are retained in an interceptor tank on each house connection.

Existing interceptor tank to open drain systems can be upgraded to SITS at relatively small expense if the existing septic tanks can be retained and improved (see Figure A2.8).

Where falls are limited, it is possible that the use of SITS will allow gravity discharge to an existing disposal point where conventional sewerage would require the inclusion of a pumping station.

Advantages. The sewered interceptor tank system has three potential benefits compared with conventional sewerage systems.

○ It allows flatter sewer gradients than those required for conventional sewers (some systems have been laid with gradients as low as 1 in 500 as opposed to the 1 in 150 that is theoretically required at the head of a conventional sewer.

○ Attenuation of flow in the interceptor

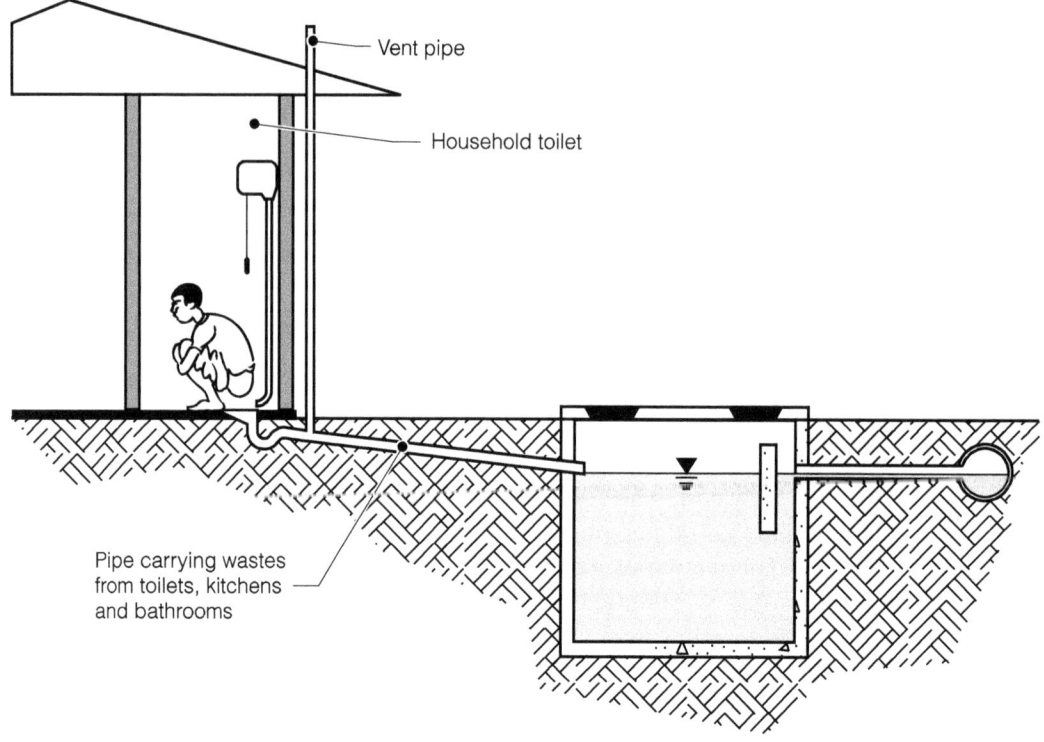

Figure A2.8 Sewered interceptor tank system

tanks reduces peak flows and allows the use of smaller sewer diameters, particularly near the head of the system (SITS have been installed with sewer diameters as small as 50 mm, compared with a minimum diameter of 100 mm for conventional sewers.

o The possibility of blockages in the sewers is reduced because gross solids are removed in the interceptor tanks. This means that the number of manholes and chambers can be greatly reduced, which has the added benefit of reducing the possibility of unwanted solids entering the sewer directly after covers have either been broken or removed. This benefit will only be realized if everyone provides an interceptor tank on his or her house connection.

Disadvantages. SITS remove wastewater from the plot but the need for disposal remains. In most cases, this will involve some form of treatment. Theoretically, the interceptor tanks will remove floating solids and grit and reduce the strength of the sewage by at least 30% and probably more in hot climates, but this will rarely be enough to remove the need for treatment.

The other potential disadvantage of SITS is that the interceptor tanks will have to be desludged from time to time. Normally, hygienic desludging will be dependent on the use of appropriate equipment, ideally some form of tanker incorporating a suction pump. There are few places at present where such equipment is available.

Wet off-site systems – sewerage

The high cost of 'conventional' sewerage is likely to make it unaffordable to low-income people and thus inappropriate for use in the areas where they live. In practice, many people living in low-income areas do use simple forms of sewerage to deal with their liquid wastes. The cost of these is often comparable with that of other sanitation systems. For instance, tertiary sewers and house connections have been built in Pakistan and Indonesia for less than the equivalent of US$40 per household.

When to use? Consider sewerage when water use is greater than at least 60 litres per person per day and housing densities make it difficult to dispose of wastewater on or near plots. This will typically be at population densities greater than about 200 people per hectare. If possible, sewerage should be avoided where the lack of fall means that pumping is necessary. There are two reasons for this. Pumps use energy, which can be expensive, and they require maintenance, which may be difficult to arrange. If pumping is unavoidable, make sure that the financial and management arrangements required to support it are in place.

Advantages. Sewerage is an attractive option for users because it removes problems from their doorsteps, at least as long as it operates as intended. It deals with both faecal wastes and sullage water and can also be used to deal with storm water.

Disadvantages. Sewerage does not solve waste disposal problems. It only moves them to another place, further removed from the households that created them. There will usually be a need for treatment to prevent deterioration of the environment. Experience suggests that sewers in low-income areas often require high levels of maintenance. There are several reasons for this, not least the discharge of silt-laden storm water run-off to sewers and use of sewers as receptacles for solid waste in areas where solid waste collection is deficient or non-existent.

Key design features. These are intended to reduce costs and improve operation.

1. Limit the sewer depth where possible. Do this by routing sewers through gardens and yards, beneath sidewalks and/or in narrow lanes, thus avoiding heavy traffic.

2. Where the sewer depth to invert is less than about 1.25 m, use small inspection chambers designed for access from ground level rather than man-entry manholes. Provide benching up to the crown level of the pipe in manholes and chambers.

3. Use appropriate locally available materials. Spun concrete pipes can be appropriate in some circumstances but may suffer corrosion if there are blockages and/or insufficient slope, so that sewage stays in the sewer for a long time, becomes septic (anaerobic) and produces hydrogen sulphide.

4. Pay particular attention to the design of manhole covers and make sure that covers can be replaced if they break. Solid waste and silt are likely to enter sewers through broken manhole covers and cause blockages.

Seek advice when contemplating the use of sewers. Look at what others have done but look for the weaknesses as well as the advantages of their schemes.

APPENDIX 3
Participatory methods for assessing sanitation conditions

This appendix provides basic information on participatory methods that can be used to assess local sanitation conditions and the possibilities for improving those conditions. The methods described can be used in local planning exercises and to obtain information about conditions in representative areas as part of a municipal or regional assessment and to assess the impact of a completed project or programme.

The assessment methods described in this appendix are introduced below in the order in which they are likely to be useful. Brief descriptions of the various methods follow.

○ Transect walks can be used to obtain an initial impression of sanitation problems and how people react to them. Informal interviews with community members in the course of such walks will help you to understand what you see and may provide information on what you cannot see.

○ Semi-structured interviews, structured observation, focus group discussions and timelines can help you to understand what has happened in the past, what is happening now and what could happen in the future.

○ Questionnaire surveys and participatory mapping can provide a more detailed understanding of the present situation. Focus group discussions and structured interviews can be used to explore specific issues arising from surveys and participatory mapping in more detail. Sanitation ladder exercises can be used to obtain an understanding of the assumptions and preferences of local people, at the same time providing opportunities for the introduction and discussion of new ideas and helping to inform demand.

Transect walks

At its most basic, a transect walk involves nothing more than walking through an area, observing and recording what you see. However, it will be better if a group of people, including men and women from both within and outside the community and with different areas of expertise and knowledge, make the walk together. Different people will see different things. Women may point out problems that are not obvious to men. Engineers may notice features of physical facilities that are missed by others. Similarly, sociologists may observe behavioural patterns that might be missed by those with a more technical background. People from the community may point to problems and issues that may not be obvious to an outsider. Local people will also enable the group to gain access to houses to observe the facilities that are available inside. The group should not be too big and group members should be encouraged to give individual team members the time and space to break off from the main group in order to explore issues with community members.

Transect walks should be timed to provide the maximum amount of information. For example, people are most likely to

Box A3.1 Examples of what you might observe in the course of a transect walk

- Young children defecating in the open provide an indication that there is a need to improve awareness of the health implications of poor sanitation. It may also point to deficiencies in latrine design, which discourage children from using latrines.
- The appearance of the outlet from a septic tank discharging to an open drain may provide guidance as to whether the septic tank is being desludged regularly. A build up of organic material around the outlet suggests that solids are being discharged and this in turn suggests that desludging is being neglected.
- Manhole covers missing on sewers, suggesting that maintenance is less than adequate.
- Solid waste dumped in open plots and drains indicate that the collection service is inadequate but possibly also that people need to develop greater awareness of the need for improved solid waste collection.
- Solid waste spread around bins suggesting that the bin is too small, the collection service is irregular, people do not bother to throw waste into the bin or some combination of the three.

use communal and shared latrines in the early morning while open defecation usually takes place after dusk. Transect walks at these times will provide information on people's habits that would not be obvious at any other time.

Informal interviews

In the course of initial transect walks, you can talk to people about their concerns and find out more about the area. Informal interviews during such walks can provide you with information on:

- what people think
- who they perceive to be their leaders and 'activists' within the community
- aspects of their day-to-day life that you cannot see.

The most important thing to remember when conducting such interviews is that you should try not to influence people by suggesting to them what you think the answers to questions should be.

Before talking to people, you should have given some thought to the issues that interest you and the ways in which you might introduce discussion of these issues. It will normally be best to start by asking some fairly general questions and guide the interviewee on to more specific issues as the interview progresses.

At a later stage in the process, efforts should be made to talk to people who may lack either the opportunity or the confidence to speak in more formal meetings. These may include women and people from minority groups. In the case of women, informal interviews conducted by other women may provide information and reveal attitudes and interests that would otherwise stay hidden.

Encourage those who carry out reconnaissance surveys to discuss their findings with colleagues from different backgrounds and professional disciplines. This will help them to 'triangulate' their interpretation of their findings. In particular, it may be instructive for men to explore the implications of their findings with women and vice versa.

Focus group discussions

Focus group discussions can be used to obtain an initial idea of a community's concerns and priorities. All that is required is to bring together a representative group or groups from the community and encourage them to talk about their concerns, preferences, hopes and fears. In some societies, it will be best to hold separate focus group discussions for men and women.

Focus groups can also be used to explore specific issues that have arisen in the course of questionnaire surveys and other general information generation methods.

One person should facilitate the discussion, with a second person taking notes of what is said. The facilitator will usually be a person from the group that is leading the process of information collection and analysis. Ideally, the meeting recorder should be from the community although this is not essential.

The facilitator should aim to:

○ ensure that no individual dominates the discussion

○ make sure that the discussion covers issues of concern.

In early focus group discussions, areas of concern should include anything relating to sanitation, drainage, solid waste disposal and associated subjects. In later focus group discussions, the discussion may need to be much more focused and this may require a greater degree of intervention on the part of the facilitator.

It will often be best to hold a series of focus group discussions, each attended by representatives of a different group within society. The aim should be to explore as wide a range of viewpoints and concerns as possible, obtaining the views of people from different genders, ages, social groups and income levels. Pay particular attention to the needs of the old and young, who may have special sanitation-related needs.

The facilitator will find it easier to guide discussion if he or she prepares a checklist of subjects to be covered before start of the focus group discussion.

Do not expect focus group discussions to give you accurate quantitative information. Rather, use them to obtain an overall impression of problems and then, if necessary, use other methods to obtain more accurate information. For instance, a focus group discussion may well lead to the conclusion that shared toilets are being used by large numbers of people but it is unlikely to tell you exactly how many people, on average, are using one latrine.

Semi-structured interviews with key informants

Informants with special knowledge or who are representative of specific groups within the community can provide much useful information. The normal approach to key informant interviews is to prepare a checklist of the points upon which you require information and to make sure that those points are raised in the course of the interview. Whenever possible, the information obtained from key informant interviews should be checked by interviewing other people who may have a different viewpoint and cross-checking specific points against other sources of information.

Key informants might include:

○ local masons who have been involved in aspects of sanitation provision (latrine construction, sewer laying, etc.)

○ employees of sanitation providers (including local authorities, specialist line agencies and, where appropriate, NGOs and CBOs)

○ women, who may face sanitation-related difficulties that are overlooked by men

○ those who have taken action to improve the sanitation facilities available to them

○ those who appear to be content with the status quo.

The information provided by different informants should be cross-checked. It may be, for instance, that comparison of the answers given by those who have and have not invested in improved sanitation facilities will provide useful information on factors that lead to increased demand for improved sanitation services.

Government employees working at the local level should be included for two reasons.

1. They should have useful insights and information, based on their work in an area
2. They are likely to be involved in the implementation of decisions made in the course of the planning process.

It is also possible that some local government representatives (e.g. school teachers) will take a leading role in planning and implementation at the local level.

Structured observations take a similar approach in that the aim is to observe a particular activity, for instance the way in which people deal with solid waste or problems that they encounter when using a communal latrine. The person or team conducting the structured observation should prepare a checklist of key points to be noted beforehand. Where the activities being observed are mainly undertaken by women, the observer or observers should also be women.

Timelines

People who have lived in an area for a number of years will have information on the way in which that area, the facilities provided to it and the problems encountered by the population have developed over time. This information should be useful in a number or ways.

○ It may reveal the resources available within the community, in particular, who has taken the lead in trying to address sanitation and drainage problems in the past.

○ It may provide information on previous attempts to solve sanitation and drainage problems. An understanding of what has gone wrong in the past will help to ensure that similar problems are avoided in the future.

○ It may reveal social factors that may be important for sanitation provision. Was everyone involved in attempts to improve sanitation? Did some people resist or did some attempt to 'highjack' the process and its benefits.

○ It may reveal changes in the overall situation. For instance, it may be that drainage problems got worse when the water supply to a settlement was improved.

Like other methods, timelines can be used at various stages in the planning process. They may be used to bring people into the process. However, they are likely to be most useful once a basic rapport has been developed between the planning team and the local community. Timelines can be particularly useful in making sure that the knowledge of older people is taken into account in sanitation plans.

While information about what has happened in the past can be obtained from individuals, it will be better to bring people together in groups to think about the past. This will enable the different people in the group to reinforce and correct each other's memories. Speak to local people to identify those who have knowledge of the history of the settlement and ask these people to be part of a timeline discussion. As with other participatory methods, consider working separately with groups representing different sectors within society to make sure that everyone's viewpoint is taken into account.

The timeline exercise itself will require a facilitator and a recorder. The facilitator should explain the purpose of the exercise. He or she should have a basic list of questions and issues to be raised. These might include the following.

o When was your settlement developed?

o What services are available and when were they provided?

o What attempts have been made to improve sanitation, who made them, when were they made and what were their results?

o Have there been any changes in the legal status of your settlement over the years? If so what were they and what results did they have?

The facilitator should allow the participants considerable freedom to introduce their memories and discuss the history of their settlement. The checklist questions should be used sparingly and the facilitator should aim to guide rather than direct the discussion. It may be useful to record information provided in the course of the discussion on a map of the settlement.

Questionnaire surveys

Questionnaire surveys have been criticized on the grounds that they tend to reflect the biases of the professionals who prepare them, they require considerable resources and are not really suitable for measuring differences from the norm (Chambers, 1983) The last two criticisms are not necessarily correct. It is true that surveys intended to produce results for inclusion in 'scientific' papers have to be sufficiently large to ensure that meaningful statistical conclusions can be drawn. However, much smaller samples can produce sufficient information on the existing situation for decisions to be made and action plans to be formulated. For instance, if a sample of 50 households from a total of 500 shows that only 10% have any form of sanitation, it is unlikely that the figure for the total population will be very different provided that the sample is reasonably representative. Whether the population with sanitation is 5% or 15% of the total is immaterial when it comes to planning the way forward.

Similarly, it is not necessarily the case that conventional socio-economic surveys do not reveal differences. It is true that the results of these surveys are usually presented in averaged form, which automatically eliminates differences. However, Box A3.2 illustrates that it is possible to obtain information on difference from the raw data.

Participatory mapping

Participatory mapping is a PRA (Participatory Rapid or Rural Appraisal) technique. In its pure PRA mode, people are asked to draw a map on the ground showing their locality and the features that are important to them. The theory is that by asking people to draw on the ground, everyone feels comfortable and is willing to participate. Experience suggests that this is not necessarily the case in urban areas, where most people may feel more comfortable drawing on paper.

This essentially open-ended approach to mapping can help to establish what is important to people and can also be very effective in drawing women into the planning process. However, it will often be of limited use in developing a detailed understanding of sanitation, drainage and solid waste management issues. When looking at these specific services, it may be better to provide people with rather more guidance as they are preparing the map. The facilita-

Box A3.2 Assessing differences through conventional surveys

In Juba, Southern Sudan, a survey of existing sanitation facilities was carried out in the early 1980s. It involved the use of a conventional socio-economic questionnaire, administered by local enumerators, trained by the team responsible for developing and managing the survey process. At the beginning of the survey, the management team was aware that some people within Juba had installed on-site pit latrines but that these pit latrines involved the use of expensive materials and usually cost over three times the average monthly salary in the town. It thus appeared that they were too expensive for general use. The survey revealed that around 20% of householders already had on-site sanitation and that a further 20% had tried to provide sanitation but had failed for one reason or another. Beyond these general conclusions, the survey results revealed some interesting facts. A small number of people claimed to have pit latrines that had cost either nothing at all or very little. Further investigation revealed that these used a variety of locally available materials, including mud and sticks and scrap taken from old cars. Further, it seemed that a common reason for the failure of attempts to build latrines was that the pit was made too large so that the cost and technical difficulty of covering it proved beyond people's resources. In both cases, it was possible to obtain useful information from individual questionnaires.

In Juba, the ability to use individual questionnaires to obtain information about differences from the norm was dependent on:

o the ability of those who debriefed enumerators to ask the right questions about what might be important
o the corresponding ability and willingness of the enumerators to notice interesting things and report them at the end of each day's survey.

If this was possible in the early 1980s, without recourse to computer analysis of data, it should be much easier with the data analysis capacity that is now available.

---

tor can provide this guidance by:

o asking questions about key points about their map, for instance which drain connects to which at a street intersection
o making suggestions as to the information that might usefully be recorded.

An example of the second would be information on details of on-site sanitation arrangements. This could be recorded house by house in what would be in effect a local community-conducted census of on-site facilities. (In many cases, local people will hold this information in their heads and will not need to go house to house to check it.) The challenge for the facilitator in such exercises will be to provide guidance while leaving space for the community to come up with their own ideas and suggestions.

Sanitation ladders

A sanitation ladder exercise can be used for hygiene education and to help users make informed choices and/or to help with planning. It involves a facilitator working with a group of community members to assess different sanitation practices and options. As with other participatory methods, it may be best to carry out the sanitation ladder exercise with representatives of different groups within society so as to capture their diverse viewpoints. The stages in the exercise are as follows.

1. Develop a series of pictures, showing different sanitation practices and options. Then bring together the group of community members and show them the pictures. Only use pictures that are relevant to the local situation. Ask the group to look through the pictures and make sure they understand what each picture represents.

2. Ask the group to rank the pictures from the worst to the best, by laying them out in a line. The group has to reach consensus on the final ranking and this should prompt discussion on what are 'good' and 'bad' practices or designs.

3. Ask the group why they ranked certain pictures as they did. For example, why did they consider a septic tank to be better than a leach pit or a pit latrine? The resulting discussion will provide the facilitator with opportunities to fill gaps in users' understanding and/or discuss hygienic aspects of the different options, thus helping to inform demand.

4. Now ask the group which picture(s) represent the typical situation in their community at present. If they cannot agree, invite them to 'vote' for the most common option. Use a pocket chart for privacy if people are uncomfortable with discussing the issue openly. A pocket chart consists of a number of rows of pockets, above each of which is fixed one of the pictures showing sanitation practices and/or options. This can be hung in a place where people can vote in privacy by placing one or more voting slips in the pockets below the pictures they believe represent the situation in their community. When everyone has voted, the pockets are emptied, usually by a community member, the votes are counted and the findings discussed.

5. Ask the group which type of sanitation they would like to have in an ideal world and which they think would be realistically achievable given local circumstances. This again provides an opportunity to help the group make an informed choice, by correcting any technical misunderstandings, making them aware of operation and maintenance requirements and costs, etc.

6. Now ask the group how they could move from 'where we are now' to 'where we want to be'. This should open the way for practical planning for local improvements.

Care should be taken when preparing the picture cards to ensure that they show realistically achievable options and that they are understandable to those who will be working with them. One way to ensure the first will be to develop your system of cards over time, adding new cards based on the ideas and suggestions that have emerged in past sanitation ladder exercises.

The most important rule for ensuring that community members understand what is shown on cards is to keep them simple. Do not show unnecessary detail but put all your efforts into ensuring that the main points are clearly and simply illustrated.

APPENDIX 4
Sources of further information

This appendix provides sources of additional information on the subjects covered by the book. The publication references are laid out following the chapter structure of the guide in order to help you identify the most relevant source for your particular purpose.

The appendix also provides contact details for:

o key international organizations in the fields of water supply and sanitation

o specialist advisory services.

The internet is a increasingly versatile dissemination and communication tool. Through e-mail networks and electronic publishing, it is a useful starting point for finding out about new publications and recent developments. Therefore, the appendix also provides information on:

o internet information networks

o mailing lists and discussion groups.

If you are unfamiliar with using the internet, the ELDIS Gateway to Information Sources on Development and the Environment offers some excellent and user-friendly guidance on where to search for further information and to keep up-to-date with new publications. It also includes a training guide and set of tools on how to use the world-wide web. 'SOURCE Water and Sanitation News', produced by the International Water and Sanitation Centre, provides an accessible option for keeping informed about new policies, projects and publications related to water and sanitation throughout the world.

Useful Publications

Chapter 1: Urban sanitation – problems and responses

Global Water Supply and Sanitation Assessment 2000 Report. WHO/UNICEF (2000) Geneva, Switzerland.

A Review of Sanitation Program Evaluations in Developing Countries. A. LaFond (1995) United States Agency for International Development (USAID) Environmental Health Project, Activity Report 5, Arlington, Virginia, USA.

Learning What Works: A retrospective view on international water and sanitation cooperation, 1978–1998. M. Black (1999) UNDP–World Bank Water and Sanitation Program, Washington DC, USA.

The Citizen at Risk: From urban sanitation to sustainable cities. G. McGranahan, P. Jacobi, J. Songsore, C. Surjadi and M. Kjellen (2001) Earthscan, London.

Constraints in Providing Water and Sanitation Services to the Urban Poor. S. Joyce, T. Solo, and E. Perez (1993) Water and Sanitation for Health Project: WASH Technical report No.85. USAID, Arlington, Virginia, USA.

The Poor Die Young: Housing and health in third world cities. S. Cairncross, J. Hardoy and D. Satterthwaite (1990) Earthscan, London, UK.

Mega-Slums: The coming sanitary crisis. M. Black (1994) WaterAid, London, UK.

Water and Sanitation in the World's Cities: Local action for global goals. United Nations Human Settlements Programme (UN-HABITAT) (2003) Earthscan, London, UK.

Integrated Water Resource Management in Water and Sanitation Projects: Lessons from projects in Africa, Asia and South America. J.T. Visscher, P. Bury, T. Gould, and P. Moriarty (1999) Occasional Paper Series 31, IRC International Water and Sanitation Centre, Delft, The Netherlands.

Global Freshwater Quality: A first assessment. Edited by M. Meybeck, D. Chapman, and R. Helmer (1989) United Nations Environment Programme and World Health Organization, Geneva, Switzerland.

The Global Burden of Disease: A comprehensive assessment of mortality and disability from diseases, injuries and risk factors in 1990 and projected to 2020. Edited by C. Murray and A. Lopez (1996) Harvard School of Public Health, USA.

Sanitation and Disease: Health aspects of excreta and wastewater management. R. Feachem, J. David, G. Hemda and D. Mara (1983) The World Bank, Washington DC, USA.

On-site Sanitation: An international review of World Bank experience. A. Fang (1999) Water and Sanitation Program, Washington DC, USA.

Chapter 2: A strategic framework for urban sanitation

Strategic Planning: A practical guide. P.J. Rea and H. Kerzner (1997) John Wiley & Sons, New York, USA.

Strategic Planning for Local Government: A handbook for officials and citizens. Edited by R.L. Kemp (1996) 2nd Edition, McFarland, Jefferson, NC, USA.

The Strategic Management Approach: Practical planning for development managers. P. Kristensen and C. Rader (2001) Conservation International, PACT Publications, Washington DC, USA.

Guidance Manual on Water Supply and Sanitation Programmes. WELL Resource Centre (1999) Department for International Development, London, UK.

Urban Water Supply and Sanitation Programming Guide. PADCO Inc. (2001) Office of Environment and Urban Programs, Center for the Environment, United States Agency for International Development.

Better Sanitation Programming: A UNICEF handbook. USAID Environmental Health Project (1997) UNICEF, New York, USA.

Sharing the City: Community participation in urban management. J. Abbott (1996) Earthscan, London, UK.

Serving the Poor: How can partnerships increase access and improve efficiency? World Bank, Water and Sanitation Division (1999) Washington DC, USA.

Water and Sanitation Services for the Urban Poor: Small-scale providers – typology and profiles. S. Snell (1998) UNDP–World Bank Water and Sanitation Program, Washington DC, USA.

Designing and Implementing Decentralization Programs in the Water and Sanitation Sector. D.B. Edwards, F. Rosensweig and S. Edward (1993) WASH Technical Report No.89. Environmental Health Project, USAID, USA.

Chapter 3: Strategic sanitation planning in towns and cities

Services for the Urban Poor: Guidelines for policymakers, planners and engineers. A. Cotton and W.K. Tayler (2000) Water, Engineering, and Development Centre, Loughborough, UK.

Participation and Partnership in Urban Infrastructure Management. P. Schübeler (1995) Urban Management Programme, UN-HABITAT, World Bank, Washington DC, USA.

Municipalities and Community Participation: A source book for capacity building. J. Plummer (1999) Earthscan, London, UK.

Partnership for Local Action: A sourcebook on participatory approaches to shelter and human settlements improvement for local government officials. (1997) UN-HABITAT/CityNet, Yokohama, Japan.

Strategic Planning Guide for Municipal Solid Waste Management. D. Wilson, A. Whiteman and A. Tormin (2001) CD-ROM prepared for the World Bank, SDC and DFID, Waste-Aware. Environmental Resources Management (ERM), London, 2000.

Municipal Solid Waste Management: Involving micro- and small enterprises – Guidelines for municipal managers. H.C. Haan, A. Coad and I. Lardinois. (1998) International Training Centre, International Labour Organisation, Turin, Italy.

Guidelines for Institutional Assessment: Water and Wastewater Institutions. D. Cullivan, B. Tippett, D. Edwards, F. Rosenweig and J. McCaffery (1988) WASH Technical Report No.37. Environmental Health Project, USAID, USA.

Chapter 4: Developing a supportive context

Guidelines for the Assessment of National Sanitation Policies. M.F. Elledge, F. Rosensweig and D.B. Warner (2002) USAID Environmental Health Project strategic report, Arlington, Virginia, USA.

Water, Sanitation and Poverty. C. Bosch, K. Hommann, C. Sadoff and L. Travers (2001) *Poverty Reduction Strategy Sourcebook: Water and Sanitation*, World Bank, Washington DC, USA.

Reaching the Urban Poor with Private Infrastructure. P. Brook-Cowen and N. Tynan (1999) World Bank, Washington DC, USA.

Toolkits for Private Participation in Water and Sanitation (1997) World Bank, Washington DC, USA.

Guidelines for Improving Wastewater and Solid Waste Management. R. Andrews, W. Lord, L. O'Toole and L. Requena (1993) WASH Technical Report No.88. Environmental Health Project, Arlington, Virginia, USA.

Water for All: The water policy of the Asian Development Bank. ADB (2001) Manila, Philippines.

Capacity Building for the Urban Environment. Edited by D. Edelman and H. Mengers (1997) Institute for Housing and Urban Development Studies, Rotterdam, The Netherlands.

Building Capacity for Better Cities: Concepts and strategies. M. Peltenburg, F. Davidson, H. Teerlink and P. Wakely (1996) Institute of Housing and Development Studies, Rotterdam, The Netherlands.

Chapter 5: Developing a strategic process from the local level

Action Planning for Cities: A guide to community practice. N. Hamdi and R. Goethert (1997) John Wiley and Sons, Chichester.

Urban Development and Civil Society: The role of communities in sustainable cities. M. Carley, P. Jenkins and H. Smith (eds) (2001) Earthscan, London.

The Community Planning Handbook: How people can shape their cities, towns and villages in any part of the world. N. Wates (1999) Urban Design Group, South Bank University and the Department for International Development, London, UK.

Community Initiatives in Urban Infrastructure. A. Cotton, M. Sohail and W.K. Tayler (1998) Water, Engineering and Development Centre, Loughborough University, UK.

From Sanitation to Development: The Case of the Baldia soakpit pilot project. Q. Bakhteari and M. Wegelin-Schuringa (1992) IRC Technical Paper No.31-E, International Water and Sanitation Centre, Delft, The Netherlands.

Community-Based Sewer Systems in Indonesia: A case study in the city of Malang. S. Foley, A. Soedjarwo, and R. Pollard (1999) Learning note, Water and Sanitation Program – East Asia, Jakarta, Indonesia.

Supporting Community Management: A manual for training in community management in the water and sanitation sector. M. Lammerink and E. Bolt (2002) IRC Technical Paper No.34-E, International Water and Sanitation Centre, The Netherlands.

World Bank Sourcebook on Participation. (1996) World Bank, Washington DC, USA.

Partnership for Local Action: A sourcebook on participatory approaches to shelter and human settlement improvement for local government officials. CityNet (1997) UN-HABITAT Community Development Programme for Asia, Bangkok, Thailand.

Chapter 6: Developing demand – sanitation promotion

Designing Water Supply and Sanitation Projects to Meet Demand. P. Deverill, S. Bibbly, A. Wedgwood, and I. Smout. (2002) Water, Engineering and Development Centre. Loughborough University, UK.

Optimising the Selection of Demand Assessment Techniques for Water Supply and Sanitation Projects. S. Parry-Jones (1999) WELL Task Report No.207, Water, Engineering and Development Centre, Loughborough University, UK.

Happy, Healthy and Hygienic: How to set up a hygiene promotion programme. V. Curtis and B. Kanki (1998) United Nations Childrens Fund, New York, USA.

Sanitation Promotion. M. Simpson-Hébert and S. Wood (eds) (1998) WSSCC Working Group on Promotion of Sanitation, World Health Organization (WHO), Geneva, Switzerland.

Towards Better Programming: A manual on school sanitation and hygiene. I. van Hooff (1998) UNICEF, Water and Environmental Sanitation Section, New York, USA.

The PHAST Methodology. A step-by-step guide: A participatory approach for the control of diarrhoeal disease (1998) WHO, Geneva, Switzerland.

UNICEF Hygiene Promotion Manual. UNICEF/LSHTM (1999) UNICEF Water, Environment and Sanitation Technical Guidelines Series, New York, USA.

Manual on Communication for Water Supply and Environmental Sanitation. UNICEF (1999) UNICEF Water, Environment and Sanitation Technical Guideline Series. New York, USA.

Chapter 7: Gathering and using information for strategic planning

Methodology for Participatory Assessments: Linking sustainability with demand, gender and poverty. R. Dayal, C. van Wijk and N. Mukherjee (2000) Water and Sanitation Program, Washington DC, USA.

Participatory Evaluation: Tools for managing change in water and sanitation. D. Narayan (1993) World Bank, Washington DC, USA.

Toward Participatory Research. D. Narayan (1996) World Bank Technical Paper No.307, World Bank, Washington DC, USA.

Utility Mapping and Record Keeping for Infrastructure. D. Pickering, J. Park and D. Bannister (1993) Urban Management Discussion Paper No.10, UN-HABITAT, Nairobi, Kenya.

Chapter 8: Choosing an appropriate sanitation technology

Low-cost Sanitation: A survey of practical experience. J. Pickford (1995) ITDG Publishing, London, UK.

Guidelines for Operational and Maintenance of Public Toilets. UMP/UN-HABITAT (1995) Urban Management Programme – Regional Office for Africa, UN-HABITAT, Nairobi, Kenya.

Why a Pit Latrine: A Manual for Extension Workers and Latrine Builders. J. Mate (1991) Training Series No.8 (TS8-E), International Water and Sanitation Centre, Delft, The Netherlands.

On-site Sanitation: Building on local practice. M. Wegelin-Schuringa (1991) Occasional Paper No.16, International Water and Sanitation Centre, Delft, The Netherlands.

A Guide to the Development of On-Site Sanitation. R. Franceys, J. Pickford and R. Reed (1992) WHO, Geneva, Switzerland.

Ecological Sanitation. S. Esrey, J. Gough, D. Rapaport, R. Sawyer, M. Simpson-Hebert, J. Vargas and U. Winblad (1998) Swedish International Development Cooperation Agency (SIDA), Stockholm, Sweden.

Sustainable Sewerage: Guidelines for community schemes, R. Reed (1995) ITDG Publishing, London, UK.

Low-cost Sewerage. D. Mara (1996) John Wiley and Sons, Chichester, UK.

Design of Shallow Sewer Systems. UN-HABITAT (1986) Nairobi, Kenya.

Simplified Sewerage: Design Guidelines. A. Bakalian, A. Wright, R. Otis and J. de Azevedo Netto (1994) UNDP-World Bank Water and Sanitation Program, Washington DC, USA.

Surface Water Drainage for Low-Income Communities. S. Cairncross and E.A.R. Ouano (1991) WHO, Geneva, Switzerland.

Storm Drainage – An engineering guide to the low-cost evaluation of system performance. P. Kolsky (1998) ITDG Publishing, London, UK.

Guidelines for The Safe Use of Wastewater and Excreta in Agriculture and Aquaculture: Measures for public health protection. D. Mara and S. Cairncross (1989) WHO, Geneva, Switzerland.

Solids Separation and Pond Systems for the Treatment of Faecal Sludges in the Tropics: Lessons learnt and recommendations for preliminary design. U. Heinss, S. Larmie and M. Strauss (1998) EAWAG/SANDEC, Report No.05/98, Duebendorf, Switzerland.

Chapter 9: Guidlines for holding a participatory planning workshop

Participatory Development Tool Kit. D. Narayan and L. Srinivasan (1993) World Bank, Washington DC, USA.

Participatory Workshops: A sourcebook of 21 sets of ideas and activities. R. Chambers (2002) Earthscan, London, UK.

Building Bridges Through Participatory Planning. UN-HABITAT (2001) Part 1 and 2. Series of Urban Governance Training manuals, Nairobi, Kenya.

The Art of Building Training Capacities. Lydia Braakman (2002) The Regional Community Forestry Training Center for Asia & the Pacific, Bangkok, Thailand.

Empowering Communities: Participatory techniques for community-based programme development. Trainer and participants manuals on learning participatory techniques (1998) Centre for African Family Studies (CAFS)/Academy for Educational Development (AED), USA.

Operation and Maintenance of Rural Water Supply and Sanitation Systems: A training package for managers and planners. F. Brikké (2001) Training manual on water supply and sanitation, IRC International Water and Sanitation Centre, Delft, The Netherlands.

MAPA-PROJECT: A practical guide to integrated project planning and evaluation. U. Schiefer, R. Döbel, L. Bal (2001) Manual on MAPA participatory planning methods, Open Society Institute, Hungary.

Participatory Development Toolkit: Training materials for agencies and communities. D. Narayan and L. Srinivasan (1993) World Bank, Washington DC, USA.

Participatory Evaluation. A users' guide. J. Pfohl, S. Buzzard, D. Pietro (1989) PACT Publications, New York, USA.

A Trainer's Guide for Participatory Learning and Action. J. Pretty, I. Guijt, J. Thompson and I. Scoones (1995) IIED Participatory Methodology series. International Institute for Environment and Development, London, UK.

Chapter 10: Implementing strategic plans

Management Guide. U. Fröhlich (2001) Vol.1 of the Series of Manuals on Drinking Water Supply, SKAT, St.Gallen, Switzerland.

Financial Management of Water Supply and Sanitation: A handbook (1994) WHO, Geneva, Switzerland.

Operation, Maintenance and Sustainability of Services for the Urban Poor: Findings, lessons learned and case studies summary and analysis. M. Sohail, S. Cavill and A. Cotton (2000) Water, Engineering and Development Centre, Loughborough University, UK.

Tools for Assessing the O&M Status of Water Supply and Sanitation in Developing Countries (2000) WHO, Geneva, Switzerland.

Operation and Maintenance of Sanitation Systems in Urban Low-income Areas in India and Thailand. IRC (1997) Report on a joint research programme, 1989–1993. Project and Programme Papers 6-E, International Research Centre (IRC), The Netherlands.

Process Monitoring for Improving Sustainability – A manual for project managers and staff. M. Hosain, C. Pendley, A. Pervaiz, T. Samina and M. Akbar (1999) Water and Sanitation Program, Islamabad, Pakistan.

Where to go for further assistance

Key international organizations in water and sanitation

InterWATER
The InterWATER Internet Gateway to Water and Sanitation Organizations provides the addresses of selected organizations concerned with water supply and sanitation in developing countries.

www.wsscc.org/interwater

International Water and Sanitation Centre (IRC)

IRC aims to provide improved access to and promote the use of knowledge among sector institutions and other stakeholders and to build the capacity of resource centres for the WSS sector in developing countries.

IRC
PO Box 2869, 2601 CW Delft
The Netherlands
Tel: +31 (0) 15 219 29 39
Fax: +31 (0) 15 219 09 55
www.irc.nl

Water and Sanitation Program (WSP)

The WSP is a global partnership, which aims to assist countries with capacity building (including policy reforms), planning and implementing sustainable investments, and synthesizing and disseminating lessons relating to all aspects of water supply and sanitation. The WSP has regional offices in Latin America, Africa, South Asia, and East Asia and the Pacific.

WSP
1818 H Street, NW, F4K-172
Washington DC, 20433, USA
Tel: +1 (0) 202 4739785
Fax: +1 (0) 202 5223313
email: info@wsp.org
www.wsp.org

UNICEF: Water, Environment and Sanitation (WES)

The UNICEF WES site presents a variety of information about UNICEF's policies and activities in this sector. WES programmes focus on sanitation for rural communities and the urban poor, health and hygiene, school sanitation and children's health. The site also includes a guide to sectoral resources on the web, including a selection of full-text electronic publications available from partners and agencies.

UNICEF-WES
3 UN Plaza, New York, NY, USA 10017
Tel: +1 (0) 212 824 6000
Fax: +1 (0) 212 824 6480
email: wesinfo@unicef.org
www.unicef.org/programme/wes

Business Partners for Development – Water and Sanitation Cluster

The Water and Sanitation Cluster, one of four Business Partners for Development (BPD) initiatives, aims to improve access to safe water and effective sanitation for the rising number of urban poor in developing countries and to promote good examples of tri-sectoral partnerships that provide water and sanitation services to the urban poor.

BPD Water and Sanitation Cluster
c/o WaterAid, Prince Consort House
27–29 Albert Embankment
London SE1 7UB, UK
Tel: +44 (0) 20 7793 4557
Fax: +44 (0) 20 7582 0962
email: info@bpd-waterandsanitation.org
www.bpd-waterandsanitation.org

Water Utility Partnership (WUP)

The basic idea leading to the creation of WUP is to build a partnership among African water supply and sanitation utilities and other key sector institutions to create opportunities for sharing of experiences and capacity building.

WUP
05 B.P. 2642 Abidjan 05
Ivory Coast
email: wup@africaonline.co.ci
http://wupafrica.org

Environmental Health Project (EHP)

The EHP assists development organizations to address environment related health problems. It is funded by USAID and provides technical assistance on water supply, sanitation, wastewater, solid waste and air pollution.

Environmental Health Project
1611 North Kent St.
#300 Arlington, VA 22209, USA
Tel: +1 (0) 703 247 8730
Fax: +1 (0) 703 243 9004
email: info@ehproject.org
www.ehproject.org

World Bank – Water Supply and Sanitation

Through its lending programmes and assistance to its partner organizations, the World Bank Group aims to help its member countries ensure that everyone has access to efficient, responsive and sustainable water and sanitation services.

The World Bank
1818 H Street, N.W.
Washington, DC 20433 U.S.A.
Tel: +1 (0) 202 473 1000
Fax: +1 (0) 202 477 6391
www.worldbank.org/watsan

World Health Organization (WHO) – Protection of the Human Environment – Water and Sanitation

The water and sanitation related activities of WHO focus specifically on health-related issues for the improvement of environmental health conditions. The Division of Control of Tropical Diseases of the WHO supports treatment and prevention programmes on various water related diseases.

WHO – Water and Sanitation
Avenue Appia 20
1211 Geneva 27
Switzerland
Fax: +41 (0) 22 791 43 21
email: info@who.ch
www.who.int/water/sanitation/health

Global Water Partnership (GWP)

The GWP aims to support high quality, integrated activities at country level and, at the international level, to bring a global learning perspective to these activities.

Global Water Partnership
Secretariat, c/o Sida
S-105 25 Stockholm, Sweden
Tel: +46 (0) 8 6985000
Fax: +46 (0) 8 6985627
email: gwp@sida.se
www.gwpforum.org

Water Supply and Sanitation Collaborative Council (WSSCC)

The WSSCC was formed at the end of the United Nations International Drinking Water and Sanitation Decade (1981–1990) to provide a framework for collaboration between sector agencies in both developed and developing countries.

WSSCC
c/o World Health Organization
Avenue Appia 20
CH-1211 Geneva 27, Switzerland
Tel: + 41 (0) 22 791 3685
Fax: +41 (0) 22 791 4847
email: wsscc@who.ch
www.wsscc.org

WaterAid

WaterAid is the UK's specialist development charity working through partner organizations to help poor people in developing countries achieve sustainable improvements in their quality of life by improved domestic water supply, sanitation and associated hygiene practices.

WaterAid
Prince Consort House
27–29 Albert Embankment
London SE1 7U
Tel: +44 (0) 20 7 793 4500
Fax: +44 (0) 20 7 793 4545
email: information@wateraid.org.uk
www.wateraid.org.uk

Network for Water and Sanitation (NETWAS)

NETWAS is a capacity building and information network for Africa focusing on the water, sanitation and environment sector. It comprises resource centres in Eastern Africa (Kenya, Uganda and Tanzania) implementing capacity-building activities on training of professionals, applied research, networking and information sharing, advocacy, advisory and consultancy services.

NETWAS
PO Box 15614
Nairobi, Kenya
Tel: + 254 (0) 2 890555
Fax: + 254 (0) 2 890554
email: netwas@nbnet.co.ke or
netwas@ken.healthnet.org
www.netwasgroup.com

Department of Water and Sanitation in Developing Countries (SANDEC)

SANDEC aims to assist in developing appropriate and sustainable water and sanitation concepts and technologies adapted to the different physical and socio-economic conditions prevailing in developing countries.

SANDEC
Swiss Federal Institute for Environmental Science and Technology
Ueberlandstrasse 133
CH-8600 Duebendorf
Switzerland
Tel: +41 (0) 1 823 5020
Fax: +41 (0) 1 823 5399
www.sandec.ch

Internet information networks

The WELL Document Catalogue
www.lboro.ac.uk/well/resources/document
catalogue.htm
The WELL Document Catalogue (available online) comprises around 10 000 library records of items relating to water and environmental health in developing and transitional countries.

SANICON – Environmental Sanitation Network
www.sanicon.net
Sanitation Connection is an internet-based resource that gives access to accurate, reliable and up-to-date information on technologies, institutions and financing of sanitation systems around the world.

ELDIS Gateway to Information Sources on Development and the Environment
www.ids.ac.uk/eldis
The ELDIS gateway provides a wealth of descriptions and links to a variety of information sources for policy makers, academics and development NGOs.

IRC Database on Water and Sanitation in Developing Countries (IRCDOC)
www.irc.nl/products/documentation
Since 1984 the IRC Documentation Unit has maintained IRCDOC, a bibliographic database on water supply and sanitation in developing countries. IRCDOC includes bibliographic descriptions of documents held in the IRC Reference Library and of a growing number of documents available on the internet.

Global Applied Research Network (Garnet)
www.lboro.ac.uk/garnet
Garnet is a mechanism for information exchange in the water supply and sanitation sector using low-cost, informal networks of researchers, practitioners and funders of research.

School Sanitation and Hygiene Education
www.irc.nl/sshe
A joint UNICEF/IRC web site that provides a collection of tools and resources on sustainable approaches to improve the health of school-aged children through better hygiene behaviour and a healthy school environment.

GTZ Ecosan – Ecological Sanitation
www.gtz.de/ecosan
The further development, testing and dissemination of alternatives to conventional wastewater and sewage disposal systems is becoming more and more indispensable for both economic and ecological reasons. GTZ aims to promote strategies oriented to the material-flow recycling process in the field of wastewater management and sanitation.

Managing Water for African Cities
www.un-urbanwater.net
Managing Water for African Cities (MAWAC) is a joint initiative of the United Nations Environment Program UNEP and United Nations Human Settlements Programme (UN-HABITAT). It aims to help members adopt and adapt water management practices and will enable practitioners, managers and researchers to share data, information and knowledge.

The African Water Page
www.africanwater.org

Issues addressed include water policy, water resource management, water supply and environmental sanitation, water conservation and demand management. Primary objectives of the page are information dissemination on water issues in Africa and the exchange of views and ideas on water on the continent.

N-AERUS – Network for Research on Urbanisation in the South
www.naerus.org

N-AERUS is a network of researchers and experts working on urban issues in developing countries. Its objective is to mobilize and develop European institutional and individual research and training capacities on urban issues in the South with the support of institutions and individual researchers with relevant experience in this field.

Water for the World – A series of USAID technical notes covering all aspects of rural water supply and sanitation
www.lifewater.org/wfw/wfwindex.htm

The Water For The World Technical Notes were published in 1982 by the former Development Information Center of the US Agency for International Development (AID). The notes are targeted towards practitioners working in the field of rural water supply and sanitation, but many are also relevant to urban sanitation.

Water and Sanitation for All – A practitioners companion
http://web.mit.edu/urbanupgrading/waterandsanitation

The toolkit has been developed through the Water Utilities Partnership (WUP) supported by the World Bank's Africa Infrastructure Unit and aims to provide sector practitioners, and policy and decision makers with practical advice on the range of options for water supply and sanitation service delivery to low-income urban areas.

Urban Upgrading Communities – A resource for practitioners
http://web.mit.edu/urbanupgrading

The site is designed to promote awareness of the critical problem of providing basic services to the rapidly increasing urban poor, to capture and evaluate the growing experience from upgrading projects and programmes, and to provide a resource for practitioners for design and implementation of urban infrastructure and services for poor communities.

Environmental Strategies for Cities
http://web.mit.edu/urbanupgrading/urbanenvironment/

This web site is for cities to initiate environmental management programmes. It is targeted toward urban policy analysts, decision makers, planners and managers, as well as to the environmental community at large and international agencies.

Technical assistance

Water Help Desk – Global Water and Sanitation Advisory Service

The World Bank and the Water and Sanitation Program's Water Help Desk serves as an entry point for government officials, NGOs, the private sector and other development organizations for locating information on the sector. In addition to the Washington DC office, the advisory service has regional focus branches in New Delhi, India and in Nairobi, Kenya.
www.worldbank.org/html/fpd/water/helpdesk.html

Washington, DC
1818 H Street, NW, Washington, DC 20433, USA
Tel: +1 (0) 202 473 4761
Fax: +1 (0) 202 522 3228

New Delhi, India
PO Box 416, New Delhi 110 003, India
Tel: +91 (0) 11 469 0488
Fax: +91 (0) 11 462 8250

Nairobi, Kenya
PO Box 30577, Nairobi, Kenya
Tel: +254 (0) 2 260 317
Fax: +254 (0) 2 260386
email: whelpdesk@worldbank.org

WELL Resource Centre Network for Water, Sanitation and Environmental Health

WELL is a consortium consisting of the Water Engineering and Development Centre (WEDC) at Loughborough University, the London School of Hygiene and Tropical Medicine (LSHTM), and IRC International Water and Sanitation Centre. WELL is a resource centre network providing services and resources and technical assistance to DFID field staff and British and southern NGOs working in the water and sanitation sector in developing countries.

Water, Engineering and Development Centre (WEDC)
Loughborough University
Leicestershire LE11 3TU, UK
Tel: +44 (0) 1509 222633
Fax: +44 (0) 1509 211079
email: well@lboro.ac.uk
www.lboro.ac.uk/well

International Water Association (IWA) Water KnowHow

The service is free to water practitioners in lower-income countries for questions taking up to an hour to answer. If your question requires more work, IWA will refer you to other sources of help.

IWA Water KnowHow
Alliance House
12 Caxton Street
London SW1H 0QS, UK
email: help@waterknowhow.info
fax: +44 (0)207 654 5555

Mailing lists

SOURCE Water and Sanitation News
www.wsscc.org/source
SOURCE Weekly brings you a weekly update of short news, while the bi-monthly *SOURCE Bulletin* gives more in-depth news, news from the WSSCC and IRC.

ID21 Development Research reporting service
www.id21.org
The ID21 Development Research reporting service provide by the Institute of Development Studies Information Service, University of Sussex, offers a selection of the latest and best UK-based development research.

Discussion groups

JISCmail
www.jiscmail.ac.uk
JISCmail offers a number of email discussion groups including:

Water and sanitation applied research: a list for discussion and information exchange relating to applied research in the water supply and sanitation sector.

Urban drainage: a list for discussion and information exchange concerning the research, planning, design, operation and modelling of urban drainage systems. Topics range from urban hydrology, drainage and sewerage to treatment plants, receiving water impacts and sustainability.

Wastewater management: a list for discussion of all aspects of sustainable wastewater management, including appropriate and affordable collection, treatment and disposal technologies and practices, especially those which encourage conservation, recycling and reuse of resources; as well as issues of planning and regulation.

Hygiene-behaviour: this network is designed to facilitate the sharing of ideas, research results and new developments concerned with hygiene behaviour in relation to the water supply and sanitation sector in developing countries.

LCSEWERAGE: Discussion list focusing on the planning, design and maintenance of low-cost sewerage technologies.

OM: a list on Operation and Maintenance (O&M) of Water Supply and Sanitation Systems in Developing Countries. Intended for HE academics with input from practitioners and sector professionals.

STREAM: a discussion list on knowledge sharing and the role of resource centres in water and environmental sanitation in developing countries. Intended for academics, researchers and practitioners with input from partners of the Streams of Knowledge coalition.

Glossary

Adaptive strategy: A strategy that recognizes that all the information required to plan for the future is not available and so allows for later activities to be modified in the light of increased information availability, including the feedback from the results of earlier activities.

Aqua privy: Latrine in which excreta are deposited through a hole and a vertical pipe into a watertight chamber. The vertical pipe should extend below the water surface to form a water seal. Excess water is allowed to overflow into a drainfield or soakaway.

Bucket latrine: A latrine in which users defecate into a bucket or other receptacle that is regularly emptied.

Composting latrine: A latrine designed to receive both faeces and waste vegetable matter with the aim of reducing the moisture content of the waste and to achieve a carbon to nitrogen ratio that encourages its rapid decomposition.

Demand: Desire for a service or utility together with a willingness to pay the price of that service or utility.

Dry latrine: The term dry latrine is used to describe:

○ crude systems in which faeces are excreted on to a slab or into an improvised container, from which they are manually removed

○ a latrine from which water and urine are excluded in order to increase the rate at which excreta decompose.

Excreta: Faeces and urine.

Institution: An organizational form set up to achieve some purpose, together with the norms, rules and ways of thinking that underpin the functioning of that organizational form.

Latrine: An installation used for defecation and urination.

Livelihoods: The capabilities, assets and activities that people require as a means of living.

Overhung latrine: Latrine sited so that excreta fall directly into a lake, river or other body of water.

Market: The system of exchange through which consensus is reached on the prices of various goods and services.

Nightsoil: Human excreta, with or without anal cleansing material, which are deposited into a bucket or other receptacle for manual removal.

On-plot facilities: Sanitation facilities that are located on the householder's plot. May be an on-plot system or the on-plot components of a more extensive system.

On-plot sanitation: A sanitation system that is contained within the plot occupied by the dwelling and its immediate surroundings (for instance when disposal is to a leachpit immediately beyond the plot boundary).

On-site sanitation: On-site sanitation includes all forms of infrastructure for managing excreta in the vicinity of the locality in which it is produced. On-site sanitation differs from on-plot sanitation as it may not be located directly on the housing plot.

Pathogens: Micro-organisms such as bacteria, viruses and protozoa, that cause sickness and disease in humans.

Pit latrine: Latrine with a pit for accumulation and decomposition of excreta and from which liquid infiltrates into the surrounding soil. (The term is sometimes used for pour-flush latrines but this usage is technically incorrect.)

Pour-flush latrine: A latrine that depends on small quantities of water, poured from a container by hand, to flush faeces away from the point of defecation. The term is normally used for a latrine incorporating a water seal.

Primary facilities: Facilities such as trunk sewers and municipal sewage treatment works that are designed to serve either a whole town or a sizeable zone of a large city. (Note that the term primary is used to describe solid waste collection services at the local level. In other words, it is used in exactly the opposite way to that commonly used for other services.)

Sanitation: A system for promoting sanitary (healthy) conditions.

Secondary facilities: Facilities that serve a district within a town or city.

Septic tank: A tank or container, normally with one inlet and one outlet, that retains sewage and reduces its strength by settlement and anaerobic digestion of excreta.

Sewage: Wastewater from a community, including excreta, that is carried in a sewer.

Sewer: A closed conduit (usually a buried pipe) that is used to convey the wastewater from more than one property.

Sewerage: System of interconnected sewers.

Soakaway: Soakpit or drainage trench for subsoil percolation of liquid waste.

Soakpit: Hole dug in the ground serving as a soakaway.

Social capital: The institutions, relationships and norms that shape the quality and quantity of a society's social interactions.

Stakeholders: The people, groups and organizations with an interest in a particular subject or outcome.

Stormwater: Run-off caused by rainfall.

Strategy: An approach to achieving an objective or overcoming a problem, usually defined in terms of a series of actions to be undertaken.

Strategic plan: A written document that defines objectives and sets out the actions required to meet those objectives.

Sullage: Wastewater from bathing, laundry, preparation of food, cooking and other personal and domestic activities that does not contain excreta (sometimes known as greywater).

Superstructure: Screen or building enclosing a latrine to provide privacy and protection for users.

Tertiary facilities: Facilities that serve streets or local neighbourhoods, typically up to about 10 hectares in area.

Unbundling: When used in relation to sanitation technologies, refers to the fact that different technologies may be appropriate for use in different locations within a town or city. When used in relation to organizations, refers to the fact that different organizations may be responsible for managing services in different locations (horizontal unbundling) and at different levels within a hierarchical system (vertical unbundling).

VIP latrine: Ventilated improved pit latrine, pit latrine with a screened vent pipe and a dark interior to the superstructure.

Water closet: A pan, incorporating a water seal, in which excreta are deposited before being flushed away using water.

Wastewater: All types of domestic wastewater (sewage or sullage), commercial and industrial effluent as well as stormwater runoff.

Workshop: An event that brings together a number of stakeholders or stakeholder representatives to plan for the future or to evaluate the results of past activities in a participatory manner.

References

Abers, R. (1997) 'Learning Democratic Practice: Distributing Government Resources Through Popular Participation in Porto Alegre, Brazil', in *Cities for Citizens*, Douglas, M. and Friedmann, J. (ed), John Wiley & Sons, Chichester and New York.

Alimuddin, S., Hasan, A. and Sadiq, A. (2000) *Community Driven Water and Sanitation: The Work of the Anjuman Samaji Behbood and the Larger Faisalabad Context*, International Institute for Environment and Development (IIED), London.

Altaf, A. and Hughes, J.A. (1994) 'Measuring the Demand for Improved Sanitation Services: Contingent Valuation Study in Ouagadougou, Burkina Faso', in *International Journal for Research in Urban and Regional Studies*, University of Glasgow, Vol.31, 10, pp.1763–76.

Anand, P.B. (1999) 'Waste Management in Madras Revisited', in *Environment and Urbanization*, International Institute for Environment and Development (IIED), London, Vol.11, No.2, October 1999.

Bakhteari, Q.A. and Wegelin-Schuringa, M. (1992) *From Sanitation to Development: The Case of the Baldia Soakpit Pilot Project*, IRC Technical Paper No.31-E, International Water and Sanitation Centre, The Netherlands.

Black, M. (1994) *Mega-slums: The Coming Sanitary Crisis*, WaterAid, London.

Blumenthal, U.J., Peasey, A., Ruiz-Palacios, G. and Mara, D. (2000) *Guidelines for Wastewater Reuse in Agriculture and Aquaculture: Recommended Revisions Based on New Research Evidence*, WELL Study, Task No.68, Part 1, London School of Hygiene & Tropical Medicine and Water, Engineering and Development Centre (WEDC), Loughborough University.

Burra, S. (2001) *Slum sanitation in Pune – A Case Study*, Society for Promotion of Area Resource Centres (SPARC), Mumbai.

Cairncross, S. (1990) 'Water Supply and the Urban Poor', in Caincross, S., Hardoy, J.E. and Satterthwaite, D. (eds), *The Poor Die Young: Housing and Health in Third World Cities*, Earthscan, London, pp.109–26.

Cairncross, S. and Feachem R. G. (1993) *Environmental Health Engineering in the Tropics: An Introductory Text*, (2nd edn), John Wiley & Sons, Chichester.

Carley, M., Jenkins, P., and Smith, H. (eds) (2001) *Urban Development and Civil Society: The Role of Communities in Sustainable Cities*, Earthscan, London.

Chambers, R. (1983) *Rural Development: Putting the Last First*, Longman, Harlow.

Chambers, R. (1994) 'Participatory Rural Appraisal (PRA) – Analysis of Experience', in *World Development*, Elsevier Science, UK, Vol.22, No.9.

Cotton, A. and Saywell, D. (1998) *On-Plot Sanitation for Low-Income Urban Communities: Guidelines for Selection*, WEDC, Loughborough University.

Cotton, A.P., Sohail, M. and Tayler, W.K. (1998) *Community Initiatives in Urban Infrastructure*, WEDC, Loughborough University.

Cotton, A. and Tayler, K. (2000) *Services for the Urban Poor: Guidelines for Policymakers, Planners and Engineers*, Section 3 – Action Planning, WEDC, Loughborough University.

Dudley, E. (1993) *The Critical Villager – Beyond Community Participation*, Routledge, London and New York.

Edwards, P. (1992) *Reuse of Human Wastes in Aquaculture – A Technical Review*, Water and Sanitation Report No.2. UNDP-Water and Sanitation Program, Washington DC.

Esrey, S.A., Potash, J.B., Roberts, L. and Schiff, C. (1991) 'Effects of Improved Water Supply and Sanitation on Ascariasis, Diarrhoea, Dranculiasis, Hookworm Infection, Schistosomiasis and Trachoma', in *Bulletin of the World Health Organisation*, WHO, Geneva, Vol.69, No.5, pp.609–21.

FAO (1995) *Water Sector Policy Review and Strategy Formulation: A General Framework*, FAO Land and Water Bulletin, No.3, Food and Agriculture Organization, Rome.

Fernando, S., Gamage, W. and Dharmawansa, P. (1987) *Navagampura and Aramaya Place: Two Urban Case Studies on Support Based Housing*, NHDA, Colombo, Sri Lanka.

Hamdi, N. and Goethert, R. (1997) *Action Planning for Cities: A Guide to Community Practice*, John Wiley & Sons, Chichester.

Hamdi, N. and Goethert, R. (1988) *Making Microplans: A Community Based Process in Programming and Development*, ITDG Publishing, London.

Hardoy, A. and Schusterman, R. (1999) 'New Models for the Privatization of Water and Sanitation for the Urban Poor' in *Environment and Urbanization*, IIE,. London, Vol.12, No.2, pp.63–75.

Hasan, A. (1997) *Working with Government: The Story of OPP's Collaboration with State Agencies for Replicating its Low-Cost Sanitation Programme*, City Press, Karachi, Pakistan.

Hobson, J. (2000) 'Sustainable Sanitation: Experiences in Pune with a Municipal-NGO-Community Partnership', in *Environment and Urbanization*, IIED, London, Vol.12, No.2, pp.53–62.

Hosain, M., Pendley, C., Pervaiz, N., Tayyaba, S. and Akbar, M. (1999) *Process Monitoring for Improving Sustainability: A Manual for Project Managers and Staff*, UNDP–World Bank Water and Sanitation Program–South Asia, Islamabad.

IRC (1997) *Operation and Maintenance of Sanitation Systems in Urban Low-Income Areas in India and Thailand*, report on a joint research programme, 1989–1993, Project and Programme Papers 6-E, International Research Centre (IRC), The Netherlands.

Isaac, T.M. (1999) *Decentralisation, Democracy and Development: People's Planning Campaign for Decentralised Planning in Kerala*, Kerala State Planning Board.

Jinchang, L. (1998) *Urban Employment Guidelines: Employment-Intensive Participatory Approaches for Infrastructure Investment*, International Labour Office, Geneva.

Khalid, A. and Aiddiqui, T.A. (2000) *Upgradation/Improvement of Katchi Abadis: Departmental vs Contractors Work: A Comparative Study*, Sindh Katchi Abadis Authority, Karachi.

Khan, A.H. (1985) *Rural Development in Pakistan*, 2nd edn, Vanguard Books, Lahore.

Kneeland, S. (1999) *Effective Problem Solving*, How to Books Ltd, Oxford.

Koenigsberger, O. (1964) 'Action Planning', in *Architectural Association Quarterly*, Architectural Association, London, May 1964.

Kolsky, P. (1999) *Engineers and Urban Malaria: Part of the Solution, Or Part of The Problem? Environment and Urbanization*, IIED, London, Vol.11, No.1, pp.159–163.

Lindblom, C. (1965) *The Intelligence of Democracy: Decision-Making Through Mutual Adjustment*, Free Press, New York.

Lines, J. (2002) 'How Not to Grow Mosquitoes in African Towns', in *Waterlines*, ITDG Publishing, Vol.20, No.4, April 2002.

Marchand, R. (1999) *Marketing of Solid Waste Management Services in Tingloy, The Philippines – A Study on Affordability and Willingness to Pay*, UWEP Working Document 9, WASTE, The Netherlands.

Masser, I. and Sliuzas, R. (1999) 'The Use of Geographic Information Technologies for Urban Planning and Management in Developing Countries', in *CDSI Journal*, City Development Strategies Initiative, London, October 1999.

McGranahan, G., Jacobi, P., Songsore, J., Surjadi, C. and Kjellen, M. (2001) *The Citizen at Risk: From Urban Sanitation to Sustainable Cities*, Earthscan, London.

Mitchell, M. and Bevan, A. (1992) *Culture, Cash And Housing: Community and Tradition in Low-Income Building*, VSO Publications, London.

Morgan, P. (1990) *Rural Water Supplies and Sanitation: A text from Zimbabwe's Blair Research Laboratory*, Macmillan Education, London.

Murray, C. and Lopez, A. (eds) (1996) *Global Health Statistics: A Compendium of Incidence, Prevalence and Mortality Estimates for Over 200 Conditions*, Vol.2, Harvard School of Public Health on behalf of WHO and the World Bank, Cambridge, MA, USA.

O'Sullivan, T.P. and Partners (undated), *A Simplified System for KIP Contract Documentation*, unpublished mimeographed report.

Parkinson, J.N. and Alam, K. (2002) *Appropriate Design Standards and Construction Specifications for Tertiary Sewerage Systems*, working paper, GHK International, London, January 2002.

Pathak, B. (1999) 'Sanitation is the Key to Healthy Cities – A Profile of Sulabh International', in *Environment and Urbanization*, IIED, London, Vol.11, No.1, pp.221–229.

Paul, S. (1996) 'Report Cards: A Novel Approach for Improving Urban Services', in *Urban Age*, World Bank, Washington DC, January 1996, pp.7–16.

Rondinelli, D.A. (1993) *Development Projects as Policy Experiments: An Adaptive Approach to Development Administration*, Routledge, London and New York.

Rose, J. B., Sun, G., Gerba, C.P. and Sinclair, N.A. (1991) 'Microbial Quality and Persistence of Enteric Pathogens in Graywater from Various Household Sources', in *Water Research*, Elsevier Science, London, Vol.25, No.1, pp.37–42.

Saidi-Sharouze, M. (1994) *Ouagadougou and Kumasi Sanitation Projects: A Comparative Case Study*, UNDP/World Bank Water and Sanitation Programme-West and Central Africa, Abidjan, Ivory Coast.

Saywell, D. and Cotton, A. (1998) *Strategic Sanitation Approach: A Review of Literature*, WEDC, University of Loughborough.

Saywell, D. and Hunt, C. (1999) *Sanitation Programmes Revisited*, WELL Task No.161, WEDC, University of Loughborough.

Senge, P.M. (1990) *The Fifth Discipline: The Art and Practice of the Learning Organisation*, Century Business, London.

Shuval, H.I., Adin, A., Fattal, B., Rawitz, E. and Yekutiel, P. (1986) *Wastewater Irrigation in Developing Countries – Health Effects and Technical Solutions. Integrated Resource Recovery*, UNDP Project Management Report, World Bank Technical Paper 51, World Bank, Washington DC.

Solo, T.M. (1999) 'Small-scale Entrepreneurs in the Urban Water and Sanitation Market', in *Environment and Urbanization*, IIED, London, Vol.11, No.1, pp.117–131.

Strauss, M. and Blumenthal, U.J. (1990) 'Use of Human Wastes in Agriculture and Aquaculture', in *Utilization, Practices And Health Perspectives*, IRCWD-Report No.08/90.

International Reference Centre for Wastes Disposal, Dübendorf.

Swyngedouw, E. (1995) 'The Contradictions of Urban Water Provision: A Study of Guayaquil, Ecuador', in *Third World Planning Review*, Liverpool University Press, Vol.17, No.4, 1995.

Thomas, F.C (1999) *Calcutta; The Human Face of Poverty*, Penguin India, New Delhi.

UNICEF (2000) *Sanitation for All: Promoting Dignity and Human Rights*, UNICEF, New York.

WaterAid and Tearfund (2002) *The Human Waste: A Call for Urgent Action to Combat the Millions of Deaths Caused by Poor Sanitation*, a WaterAid/Tearfund report, London.

Watson, G. (1995) *Good Sewers Cheap: Agency–Customer Interactions in Low-cost Urban Sanitation in Brazil*, IBRD/World Bank, Washington DC.

Watt, S.B. (1984) *Septic Tanks and Aqua-privies from Ferrocement*, ITDG Publishing, London.

Weisburd, C. (2000) 'Community sanitation in Yoff', in *Waterlines*, ITDG Publishing, London, Vol.19, No.1, July 2000.

Whittington, D. et al. (1992) *Household Demand for Improved Sanitation Services: A Case Study of Kumasi, Ghana*, The World Bank, Washington DC.

Whittington, D. (1998) 'Administering Contingent Valuation Surveys in Developing Countries', in *World Development*, Vol.26, No.1, pp.21–30.

WHO/UNICEF (2000) *Global water supply and sanitation assessment 2000 Report*, Geneva.

World Bank (1994) *World Development Report 1994: Infrastructure for Development*, Oxford University Press, New York.

World Bank (2000) *Entering the 21st Century: World Development Report 1999/2000*, Oxford University Press, New York.

Wright, A.M. (1997) *Towards a Strategic Sanitation Approach: Improving the Sustainability of Urban Sanitation Planning in Developing Countries*, Water and Sanitation Program, Washington.

WSP India/DFID (1999) *Willing to Pay but Unwilling to Charge: Do Willingness to Pay Studies Make a Difference?* Water and Sanitation Program, New Delhi.

WSP-SA (2000) *Urban Environmental Sanitation Planning: Lessons from Bharatpur, Rajasthan, India*. Field Note, UNDP–World Bank Water and Sanitation Programme, South Asia Region.

WSSCC (2000) *Vision 21: A Shared Vision for Hygiene, Sanitation and Water Supply*, Water Supply and Sanitation Collaborative Council, WHO, Geneva.

Zaidi, A. (1996) 'Urban Local Government in Pakistan – Expecting Too Much from Too Little?' in *Economic and Political Weekly*, Mumbai, India, Vol.31, No.44, pp.2948–53.

Zaidi, A. (2001) *From the Lane to the City: The Impact of the Orangi Pilot Project's Low-cost Sanitation Model*, Water Aid, London.

Index

ACORD 26, 28
action planning 31, 47
activists 74–5
adaptive processes 55
administrators 7
advocacy 136
Africa 85
agencies
 bilateral 51–3, 100, 122
 government 173
 international 7, 51, 85, 100, 123, 173
 multilateral 100
 water supply 115
amoebic dysentery 179
analysis quantitative 104
Andhra Pradesh, India 54, 64, 92–3, 104, 110
 Government of 110
 Urban Services for the Poor project 101, 105
Anjuman Samaji Behbood 72
appraisal, rapid 109
appropriate designs 70
aquatic environment 3, 55
ascaris (roundworm) 180
Asian Coalition of Housing Rights 174
assessment 102, 171–2
 qualitative 123
Association pour la Promotion Economique Culturelle et Social de Yoff (APECSY) 165
attitudes and assumptions 13, 48–9, 65 67–8, 103, 142

Baldia Project, Karachi 191
barriers
 to changes in behaviour 99
 to improved sanitation 49
behaviour 13
Bharatpur 4–5, 23, 25–30, 34–5, 41, 43, 54, 95, 112–3, 118, 124
 Municipal Council 25, 28–9
 pilot project 48, 51
 plan 46
 resource analysis 114
 Sanitation Coordination Committee 36
 Workshop 37
big idea 162
blueprint approach 12
 plans 13
boundaries physical and social 76
 between responsibilities of different stakeholders 164

boundary problems 9, 143
Burkina Faso 98

capacity building 55, 62
 to deliver 16
 to produce and implement strategic plans 61
cards in participatory sessions 151
case studies 123
central planning 8
champions 20, 49, 85
 internal 52
 of change 51
Chennai, India 141
children 1, 75
children's defecation practices 93
children's faeces 93
child to child promotion approaches 95
China 132
city-wide perspective 15, 84
Civic Exnora 141
Collaborative Katchi Abadi Improvement Programme 71
Colombo Municipal Corporation, Sri Lanka 165
communication 44, 83
 skills 91, 146
 difficulties 173
 of policy 56
community
 based organisations (CBOs) 16
 contracting 168
 development councils 68
 groups 7, 9
 involvement 29, 114
 leaders 109
 organisations 108, 117
 managed schemes 167
 mapping exercise 149
 members 104, 109, 142
 members as fieldworkers 94
 mobilization 33
Community Action Programme - Faisalabad 69
composted solid waste 40
 market for 40
consensus 32
consultation 34, 162
constraints 45, 96, 161
construction details 7
contingent valuation 139–40, 142
 studies 10
contract documentation 159–60
contracts role in regulation 65

convenience 3, 128
coordination 7, 21, 44
core team 32, 76
cost
 capital 84, 130, 132
 estimation 132–4
 of networked system 133–5
 of technologies 103
 operational 84, 135–6
 recovery 44
 recurrent 130, 135–6
 reduction options 139–40, 142
 schedule 134
 unit 115, 133–4
CRESP Senegal 165

Dakar, Senegal 165
database 118, 120, 160
demand 7, 10 16, 23, 57, 75, 88–9, 110, 126
 informed 16, 35, 89
 orientation 10
 reponsive approach 10, 125
demonstration projects/initiatives 20, 56, 81–3
Department for International Development (DFID) 26, 59, 101
development goals 12
developing solutions 31, 32, 55, 80, 81, 87, 91, 105, 117, 161
 transition from 42
 stage of plan 41
devolution 10, 164
 of responsibilities 57
diarrhoea 179
diarrhoeal disease 1
drainage 81, 115, 121, 172
 basin boundaries 116
 planning 33
 schemes 2, 116
drains 5, 76, 90, 107, 109, 116
 cleaning 29
drainage survey 29
drawings requirements for 159
Durban Metropolitan Council, South Africa 168

economists 4, 17, 50
economy, the 4
elected representatives 32, 46, 90
enabling environment for sanitation promotion 99
engineering education 4
engineers 4, 7
entrepreneurs 18, 109, 168

environment 3–4, 7, 9
  degradation of 33
  impacts on 22
  improvement of 7, 9
  wider 22
Environmental Health Project 124
environmental problems 3
environmental services 7
equity 4, 23
exchange visits 61
excreta 126
  disposal 1, 89
  related diseases 3
expenditure capital 163
  recurrent 163
external agencies 51–2, 65, 100
external stakeholders 83
externally-funded projects 6, 61

'f' diagram 177–8
Faisalabad, Pakistan 72, 108, 140, 161
Faisalabad Area Upgrading Project (FAUP) 59, 140, 167
Faisalabad Water and Sanitation Agency (FWASA) 69
field observation 105
filariasis bancroftian 181
financial improvements 163–4
flooding 3
Food and Agriculture Organization (FAO) 12
focus group discussions 116, 118, 196, 197
force account methods 166
funding for promotion 100

gentrification 128
geographical information systems (GIS) 39, 118, 119
government 5–6, 11 14, 67, 143, 164
  agencies 83
  central 100
  culture of 65, 111
  departments 8, 81, 84
  employees 109
  local 7
  officials 8, 28, 108–9, 149, 164
  state/provincial 100

handwashing 93
Harare City Council 57
health 1, 3–5, 8
  benefits 128
  professionals 4
  ranking 92
  walk 92
helminths 177
  soil-based 178, 180
  water-based 178–9
hepatitis A 179
hookworm 22, 96, 180–1
household-centred approach 23
householders 122, 135
households responsibility for payment 84
  low-income 84
housing 1
human resource development 61

Hyderabad, India 54, 110
Hyderabad, Pakistan 71
Hyderabad Water and Sanitation Agency 71
hygiene 1, 22, 78–9, 89, 159
  at school 93
  barrier 178
  behaviour 92
  education 33, 88, 115
  food 93
  messages 97, 99, 101
  practice 78, 89
  promotion 34, 75, 88–91, 93, 101, 172
  promotion messages 100
  risk practices 90
hygienic practices 33

implementation responsibility for 165
incentives 7, 10, 18–9, 58, 115, 122, 162
  financial 10
incentive systems 164
India 2, 4–5, 9, 51, 105
Indian Constitution 73rd and 74th amendments to 66, 85
Indonesia 54, 195
Indonesian government 62
infections
  categories 178–81
  faecal-oral 100, 177–9
  latent 177
  transmission routes for 177–8
informal sector 1, 64
informal areas 1, 57, 68
information 124, 149
  base 37, 120, 153
  collection 39
  culture 123
  definitive 103
  for good O&M 161
  for policy development 55
  for understanding problems 108
  recognizability 103, 124
  requirements 104
  qualitative 103–4, 108, 118, 198
  quantitative 103–4, 108, 118
  secondary 105, 109
  sharing 173–4
  sources 105
  spatial 103, 107
  systems 111
  written 148
institutional structures 54
institutions 14
interviews 116, 118
  informal 196–7
  semi-structured 196, 198–9
Integrated Low Cost Sanitation programme 6, 23, 30, 40, 60, 92, 95, 105, 123

Juba, Southern Sudan 90, 201

Kampung Improvement Programme, Indonesia 176
Karachi 11, 25, 72, 138
Kerala
  People's Planning Campaign 85

Municipality Act 85
Khan Dr Akhtar Hamid 71
Kumasi, Ghana 10
key informants 11

Lahore, Pakistan 72
land tenure 122
latrines 1, 90, 93, 121, 127
  bucket 2
  dehydrating 187
  dry box 187–9
  pit 6, 22, 57
  pour-flush 125
  simple pit 183–4
  single leach pit 189
  twin leach pit 29, 190–1
  twin-pit 186–7
  Vietnamese double vault 187
  VIP 57, 131, 184–6
leach pits 81
learner-centred approach to training 56
legislation 54, 56–8, 164, 175
legislative barriers 52
Lesotho 18
level of service 17
livelihoods 4
loans for sanitation 84
local businesses 43
local collective action model 8–9, 68, 70
local knowledge 8–9
local leaders 74
Lodhran Pilot Project 86
logical frameworks as aid to monitoring and assessment 169–70
low-income areas 37, 109, 111
Lupin 26, 28, 29

maintenance 37
  health implications if neglected 89
  model' regime for 171
  user involvement in 34
manageable steps 22–3
management
  arrangements 42, 195
  community involvement in 83, 129, 165
  deficiencies 13, 24, 33, 37
  efficiency 18
  of cities 10
  of organizations 33
  of the strategic plan 44
  responsibilities 21, 56, 160
  skills 40, 131
  team 75, 201
map base 124
maps 149
  base 115–6, 118–9, 149
  overlays 149
market model 7–9, 77, 125
market forces 8–9
materials provision as incentive 60
Maseru 18
mass media 97
master plans 5–7, 12
McGranahan et al 7, 11
mental models 48

micro-planning 68, 77
Million Houses Programme 67
models of sanitation improvement 7
monitoring 102, 171
   programme for promotion 99
mosquitoes, diseases spread by 182
Mozambique 58, 60, 127
   National Programme for Low-Cost Sanitation 60
Mumbai, India 127, 129
multi-lateral agencies 53
municipal accountability 59
municipal authorities 28, 33, 43, 77
municipal leaders 50
municipal officials 32
municipal planning authorities 106

National Housing Development Authority, Sri Lanka 67
National Rural Support Programme, Pakistan 86
negotiation 5, 81, 82
neighbourhood profile 119–20, 121
networks 174–5
   drainage 116
   sewerage 116
Noma and Dombi Cleaning and Catering Services 168
non-governmental organizations 4–5, 9, 43–5, 49, 67, 70, 87, 91, 100–1, 107–9, 120, 122, 147, 164–5, 173–4, 198
   international 51, 53, 100
   local 51
   national 53, 100, 123
North-east Lahore Upgrading Project, Pakistan 176

officials 50
old people 55
organizations
   civil society 18, 55, 122, 147, 164
   community based 19, 44–5, 75–6, 163–4, 173–5, 198
   external 49
   international 19
   private sector 18, 55, 115, 122, 164, 175
open defecation 91, 93
operation and maintenance 2, 7, 33, 36, 88, 132, 142, 160–3, 166, 175
   costs 72, 97, 118
   inadequate 13
Orangi Pilot Project 11, 68, 70–4, 86–7
Ouagadougou 10, 98

Pakistan 3, 9, 11, 16, 67–8, 138, 165, 167, 195
participatory appraisal 104
participatory budgeting 85
participatory mapping 116, 196, 200–1
participatory needs assessment 91, 94, 100
pathogens 4, 130, 177
People's Dialogue, South Africa 174
Philippines 143
physical improvements, requirements for 159

pilot projects 35, 40–1, 52, 81–3, 117
plan
   city-wide 31, 42, 105
   components 43
   comprehensive 48
   framework 44
   goal 46
   implementation 158
   local 73, 80, 83, 85
   strategic 34, 55
   structure and contents 42
   written 30
planners 173
   city 104
   national 7
planning 8–10, 75
   adaptive approach to 13, 22
   central 9, 11
   committee 46
   in Bharatpur 5
   information-based 102
   model 7–8
   objectives 8
   principles 46
   process 5, 32, 42, 74, 102, 146
   process at the local level 73
   promotion campaign 94
   strategic 10, 55, 79
   strategic approach 48
pocket chart 202
policies 120
   charging 109
policy 52, 55, 104, 105, 147
   context 48, 52, 65
   development 123
   environment 48–9, 120
   makers 65, 104, 120, 138, 173
   statements 54
politicians 3–4, 6, 75
   local 51, 76, 109
   senior 51
pollution 2, 130
   of Sujan Ganga 5
popular culture promotion methods 97
Porto Alegre, Brazil 85
poverty 6, 9
   focus 60, 68
presentation options 149–50
privacy 3, 19
private sector 8, 64, 117, 163
   finance 122
   small-scale 65
private sweepers 30
problem
   analysis/assessment 78, 111
   boundary 9
   causes 79
   identification 146
   location 79
   off-site 81
   responses to 5
   tree analysis 112–3
   with programme schemes 7, 111
procedures 54, 56, 175
promotion
   materials 97
   specialists 96

programme approaches 6
programme planners 120
programmes 60, 65, 120, 122
   existing 36, 60
   national sanitation 104
   sanitation 107
project cycle 32, 173
Public Health Engineering Department 26, 28–9, 34
public health legislation 9
public officials 7
Pune, India 129, 163, 167
Pune Municipal Corporation 167

Quthbullapur, Andhra Pradesh 109, 145, 151

Rajasthan 4–5, 25, 26
   state government 48
rats, diseases spread by 182
referees 19
regulating bodies 19
responsibility for sanitation and hygiene promotion 94
rewards for good performance 19, 56
resource constraints 61
resource mapping 92
resource requirements 45
resources 8–9, 11, 28, 113, 122
   financial 9, 103, 115
   human 103, 122
   household 7
   institutional 103, 122
   internal and external 80
   organizational 113
   physical 103
roles and responsibilities 122
rules and procedures 59
rules and regulations 7, 32, 64

Saifabad 2, 69
Sana'a, Yemen 21, 187
sanctions 19
sanitation
   barrier 177
   choice 125–6
   communal 2, 128–9, 139, 166
   coverage 107
   deficiencies 1
   dry 126, 129
   ecological 132
   facilities 33
   household-level 4, 126
   hybrid systems 126, 130, 193–4
   ladder 92, 201–2
   low-cost 108, 115
   off-site 126–7
   on-site 108, 126–7, 130, 136
   programmes 116
   promotion 29, 34, 88–9, 91, 93, 96, 100–1
   services 108, 120
   shared 128, 139
   technologies 104, 126, 129
   wet 126
   wide view of 10
Schistosomiasis 1, 180, 187
school health clubs 95

sector profiles 123
septic tanks 14, 91, 111, 132, 192–3
service hierarchy 20
service providers 41, 137
services sustainable 24
  existing 36
sewage 14
  treatment 130, 181, 194–5
sewerage 2, 6, 35, 110, 125, 130, 138
  authorities 9
  condominial 140
  plan for Orangi Township 70
sewered interceptor tanks 131–2
sewers 73, 76, 79, 81, 86, 107, 109, 132, 162, 165
sharing experience 172–4
Sind Katchi Abadi Authority 71, 168
Slum Dwellers International 174
slums 25, 106
small steps approach 10, 27, 28
social capital 4
social development specialists 4
social and technical mapping 29, 118–9
solid waste 112
  collection 2, 8, 20, 76, 109, 117
  disposal 43, 92
  management 29–30, 115, 121
  transfer points 109
sound finances 10, 17, 57, 59
SPARC 129, 167, 174
specifications, engineering 58, 160
squatter settlements 106
Sri Lanka 78
stairs analogy 27
stakeholder involvement in planning 55
stakeholders 158
  external 124
  local 10, 117, 138
  primary 19, 145
  secondary 19, 109, 145
standards
  appropriate 57–8, 70, 140, 142
  technical 17, 107
state authorities 43
state. provincial government departments 115
sticky cloths 151–2
strategic approach to policy development 52
strategic decisions 104
strategic goals 15
strategic plan 12, 15
  capacity to prepare and implement 61, 66
strategic planning 12, 19, 120, 144
  support to 61
  culture 50, 52, 65
  principles 16–24, 28, 52, 61, 68, 154
  process 31, 88
Strategic Sanitation Approach (SSA) 1, 10, 26
strategic vision 15
structured observation 116, 196

subsidies 8, 17, 138
subsidy of O&M costs 35
Sujan Ganga 5, 25
Sukkur, Pakistan 73
  Municipal Corporation 73
Sulabh International 26, 29
sullage 126, 130
supervision 166, 171
supply 16
supportive context 48
surveys of existing services and programmes 116
  questionnaire 116, 118, 196, 200–1
sweepers
  municipal 109, 117
  private 117

tapeworms 180
tariffs 18, 169
technical guidance 60
technical specialists 96
technologies 103, 107
  appropriate 125, 142
tenants 77, 157
tertiary-level facilities 35
think tanks 51–2
timelines 92, 196, 199–200
training 56, 106, 164
  institutions 63–4
  linked to strategic planning 62
  materials 63
  of trainers 64
  problems relating to 63
training institutions 56
transect walks 91, 109, 123, 196, 197
triangulation 106

unbundling 21, 64, 70
  horizontal 10, 20
  of responsibilities 10
  of technology 18
  vertical 20
United Nations Centre for Human Settlements (UNCHS), best practices initiatives 87
understanding problems 31, 33–4, 77, 104, 107
UNDP-LIFE Programme 86–7
United Nations Childrens Fund (UNICEF) 1, 73, 174, 192
Urban Basic Services Program (UBSP) 73
urban growth rate 120
urbanization 1, 11
United States Agency for International Development (USAID) 124

vectors 177
vermi-composting 141
videos, use in promotion 98
  for documenting activities 118, 173
Vietnam 132

WASPOLA

wastewater 126, 130
  as a resource 40
  disposal 89
water
  black 22
  grey 22
  ground 4, 130
  surface 4
  related policies 12
WC 130
Water and Environmental Sanitation Network (WESNET) 175
Water and Sanitation Program (WSP) 1, 10, 174
Water and Sanitation Program - South Asia (WSP-SA) 5, 26, 51
Water and Sanitation Program - East Asia and Pacific (WSP-EAP) 62
water supply 121
Water Supply and Sanitation Policy Formulation and Action Planning Project (WASPOLA) 62, 66, 123
West Africa 10
western industrialized countries 4
willingness to charge 137, 142
willingness-to-pay 16–7, 103, 115, 125, 136–7
  information transfer approach to 138
  revealed preference approach to 137
  rule of thumb approach to 137
  studies 17, 137, 141
women 55, 91, 110, 145, 148, 196–201
  as entrepreneurs 168
  as field workers 91, 199
  concerns/needs 3, 55
  health issues 92
  views on sanitation 118, 126
work packages 160
workshop 27, 51–2, 56, 61, 110
  facilitation 155–6
  facilitator 27
  local 91
  logistics 148–9
  municipal level 147
  outputs 156
  participatory 144–57
  participants 39, 113
  planning 26–7, 30, 35, 42, 48, 74, 77, 111, 113
  policy 147
World Bank 62, 127, 175
World Health Organisation (WHO) 1
World Summit on Sustainable Development 2002 66
Written material 98, 173

Yoff, Senegal 153, 164, 176
Youth Commission for Human Rights (Lahore, Pakistan) 72, 175

Zimbabwe 57, 95

www.ingramcontent.com/pod-product-compliance
Ingram Content Group UK Ltd.
Pitfield, Milton Keynes, MK11 3LW, UK
UKHW050457150426
5217IPUK00025B/1726